D1134670

Skin Disease in Old Age

Skin Disease in Old Age

Second Edition

Ronald Marks, FRCP, FRCPath
Professor of Dermatology, University of Wales College of Medicine

MARTIN ■ DUNITZ

© Ronald Marks 1987, 1999

First published in the United Kingdom in 1987 by

Martin Dunitz Ltd
The Livery House
7–9 Pratt Street
London NW1 0AE

Second Edition 1999

A CIP catalogue record for this book is available from the British Library

ISBN 1 85317 227 8

Distributed in the United States by:
Blackwell Science Inc.
Commerce Place, 350 Main Street
Malden, MA 02148, USA
Tel: 1-800-215-1000

Distributed in Canada by:
Login Brothers Book Company
324 Salteaux Crescent
Winnipeg, Manitoba, R3J 3T2
Canada
Tel: 204-224-4068

Distributed in Brazil by:
Ernesto Reichmann Distribuidora de Livros, Ltda
Rua Coronel Marques 335, Tatuape 03440-000
Sao Paulo,
Brazil

Composition by Scribe Design, Gillingham, Kent, UK
Printed and bound in Singapore by Kyodo Printing Co (S'pore) Pte. Ltd

CONTENTS

INTRODUCTION

The elderly are not merely weaker versions of the young or mature. There are marked differences in the structure, function and responses of their tissues to damage and injurious environmental influences. There are also major age-related differences in the incidence of, susceptibility to and expression of disease and in the attitudes to bodily disorder. Of equal importance is the altered social milieu of the elderly patient. The differences between the age groups are particularly obvious in the skin, and, surprisingly, comparatively few researchers have worked on the problems of cutaneous ageing until recently. The well-known shift in the age structure of the population of the industrialized West in the past two decades has now stimulated many researchers to study the skin in old age. Although there are still gaps in our knowledge, we have a much better understanding of what makes skin function at a slower pace as it grows old.

None of the human anatomical parts or functions studied to date suddenly ages at 65 years old. There seems to be a gradual decrease in size of the organs and a slow drop in the rate of and/or efficacy of function during ageing. These observations have a particular biological significance for the future as, although the proportion of people of pensionable age is not now increasing, the numbers of the very old are.[1] This implies that we will all see an increase in the social and medical problems associated with ageing in the next few years and that this will require different skills and a change in the prevailing attitudes of indifference and disinterest. The very old tend to be less demanding than other age groups but they have more and different problems.

Growing old is a very personal affair. We are all aware that some sprightly 70- or even 80-year-olds do not look or behave according to their age whereas other people seem worn, haggard and sluggish at 35. We do not have an explanation for this large intersubject variability in ageing, any more than we know about the nature of the ageing process itself. Do these variable outer evidences of ageing have any significance for longevity? This fascinating question is not completely answered, but the indications are that it will be possible to predict lifespan using a battery of tests. This was certainly the case in a study of the survivors of Hiroshima, although the specialized circumstances of this investigation make generalizations from it difficult.[2] The different pace of ageing makes a study of the processes involved difficult. There is no problem with mice—a population can be watched and studied over their entire lifespan of about 2 years without difficulty. With humans this cohort type of study is not possible, and the alternative approach of cross-sectional sampling has to be adopted. Because intersubject differences are large, observations give a wide scatter of results and drawing valid statistical conclusions is difficult—facts which should be borne in mind in the assessment of the results of any study of ageing in humans. In recent years many new ideas have emerged about the biological significance of the ageing process, and I would recommend further reading on this topic.[3,4,5] Although much is in doubt, all are agreed that careful distinction must be made between the effects of 'intrinsic ageing' itself and the effects of cumulative environmental trauma. Skin is at the interface between the variably noxious environment and the vulnerable internal tissues. Although the skin is designed to protect, it is itself gradually damaged by the combined forces of climate and human activity. Most of what is popularly thought of as the effects of age on the skin are in fact attributable to various sorts of weathering.

There are very few disorders that affect only one age group. Most have a predilection for a specific group but can, rarely, affect another. Interestingly, the prevalence of skin complaints increases with age and the skin is often a source of severe discomfort and distress in the elderly.[6] Inevitably there has to be a somewhat arbitrary decision as to the inclusion of certain disorders in a book such as this. I hope readers will not be irked at my pragmatic approach. The book has been aimed at those who want to know more about what happens to the skin in old age. It is not an encyclopaedia but a commentary and guide for those who will look after the skin of the elderly.

References

1   Office of Population Censuses and Surveys. Population Projections 1978–2018 (H M Stationery Office: London.)

2   Hollingsworth J W, Hashizume A, Hablon S. Correlations between tests of ageing in Hiroshima subjects: an attempt to define "physiological age". *Yale J Biol Med* (1965) **38**:11–26.

3   Comfort A. *The Biology of Senescence*, 3rd Edn (Churchill Livingstone, Edinburgh, 1979).

4   Hart R W, Turturro A. Theories of ageing. *Rev Biol Res Ageing* (1983) **1**:5–17.

5   Dice J F. Cellular and molecular mechanisms of ageing. *Physiol Rev* (1993) **73**:149–59.

6   Fleischer A B Jr, McFarlane M, Hinds M A, Mittelmark M B. Skin conditions and symptoms are common in the elderly: the prevalence of skin symptoms and conditions in an elderly population. *J Geriat Dermatol* (1996) **4**:78–87.

1
Structure and function of aged skin

The most obvious outward signs of 'getting old' reside in the skin. However, the majority of these stigmata are the result of cumulated environmental damage and not due to intrinsic ageing (see Chapter 2). Alterations that take place in non-sun-exposed skin as it ages visibly change its appearance and function, but these changes are more subtle than those due to climatic exposure.

The skin surface and the stratum corneum

Poets talk of the 'bloom of youth' and, difficult though it is to define, it does seem to exist; even non-sun-exposed skin looks and feels different in old age. It seems that the changes in appearance are primarily the result of altered optical properties of the stratum corneum and the skin surface. Although facial wrinkle lines increase in numbers, depth and prominence, the normal fine surface markings of the skin decrease with age. This change is more prominent in sun-exposed sites but is also seen in covered parts. In fact a recent study indicated that in non-exposed skin there was, if anything, an increase in the degree of roughness compared to a decrease in the usually exposed sites.[1] The furrows are narrower and the lines intersect at less acute angles in sun-exposed skin. Other authors have reported different observations,[2] but the discrepancies seem more attributable to differences in the methodology and the magnification scale of the parameters discussed rather than to any fundamental differences. The stratum corneum itself changes little if at all in thickness during ageing but its component horn cells—the corneocytes—increase in surface area[3,4] (Figures 1.1 and 1.2). Whether this increase in area is accompanied by a change in corneocyte thickness is uncertain, though it seems likely that the cells do become thinner.

The change in mean corneocyte area may have implications for stratum corneum function because of the decreased volume of intercorneocyte space per unit volume of stratum corneum compared with a horny layer containing smaller corneocytes.[5] If, as is believed, the intercorneocyte space is important in percutaneous penetration, the movement of water vapour (transepidermal water loss) and in cell-to-cell cohesion, decrease in this structure owing to ageing may be expected to result in changes in these functions. Observations suggest that although there is indeed a drop in transepidermal water loss and cell-to-cell binding forces;[6] the changes recorded are small and at the limit of the sensitivities of the monitoring techniques currently in use. The same may apply to the rate of percutaneous penetration of topically applied substances, although there is scant published evidence to support this contention. Indirect supporting evidence is found in the increased time taken for the skin of the elderly to blister after the application of ammonium hydroxide and in the decreased reaction noted in aged skin after application of a variety of irritating substances.[7] It is quite clear that during the ageing process the permeability barrier is considerably altered and takes much longer to be repaired after damage.[8]

Recent studies indicate that although there are few significant changes in the structure or function of the stratum corneum under basal conditions, the situation is altered after perturbation. Studies have shown that adhesive tape stripping or acetone treatment disrupted the permeability barrier for much longer in the elderly compared to the young.[9] Furthermore, there was a comparative reduction in the lipid lamellar bilayers of the stratum corneum in elderly subjects.

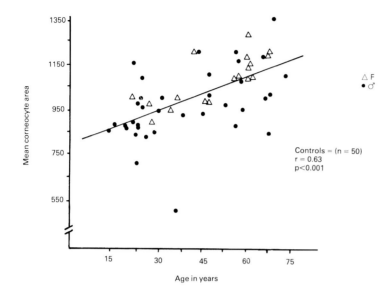

Figure 1.1

Relationship between mean corneocyte area and age in 50 subjects of both sexes.

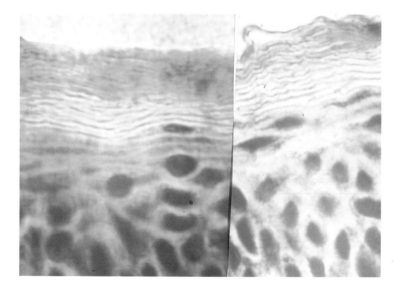

Figure 1.2

Stratum corneum. This composite photomicrograph shows the stratum corneum from a man aged 21 on the left and the same area of skin from a man of 91 on the right. There is no obvious morphological difference between the two horny layers (methylene blue and alkaline swelling technique H & E; ×150).

The rate of renewal of the stratum corneum is undeniably altered in the elderly. Measurements taken with the fluorescent dyes tetrachlorsalicylanide and dansyl chloride indicate that the rate of loss of corneocytes at the surface progressively decreases with age.[10,11] In these tests the marker substances are placed on the skin surface occlusively and penetrate the stratum corneum. The time to disappearance of the fluorescence (extinction time) is the time taken for renewal of the stratum corneum and parallels the rate of epidermal cell production. The decreased rate of desquamation may give rise to an altered pattern of cell loss and could partly account for the changed appearance of the skin surface.

There appears to have been relatively little investigation of any change in the mechanical properties of the stratum corneum that occur as

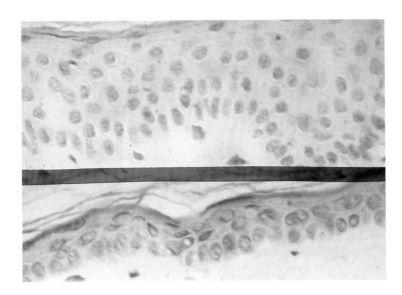

Figure 1.3

This composite photomicrograph is taken from forearm skin biopsies of a man aged 20 (top) and a man aged 84 (bottom). The epidermis is much thinner in the specimen from the older subject and the individual epidermal cells seem smaller too (H & E; ×90).

a result of age. Observation would suggest that there is decreased elasticity and breaking strength resulting in an increase in fragility. This would explain the ease with which superficial fissuring occurs in the skin of the elderly when it is inflamed. It is often suggested that these altered physical properties are a result of a decreased stratum corneum water content in old age, but there is sparse evidence to support this suggestion. The propagation and attenuation of low frequency shear waves in human skin have been found to be highly dependent on the water content of the stratum corneum. The results in different age groups indicated a reduced water content in the skin of the older individuals.[12] Studies[13] conducted in vivo using specially constructed measuring devices to detect alterations of the mechanical properties of skin with increasing age have recorded a variety of changes. A proportion of the changes recorded are probably due to the effects of age on the stratum corneum.

Epidermal changes

The epidermis becomes thinner and loses its undulating rete pattern with increasing age (Figure 1.3). The degree of epidermal thinning that occurs is extremely variable,[14] as are most age-related structural changes if examined in cohorts rather than sequentially in the same population.[15] In the young adult the mean epidermal thickness of limb and trunk skin is 35–50 μm. At the age of 70 years the mean thickness is 25–40 μm. Of greater interest is the shrinkage of the epidermal cells themselves. The decrease in size seems to be linearly related to age and observed equally at all sites (non-sun-exposed) examined (Figure 1.4); it is seen equally in both sexes. The shrinkage appears to take place at all stages of epidermal differentiation and in all dimensions, that is, there is a volume decrease. There is no information available on the structural factors underlying the decrease in epidermal cell size, but our own preliminary studies indicate that all parts of the cell decrease equally in size.

The decrease in epidermal cell size is difficult to reconcile with the increase in corneocyte area mentioned earlier, but several explanations are possible. The simplest is that although there is an increase in mean corneocyte area, there is actually a decrease in corneocyte volume. The decrease in corneocyte thickness needed to 'match up' corneocyte volume with the decrease in epidermal cell volume, despite an increase in

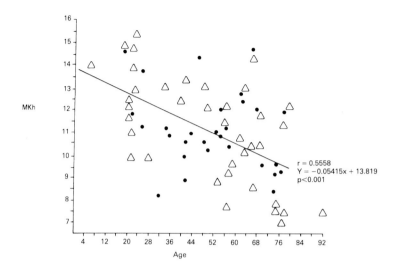

Figure 1.4

Relationship between epidermal cell size measured as mean keratinocyte height (MKh) and age. Although there is a wide scatter of observations, it can be seen that there is a significant relationship between epidermal cell size and age. Skin samples were taken from the non-exposed site of the flexor aspect of the forearm.[14]

corneocyte area of the magnitude seen, seems more than possible. Unfortunately sufficiently accurate measurements of corneocyte thickness cannot yet be made to test this hypothesis.

The increase in stratum corneum renewal time discussed earlier might be expected to be the result of a decrease in the rate of epidermal cell production. Although it has been disputed,[16] the limited evidence available does indeed favour an age-related decrease in this activity.[7] Regrettably the available techniques are not sufficiently precise to determine at which stage or stages the process is slowed. Studies in which the number of cells in DNA synthesis are counted after exposing the tissue to the tritiated DNA precursor thymidine and then preparing the tissue autoradiographically, only provide limited information. Such studies cannot reveal alterations in the number of cells capable of cell division (germinative population) or the proportion of these cells that are in the growth cycle (growth fraction) or any change in the rate of DNA synthesis.

Pigmentation

Persistently and heavily sun-exposed skin may become hyperpigmented. The colour change may be permanent and is more of a mahogany colour than the sun-tanned skin of younger individuals. The non-exposed sites are by contrast often less pigmented than in younger subjects.

Skin colour is a complex amalgam of the number and synthetic activity of melanocytes, the number and size of melanosomes, the number, depth and dilatation of the blood vessels, the state of oxygenation of the blood in the vessels, the presence of abnormal pigments and the optical properties of all the skin structures. Ageing may involve changes in several of these and partially account for the 'loss of bloom' and altered pigmentation of old skin. Melanocytes participate in the ageing process. Studies in which dopa (dihydroxyphenylalanine) positive dendritic cells have been counted in whole epidermal mounts (after splitting the dermis from the epidermis) have demonstrated a linear reduction of the numbers of melanocytes per square millimetre with age. The decrease found has amounted to 10–20% per decade.[17–19] Gilchrest's group,[20] who have taken particular interest in the relative effects of ageing and chronic solar damage on the skin, have confirmed the decreased melanocyte population in non-exposed ageing skin and found that there is an increase in sun-damaged areas. Increased pigmentation of exposed skin as a function of age has also been found in New Guinea natives; and some authors have commented on the decreased dopa reactivity of melanocytes although this is intrinsically more difficult to quantify.

Langerhans cells

These intra-epidermal dendritic cells are now recognized to be of prime importance to the immune defences as 'antigen presenting cell'.[21,22] In reality they belong to the reticuloendothelial system and originate in the bone marrow. After topical application of an antigen-containing substance the antigen is found on the surface of the Langerhans cells. The antigen-bearing Langerhans cells then 'process the antigen', migrate into the dermis and 'transmit' their message to T lymphocytes, setting in motion the cell-mediated hypersensitivity response.

There is a reduction in the Langerhans cell population in elderly subjects. There were about 15% fewer Langerhans cells in the buttock skin of subjects aged 65 or more compared with a control group of less than 24 years in age in a study by Thiers and others.[23] In contrast to the situation with melanocytes, chronically sun-damaged skin showed an even greater reduction in Langerhans cell numbers in this investigation. There were only about two-thirds as many Langerhans cells in arm skin from the older group compared with the young controls. Other studies have demonstrated a decrease in the Langerhans cell population after acute exposures to ultraviolet radiation (UVR). The functional consequence of the reduction in this vitally important cellular link in the immune defence chain has not been confirmed, but has led to some interesting speculation. In particular the relationship of the reduction in number to the development of neoplastic disease has been mooted. The reduction in the sensitizing capacity of potent antigens such as DNCB (dinitrochlorobenzene) in the elderly also may in part be due to the reduced number of Langerhans cells.

Age changes in dermal connective tissue

As detailed in Chapter 2, many of the clinical changes in the skin of our senior citizens are the result of the cumulative damage from environmental traumata. The wrinkling and leathery appearance of the skin of the face is due to solar elastotic degenerative change as are the odd angulated scars and ecchymotic spots on the backs of the hands and forearms. However, changes do take place in dermal connective tissue as a result of intrinsic ageing. They are seen in their 'purest' form in the covered skin of elderly black individuals but are also found in the covered areas of Caucasians. The clinical sequelae of pure 'dermal ageing' are less obvious than the changes of chronic actinic damage. They consist of loss of elasticity and palpable thinning. There is also a loss of resistance to the indenting finger and a loss of rebound of a pinched fold of skin, which are crude tests of many mechanical features of skin that in part monitor dermal hydration and in part reflect alterations in the fibrous structure of the connective tissue framework.

The dermis becomes thinner in old age. This was first detected using a radiological method and later confirmed and the data extended using a special ultrasound device.[24,25] The latter study showed that skin thickness gradually increased up to the age of 20 years, remained constant between 20 and 40, and then gradually declined in an age-related manner. These findings have for the most part been confirmed by Léveque and his co-workers, although they suggest that the decline in thickness is not exactly linear and shows a more rapid decline in the last two decades of life.[26] As so often appears to be the case, men fare worse than women in the attrition of ageing and the rate of decline of total skin thickness (of which dermis accounts for the major part) is greater in men than in women (Figure 1.5). The normal total skin thickness in maturity in men is 1.0–1.2 mm and in women is 0.8–1.0 mm.[25] At the age of 70 the measurements are similar in both sexes, from 0.7 to 0.9 mm. As with all biological measures of ageing in populations there is marked variability in the observations but the tendency to thinning is undeniable. The loss of dermal substance seems to be from all parts of the dermis but may be particularly marked from the papillary dermis. Not only does the dermis feel thinner, but it also looks less substantial and may be optically more transparent—allowing veins, tendons and muscles to be more easily

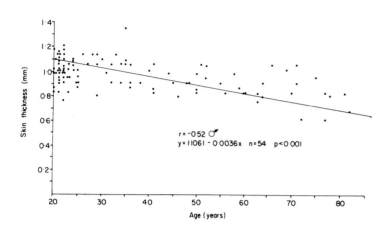

Figure 1.5a

Skin thiskness as measured by ultrasound in 54 men of different ages. It can be seen that there is a significant relationship between age and skin thickness.[25]

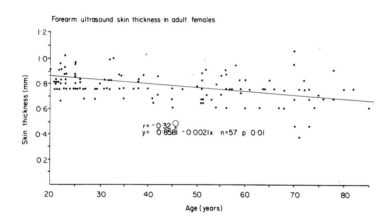

Figure 1.5b

Skin thickness as measured by ultrasound in 57 women of different ages. Again it can be seen that there is a significant relationship between age and skin thickness.[25]

seen (Figure 1.6). If the individual has senile or 'postmenopausal' osteoporosis, the tendency to dermal thinning is even more marked, as was noted by McConkey.[27] Interestingly, the depressed collagen content can be restored in postmenopausal women by hormone replacement treatment.[28]

The dermal thinning accompanying senescence seems to be mainly the result of loss of proteoglycan, although there is also a decreased amount of total collagen when the results are expressed per unit surface area.[24] Strangely, the water content of the skin seems greater with increasing age when expressed per unit weight.[5] The various

alterations to the molecular structure of collagen during ageing have been well reviewed by Hall.[29] In summary, the number of stable intermolecular cross links increases with age and the proportion of insoluble collagen increases while that of soluble collagen decreases. Recent studies suggest that elastic fibres are not immune from the ageing process (independent of any additional solar effect). Ultrastructurally the elastic fibres appear broader and more 'ragged' at the margins in skin from elderly subjects. They are also irregularly distributed, looser in texture and more easily dissociated by enzymes.[30,31] These biochemical and structural changes are almost certainly

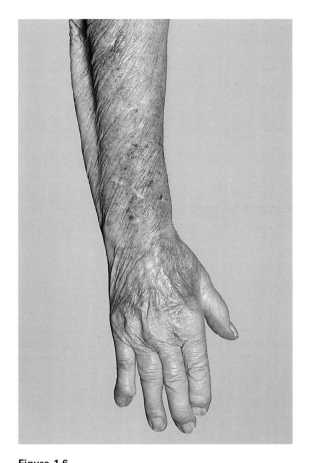

Figure 1.6

Thin skin of back of hand in elderly woman.

contact of fibroblasts with the connective tissue framework.[34]

Studies of the mechanical properties of skin have been bedevilled by the great variety of methods used and the difficulties in comparison of results from different laboratories as well as interpretation of these in functional terms. It is hardly surprising that force extension measurements made *in vitro* on rat skin do not match up to 'suction cup' measurements made *in vivo* in humans.[35] Table 1.1 summarizes a selection of the investigations of the 'viscoelastic' properties of aged skin in humans. Among the most rigorous of studies are those of Vogel[36,37] who has meticulously documented the alterations due to ageing in rat skin *in vitro*. He has employed the classic technique of stretching the skin in an extensometer (an Instron device) to obtain data on the force–extension relationships. Results with this technique indicate that the skin is less extensible when taken from older rats (ie, is stiffer), it relaxes after stretching with greater difficulty, and it is more fragile (ie, there is a decreased load to 'break point'). This type of experiment, while a long way from intact human skin, does teach us something of the changes that take place in skin in absolute terms. It should be noted that skin is anisotropic—it does not function identically in all spatial orientations—and results obtained in the longitudinal body axis may differ markedly from those obtained when observations are taken at 90 degrees to the long axis.

Studies performed in humans have used a variety of techniques that have included suction cup measurements,[35,38] torsion devices[39] and indentation and distortion measurements,[40,41] as well as devices that tap[42] and pinch[43] the skin. Most record a degree of alteration in the physical characteristics of aged skin but differ greatly as to the extent of these changes. In general there is a decrease in breaking strength, elasticity and in rebound after deformation.

Another interesting approach to the characterization of the effects of ageing on dermal connective tissue was that of Bhagat and Kerrick[44] who used an ultrasound technique in mice of different ages. They found a decreased velocity in the aged mice they tested and suggested that there was a decrease in a 'resilience factor'.

responsible for the biomechanical profile of aged skin. Oikarinen[69] has reviewed the biochemical properties of ageing dermal connective tissue and their measurement.

Fibroblasts appear to decrease in number and size with age. The replicative ability of fibroblasts *in vitro* appears to be finite and not unlimited.[32] The fact that the cells are capable of only a certain number of cell divisions suggests that there is programmed senescence in tissues and has led to considerable speculation as to the nature of the ageing process. Other studies emphasize the decreased replicative ability of fibroblasts in old age[33] and suggest decreased

Table 1.1   Some of the results of investigation of the mechanical properties of elderly skin

Technique	Main findings	References
Suction cap	Increase in elastic modulus with age	Grahame[a]
Pre-tension and suction cap	Increase in elastic constant relating to ground substance and elastic fibre components with age	Alexander and Cook[b]
Rotating disc and guard ring torque measurement	Increase in Young's modulus with age	Agache et al[c]
In vitro extensometry	Thickness decrease, reduced rupture strength, reduced elasticity, reduced tensile strength	Holzmann et al[d]

[a] Grahame R. A method for measuring human skin elasticity in vivo with observations on the effects of age, sex and pregnancy. *Clin Sci* (1970) **39**:223–238.
[b] Alexander CH, Cook TH. Accounting for the natural tension in the mechanical testing of human skin. *J Invest Dermatol* (1977) **69**:310–314.
[c] Agache P, Leveque JL, De Rigal J *et al*. Biomechanical properties of the human skin in vivo, and ageing. *Bioengineering Skin* (1980) **2**:20–30.
[d] Holzmann H, Korting GW, Kobett D *et al*. Studies on mechanical properties of human skin in relation to age and sex. *Arch Klin Exp Dermatol* (1971) **239**:355–367.

Age-related changes in hair

Changes in hair are among the most obvious effects of growing old. Androgenic alopecia has been extensively investigated. Indeed, there have been several comprehensive monographs published on this topic alone (eg, Baccaredda-Boy et al[45]). As the term implies, androgenic alopecia is not purely age related. It is dependent on two other variables. It is first dependent on a dominantly inherited tendency to develop the condition and second on the influence of male sex hormone. Thus the condition is not seen in some families unless the gene responsible is introduced, and it does not develop in eunuchs even if they possess the gene unless they receive supplements of testosterone. However, once started, the process is progressive and worsens with the passing of the years—as the author will vigorously testify. Although the process is often called male pattern baldness or androgenic alopecia, it occurs in some women as well and is a trying cosmetic problem for these individuals.

Clinically the condition starts in the temporal regions as a recession of the hair line (the so-called bitemporal recession or 'widow's peak'). A little later, thinning over the vertex occurs, and later the process spreads to include, in the most severe cases, most of the crown, giving the typical 'billiard ball' appearance. In women there may be a different pattern; it is true that bitemporal loss and thinning of the hair of the vertex are quite often seen but in a proportion of affected women there is also a marked diffuse loss of hair. As close inspection of the bald scalp will confirm, the pigmented terminal hair gives way to a sparser 'fuzz' of vellus hair. After many years even this is lost and the skin becomes perfectly smooth and atrophic.

Mirroring the clinical appearance of atrophy, the hair follicles themselves gradually become smaller and fewer. Other changes are described histologically in the scalp of patients with long-standing male pattern alopecia including a reduction in the capillary vasculature, chronic inflammatory cell infiltrate and fibrosis. Whether these changes are primary and central to the pathogenesis or secondary to the loss of protection from the loss of hair is uncertain.

Androgenic alopecia aside, there is a gradual loss of hair as part of the ageing process. The loss is not confined to the scalp but includes all body hair. The hair shaft diameter decreases and the anagen phase shortens, so that hair density decreases. In addition the rate of hair growth decreases.

It may not be generally appreciated just how disabling loss of scalp hair can be. The loss of self esteem on account of the altered appearance is variable but extremely distressing for some who will embrace any measure to stimulate regrowth or replace or disguise the loss of hair. The loss of hair is not only a cosmetic issue. Bald-headed individuals injure their scalps more readily after minor bumps and scrapes. Exposure of scalp skin to solar radiation results in the development of rosacea on the bald part.[46] Solar keratoses also arise on the area of hair loss—in one study after a mean period of 33 years following loss of hair.

Treatment of male pattern alopecia

Sadly there is no ideal method for restoring the hair after loss in male pattern alopecia. Minoxidil is a drug that was used extensively in the treatment of hypertension and was found to result in generalized hirsutism. Subsequently a topical form was developed (as a 2% lotion) and promoted to stimulate hair growth. It is effective in 25–30% of cases, but has to be used continuously. It is clearly far from ideal and it is hoped more effective alternatives will be available soon.

Hair transplantation in which 'plugs' of hair bearing skin are transferred from the sides of the scalp where hair is still growing to the bald central parts of the scalp may be successful, but is dependent on the skill and experience of the surgeon responsible. Rows of cylinders of hair follicle bearing skin are placed at the front of the skin at first. Later the 'gaps' are filled in. The cylindrical plugs are taken at an angle so as not to injure the follicles they contain (Figure 1.7). Further details are found in several reviews (eg, Marritt and Dzubow,[47] Biscaccia[48]). Other surgical manoeuvres include scalp recession.[49] Those who can't afford such cosmetic surgery or are fearful of them often resort to hair pieces (wigs, toupees).

The greying of hair is among the popularly recognized signs of growing old. The time of its onset is variable and 'premature' greyness is not at all uncommon. However, advancing age does produce more grey hairs due to decreased melanin synthesis by the melanocytes of the hair bulb.

Sebaceous glands

Sebaceous glands do not appear to diminish noticeably with age. Indeed, in some individuals, particularly elderly men, the sebaceous glands on the face and upper back are paradoxically hypertrophied (see page 189). Clinically the hypertrophied glands are obvious as small yellow nodules. They are not infrequently mistaken for basal cell carcinoma lesions or even non-pigmented dermal cellular naevi. Histologically, sebaceous gland hyperplasia may be distinguished from other conditions with overgrowth of sebaceous tissue such as naevus sebaceous and sebaceous adenoma by the regularity of the differentiation and the normality of the hypertrophied glands (Figure 1.8). The condition has been extensively studied.[50–52] The sebaceous gland cells appear to mature and

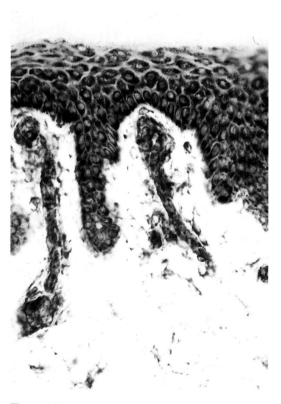

Figure 1.7

Papillary capillaries are demonstrated in this enzyme histochemical preparation of hypertrophied skin. The enzyme histochemical test is nicotine adenosine diaphorase (×150).

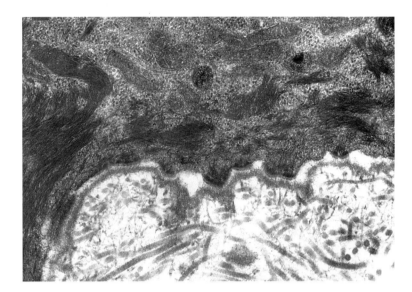

Figure 1.8

Electron micrograph to show dermo-epidermal junction. The lamina lucida and lamina densa of the basal lamina, hemidesmosomes and anchoring fibrils are well shown (original magnification ×46,000).

migrate more slowly than in normal glands but the cause of sebaceous gland hyperplasia remains mysterious. The rate of sebum secretion does not decrease in elderly men until the age of 80 but does decrease in women after the menopause.[53] In Parkinsonism there is an increased rate of sebum secretion. It is of considerable interest that despite the maintenance of sebum secretion in old age, acne is less common than in younger age groups, but by no means unknown. The author has recently studied 10 male patients in whom acne developed for the first time after the age of 60.

The nails

As may be expected, the nail plates grow less rapidly in the elderly. Bean measured his own rate of nail growth throughout life and found that it decreased from 0.83 mm per week in the third decade to 0.52 mm per week in the eighth decade.[54] The fingernails also become thinner, less flexible, more brittle and may develop fine longitudinal striations in old age. The toenails unlike the fingernails often seem to become thicker in old age. As they also take on a yellowish hue care must be take to rule out a ringworm infection.

Sweat glands

The eccrine sweat glands seem to diminish in size in old age and secrete less sweat than in younger individuals in response to stimuli.[55] Occasionally yellowish granules of lipofuscin of unknown significance are found within the glandular epithelium. The apocrine glands also become smaller and their ability to secrete is also reduced.

The dermal vasculature

There are no capillary vessels in the epidermis, and this part of the skin is supplied with oxygen and nutrients by capillary vessels in the dermal papillae. These arise from vascular plexuses arranged horizontally in the dermis. There are also rich plexuses of blood vessels that ramify around the hair follicles and to a lesser extent the sweat glands. The arterial vessels tend to thicken in older individuals and there is a reduction in the number of capillaries. The capillaries of non-exposed skin become thinner, probably owing to decreased synthetic activity and the number of investing fibroblasts (Veil cells).[56] Vascular response to all types of stimuli also tends to be muted in old age and this is one explanation for the apparent decreased response to chemical and mechanical trauma and the complaint of elderly subjects that they feel the cold. Materials injected intracutaneously, such as saline or fluorescein solutions, take longer to clear from the injected site in the elderly.[57]

Neural structure and function

Neural structures are embryonically derived from the embryonic neural crest and include the nerves, nerve fibres and end organs.[58] Discriminative tactile ability is decreased in the elderly but little in the way of structural alterations has been recorded.

The dermo-epidermal junction

This is an extremely complex zone that is important for skin function and is frequently involved in disease.[59] It can be adequately visualized only by ultrastructural techniques. It consists of a basal lamina on which rest the epidermal cells and which itself consists of an upper lamina lucida and a lower lamina densa. Dermal microfibril bundles and anchoring fibrils link the dermal elastic fibre network to the lamina densa. Anchoring filaments composed of type VII collagen join the lamina densa to the epidermal cells at the sites of hemidesmosomes. The lamina densa is composed of type IV collagen, while the lamina lucida contains, amongst other things, glycoproteins (170 kDa and 230 kDa) important in bullous pemphigoid. Numerous proteins are associated with the region and seem vital to the integrity of the structure. Detailed ultrastructural studies have shown that at least up to the age of 60 there is no alteration in width of the basal lamina, but that there is a decrease in the number of dermal microfibril bundles.[60]

Wound healing in the elderly

The sequence of events following wounding is complex but similar in outline whether the wound is caused by a knife, by a burn or by a destructive disease process. Haemostasis and vasoconstriction are the initial 'emergency measures' in an incisional wound. Within the first few hours the wound cavity becomes filled with blood clot, inflammatory cells and tissue debris. Re-epithelialization begins some time between 12 and 24 hours later and continues until the breach in the skin surface is repaired. The new epidermis burrows between the slough and the viable dermal tissue beneath, using its own fibrinolytic and collagenolytic activities. The migrating epidermal cells are actively motile and bursts of mitotic activity are not seen until some 72 hours after wounding.

While re-epithelialization proceeds, damaged dermal elements are removed by macrophages and new collagen is laid down from the third or fourth day after wounding. The new collagen takes up the orientation of the surrounding dermis and becomes functionally protective only some weeks or even months later. In addition to these processes, wound contracture occurs from the third or fourth day after wounding. Fibroblasts develop an ability to contract (myofibroblasts) and draw the edges of the wound together.

Everyone who has studied the subject of wound healing in the elderly agrees that the process is slower and less efficient in old age.[61] These opinions are, however, based mainly on clinical evidence, there being a deficiency of studies on the effects of ageing on the wounding process in humans. Early studies on the healing of war wounds demonstrated that wounds decreased in area as a consequence of age but that there was considerable variability— leading to the concept of biological ageing.[62] More recently blister bases were found to re-epithelialize at a slower rate in the aged.[63]

This aspect of the skin in old age must be appreciated for its influence both on the clinical features and on the response to treatment of all skin disorders in the elderly patient.

Premature ageing

A look around a peer group will confirm that the rate at which the signs of ageing are developed is remarkably variable. This variability appears to be independent of the differing experience of environmental injury and as with other aspects of true ageing, is unexplained. Apart from the inherent differing rates of senescence, whether the process of ageing can be accelerated or not is a moot point.[64] It is clear that some of the skin signs of ageing can be simulated. Radiation and corticosteroids thin the epidermis, slow its rate of growth, decrease the size of epidermal cells and thin the dermis—all changes observed in the ageing process. However, it seems likely that this similarity is merely the result of the limited range or response of the skin to 'suppressive' stimuli.

Premature ageing syndromes are those disorders in which the signs of ageing appear very early in life. Progeria is the archetypal example of this group of diseases and the results of its investigation highlight the discussion concerning the possibility of there being a true acceleration of the process of ageing.[65] It is an extremely rare disorder characterized by loss of hair, thinning of the skin and loss of subcutaneous fat. The skin becomes brownish in colour, bound down and scleroderma-like. These signs develop in the first years of life, or even the first few months, and are accompanied by skeletal hypoplasia and cataracts. A rare condition in which the changes of ageing are confined to the extremities has been described and is termed acrogeria.

Werner's syndrome (adult progeria)[66] is less rare but still very uncommon, there being some 200 cases described in the literature. The disorder is characterized by sclerodermatous and poikilodermatous changes developing in the skin, as well as loss of hair and cataracts. The skin atrophy results in intractable ulcerations. Many other abnormalities are present, including short stature, hypogonadism and predisposition to diabetes, atherosclerotic disease and malignancies. A further similar disease, termed metageria, has also been described.[67]

There is considerable confusion in the literature concerning the identities and similarities within this odd group of tragic diseases, and there is virtually no information available as to whether or not they represent the same underlying metabolic (or immunological) abnormality. To add to the confusion there are several syndromes in which there are some of the signs of premature ageing but which for other reasons can be differentiated. One such disorder is the Rothmund–Thomson syndrome (poikiloderma congenitale) which is characterized by the presence of mottled pigmentation, telangiectasia and atrophy, as well as hyperkeratotic lesions and a predisposition to cutaneous malignancies. The distinguishing features of this and other similar diseases are well described by Rook et al.[68]

References

1   Edwards C E, Heggie R H, Marks R. A study of differences in surface roughness between exposed and unexposed skin with age. *Arch Dermatol* (in press).
2   Lavker R M, Kwang F, Kligman A M. Changes in skin surface patterns with age. *J Gerontol* (1980) **35**:348–54.
3   Plewig G, Marples R R. Regional differences of cell sizes in human stratum corneum. Part II. Effects of age and sex. *J Invest Dermatol* (1970) **54**:19–23.
4   Grove G, Lavker R M, Holzle E, Kligman A M. Use of non intrusive tests to monitor age associated changes in human skin. *J Soc Cosmet Chem* (1981) **32**:15–19.
5   Marks R, Barton S P. The significance of the size and shape of corneocytes. In: Marks R, Plewig G, eds *Stratum Corneum* (Springer Verlag: Berlin, 1983).
6   Wilhelm K P, Cua A B, Maibach H I. Effect of transepidermal water loss, stratum corneum hydration, skin surface pH and casual sebum content. *Arch Dermatol* (1991) **127**:1806–9.
7   Kligman A M. Perspectives and problems in cutaneous gerontology. *J Invest Dermatol* (1979) **73**:39–46.
8   Ghadially R, Brown B E, Sequeira-Martin S M, Feingold K R, Elias P M. The aged epidermal permeability barrier: Structural, functional and lipid biochemical abnormalities in humans and a senescent murine model. *J Clin Invest* (1995) **95**:2281–90.
9   Elias P M. Decreased epidermal lipid synthesis accounts for altered barrier function in aged mice. *J Invest Dermatol* (1996) **106**:1064–9.
10 Baker H, Blair C P. Cell replacement in the human stratum corneum in old age. *Br J Dermatol* (1968) **80**:367–72.
11 Roberts D, Marks R. Determination of regional and age variations in the rate of desquamation. A comparison of four techniques. *J Invest Dermatol* (1979) **74**:13–16.
12 Potts R O, Buras E M, Chrisman D A. Changes with age in the moisture content of human skin. *J Invest Dermatol* (1984) **82**:97–100.

13 Marks R. Techniques for measuring mechanical properties of skin. *J Soc Cosmet Chem* (1983) **34:**429–37.

14 Marks R. Measurement of biological ageing in human epidermis. *Br J Dermatol* (1981) **104:**627–33.

15 Comfort A. Measuring the human ageing rate. In: *The Biology Of Senescence*, 3rd Edn (Churchill Livingstone: Edinburgh, 1979).

16 Epstein W I, Maibach H I. Cell renewal in human epidermis. *Arch Dermatol* (1965) **92:**462–8.

17 Fitzpatrick T B, Szabo G, Mitchell R E. Age change in the human melanocyte system. In: Montagna W, ed. *Advances In Biology Of The Skin* (Pergamon Press: Oxford, 1964).

18 Quevedo W C, Jr, Szabo G, Virks J. Influence of age and UV on the population of dopa-positive melanocytes in human skin. *J Invest Dermatol* (1969) **52:**287–90.

19 Snell R S, Bischitz P G. The melanocytes and melanin in human abdominal wall skin. A survey made at different ages in both sexes and in pregnancy. *J Anat* (London) (1963) **97:**361–76.

20 Gilchrest B A, Blog F A, Szabo G. Effects of ageing and chronic sun exposure on melanocytes in human skin. *J Invest Dermatol* (1979) **73:**141–3.

21 Rowden G. The Langerhans cell. *CRC Crit Rev Immunol* (1981) **3:**95–180.

22 Hunter J A. The Langerhans cell: from gold to glitter. *Clin Exp Dermatol* (1983) **8:**569–92.

23 Thiers B H, Maize J C, Spicer S S et al. The effect of ageing and chronic sun exposure on human Langerhans cell population. *J Invest Dermatol* (1984) **82:**223–6

24 Shuster S, Black M M, McVitie E. The influence of age and sex on skin thickness, skin collagen and density. *Br J Dermatol* (1975) **93:**639–43.

25 Tan C Y, Statham B, Marks R et al. Skin thickness measurement by pulsed ultrasound: Its reproducibility, validation and variability. *Br J Dermatol* (1982) **106:**657–67.

26 De Rigal J, Escoffier C, Querleux B, Faivre B, Agache P, Léveque J L. Assessment of skin ageing of human skin by in vivo ultrasonic imaging. *J Invest Dermatol* (1989) **93:**622.

27 McConkey B, Walton K W, Carney S A et al. Significance of occurrence of transparent skin. A study of histological characteristics and biosynthesis of dermal collagen. *Ann Rheum Dis* (1967) **26:**219–25.

28 Brincat M, Moritz C F, Studd J W W et al. Sex hormones and skin collagen content in postmenopausal woman. *Br Med J* (1983) **287:**1337–8.

29 Hall D A. *The Ageing of Connective Tissue* (Academic Press: London, 1976).

30 Tsuji T, Hanada T. Age related changes in human dermal elastic fibres. *Br J Dermatol* (1981) **105:**57–63.

31 Braverman I M, Fonferko E. Studies in cutaneous ageing I. The elastic fiber network. *J Invest Dermatol* (1982) **78:**434–43.

32 Hayflick L. The limited in vitro lifespan of human diploid cell strains. *Exp Cell Res* (1965) **37:** 615–35.

33 Schneider E L. Ageing and cultured human skin fibroblasts. *J Invest Dermatol* (1979) **73:**15–18.

34 Pieraggi M T, Julian M, Bouissou H. Fibroblast changes in cutaneous ageing. *Virchows Arch* (1984) **402:**275–87.

35 Ishikawa T, Ishikawa O, Miyachi Y. Measurement of skin elastic properties with a new suction device (1): Relationship to age, sex and the degree of obesity in normal individuals. *J Dermatol* (1995) **22:**713–17.

36 Vogel H G. Directional variations in mechanical parameters in rat skin depending on maturation and age. *J Invest Dermatol* (1981) **76:**493–7.

37 Vogel H G. Influence of maturation and age and of desmotropic compounds on the mechanical properties of rat skin in vivo. *Bioeng Skin* (1985) **1:**35–54.

38 Grahame R, Holt P J L. The influence of ageing on the in vivo elasticity of human skin. *Gerontologica* (1969) **15:**121–39.

39 Léveque J L, Rigal J de, Agache P G et al. Influence of ageing on the in vivo extensibility of human skin at a low stress. *Arch Dermatol Res* (1980) **269:**127–35.

40 Pierard G E, Lapiere Ch M. Physiopathological variations in the mechanical properties of skin. *Arch Dermatol Res* (1977) **260:**231–9.

41 Oikarinen A. Ageing of the skin connective tissue: How to measure the biochemical and mechanical properties of ageing dermis. *Photoderm Photoimmun Photomed* (1994) **10:**47–52.

42 Tosti A, Compagno G, Fazzini M L et al. A ballistometer for the study of the plasto-elastic properties of skin. *J Invest Dermatol* (1977) **69:**315–17.

43 Marks R, Edwards C, Caunt A et al. Turgometer— a novel device for the assessment of skin turgor and regional mechanical function. *Paper presented at Vth International Symposium, International Society For Bioengineering and the Skin.* Aug–Sept 1985, San Francisco.

44 Bhagat P K, Kerrick W. Ultrasonic characterisation of ageing in skin tissue. *Ultrasound Med Biol* (1980) **6:**369–75.

45 Baccaredda-Boy A, Moretti G, Frey J R. *Biopathology of Pattern Alopecia* (Karger: Basel, 1968).

46 Gojewksa M. Rosacea on common male baldness. *Br J Dermatol* (1975) **93:**63–6.

47 Marritt E, Dzubow L. A redefinition of male pattern baldness and its treatment implications. *Dermatol Surg* (1995) **21**:123–35.

48 Bisaccia E, Scarborough D. Hair transplant by incisional strip harvesting. *J Dermatol Surg Oncol I* (1994) **20**:436–42.

49 Seery G E. Anchor scalp reduction. *Dermatol Surg* (1997) **22**: 1009–13.

50 Luderschmidt C, Plewig G. Circumscribed sebaceous gland hyperplasia: autoradiographic and histoplanimetric studies. *J Invest Dermatol* (1978) **70**:207–9.

51 Plewig G, Kligman A M. Proliferative activity of the sebaceous glands of the aged. *J Invest Dermatol* (1978) **70**:314–17.

52 Braun-Falco O, Thianprasit M. Uber die circum-skripte senile talgdrusenhyperplasie. *Arch Clin Exp Dermatol* (1965) **221**:207–31.

53 Pochi P E, Strauss J S, Downing D T. Age related changes in sebaceous gland activity. *J Invest Dermatol* (1979) **73**:108–11.

54 Bean W B. Nail growth. Twenty five years observation. *Arch Int Med* (1968) **122**:359–61.

55 Silver A F, Montagna W, Karacan I. The effect of age on human eccrine sweating. In: *Advances in Biology of Skin*, Vol IV, Ageing (Pergamon Press: Oxford, 1995) 129–50.

56 Braverman I M, Fonferko E. Studies in cutaneous ageing II. The microvasculature. *J Invest Dermatol* (1982) 444–8.

57 Harvell J D, Maibach H I. Percutaneous absorption and inflammation in aged skin: A review. *J Am Acad Dermatol* (1994) **31**:1015–21.

58 Reed M L, Jacoby R A. Cutaneous neuroanatomy and neuropathy. *Am J Dermatopathol* (1983) **5**:335–62.

59 Katz S I. The epidermal basement membrane zone structure, ontogeny and role in disease. *J Am Med Assoc* (1984) **11**:1025–37.

60 Tidman M J, Eady R A J. Ultrastructural morphometry of normal human dermal epidermal junction. The influence of age, sex and body region on laminar and non laminar components. *J Invest Dermatol* (1984) **83**:448–53.

61 Goodson W H, Hunt T K. Wound healing and ageing. *J Invest Dermatol* (1979) **73**:88–91.

62 Du Nouy P L. *Biological Time* (Macmillan: New York, 1937).

63 Grove G L. Age related differences in healing of superficial skin wounds in humans. *Arch Dermatol Res* **272**:381–5.

64 Comfort A. Ageing and the effects of ionising radiation. In: *The Biology of Senescence*, 3rd Edn, (Churchill Livingstone: Edinburgh, 1979) 239–50.

65 Kaloustian V M der, Kurban A K. Syndromes with premature ageing. In: *Genetic Disease Of the Skin* (Springer Verlag: Berlin, 1979) 116–22.

66 Epstein C J, Martin G M, Shultz A L, Motulsky A G. Werner's syndrome. Review of its symptomatology, natural history, pathologic features, genetics and relationship to natural ageing process. *Medicine* (Baltimore) (1966) **45**:177–221.

67 Gilkes J J H, Sharvill D E, Well R S. The premature ageing syndromes. *Br J Dermatol* (1974) **91**:243–62.

68 Rook A, Davis R, Stevanovic D. Poikiloderma congenitale Rochmund–Thomson syndrome. *Acta Dermato-Venereol* (1959) **39**:392–420.

69 Oikarinen A, Kallioinen M. A biochemical and immunohistochemical study of collagen in sun exposed and protected skin. *Photo-Dermatology* (1989) **6**:24–31.

Protection (
clothing

Artificial protect
be more appar
the shade unde
day may seem
protection as U
surfaces. Simil
protective; it
sunburn throug
thicker clothing
completely imp
hat (such as a
some protectio
foolish to rely (

Sunscreens

Sunscreens are
designed to abs
damage to the s
sunscreens con
the erythematog
opaque suncre
used, protect a
Table 2.1). Their
sunburn wavele
expressed as a
This is a ratio of
cial UVR to pr
sunscreen prof
required withou
debate as to v

Table 2.1 Main a

Ingredients

Para-aminobenzoic
esters, eg, padima
PABA
Cinnamates, eg, o
Benzophenones, e
Anthranilates
Camphor derivative
Opaque sunscreer
veterinary petroleu
dioxide, zinc oxide

2
Environmental considerations

Skin differs in one major and obvious way from all other organs—it is directly exposed to all the rigours and hazards of the environment. Our continued survival on this planet has been possible only because protective mechanisms have evolved. Two adaptations of the skin to the hostile environment are of particular importance: first, the mechanically protective and partially permeable outer horny covering to the skin—the stratum corneum; second, the photo-absorptive melanin pigment system. Even though both adaptations are efficient, they cannot prevent the barrage of climatic insults from causing some permanent damage to the skin's structure.

The degree of damage sustained by the skin is dependent on the type and intensity of the injurious insult and on the susceptibility of the individual. Usually the damage sustained is permanent and accumulates—the older the individual, the more the cumulated damage from climatic exposure. Since the clinical sequelae of cumulative environmental injury are visible on the exposed parts of the skin, they are difficult to distinguish from authentic intrinsic ageing. Indeed, the popular view is that these signs of climatic injury are due to ageing and are therefore unavoidable. As repeated environmental injuries are very common and eminently preventable, a detailed discussion of their effects and of the stimuli that cause them is worth while.

Sites of environmental damage

Climatic, cultural, religious and even political factors may have an influence on the skin sites affected by sun exposure. The face and the backs of the hands are the areas of skin most consistently affected by environmental damage. The 'V' of the neck is also frequently affected, especially in women and manual workers. The scalp skin is subject to solar damage in bald-headed men, adding environmental injury to biological insult. The lower legs, particularly the lower shins, are frequently the site of solar damage in women and of thermal injury from focal heating in both sexes. The back of the neck seems peculiarly prone to solar damage in very sunny climates, especially in outdoor manual workers—giving rise to the expression 'rednecks' to describe the most prominent clinical change at this site in this particular social group.

Not all parts of the face are equally affected by solar injury. The forehead, nose and cheeks receive the greatest dose of solar irradiation and are the areas worst affected. The periocular and perioral areas are much less subject to environmental damage being shaded by bony prominences; the submental area is also relatively spared.

The palms and soles undergo perpetual mechanical trauma and may show permanent evidence of this. The hands, feet and face are the areas most subject to cold injury, although chilblains have been described on the loins, thighs and buttocks as well. The hands are also the sites most frequently affected by toxic chemical injury.

Effects of long-term exposure to the sun

Solar ultraviolet radiation

The ultraviolet portion of the solar spectrum is responsible for most of the damaging effects of solar exposure. The visible part of the spectrum is harmless, but infrared radiation can be damaging. The sun's ultraviolet radiation (UVR) is

700

convention
UVA, UVB
('UVA' or
wavelengtl
wave UVR
spectrum)
between :
('UVC') cor
280 nm.
  UVC is c
little, if any
surface, mo
layer and 1
most impo
cause mos
exposure.
penetrates
penetrate
seems, hov
have a bio
approximat
is needed 1
may be cor
to produc
erythema.
  In recent
divide UV
(350–400 nr
seems to h

keratoses compared to no change in a control group using 'vehicle alone' control in a study by an Australian group.[6] Regular use of sunscreen has also been shown to reduce the amount of solar elastosis in skin as measured by image analysis methods.[7]

Lifestyle

One of the most important measures for protection against damage from UVR is education. While white Caucasians believe that to be chic, healthy and attractive is to be bronzed, we must expect to see young and middle-aged people with signs of severe solar damage to the skin. The advent of the cheap package holiday to the sun-drenched playgrounds of the Mediterranean, and the increasing amount of leisure time and emphasis on outdoor activities has ensured that the average citizen of Western industrialized communities has experienced a high cumulative dose of UVR in recent years. In fact, it has been estimated that those who have a 2–week holiday in the sun receive three times more UVR than their usual annual dose.[6]

Sunbeds and solaria add to the overall UVR dose and therefore they must be considered undesirable. That such artificial sources of UVR irradiate at low dose rates cannot be considered reassuring as there is evidence to suggest that, if anything, low dose rates of UVR are just as dangerous for some types of skin damage as high dose rates.

UVR-induced changes in dermal connective tissue

When skin from chronically sun-exposed areas is inspected microscopically after routine histological preparation, the upper dermis is obviously abnormal (Figure 2.2). The usual fibrillar structure has largely disappeared and the connective tissue is arranged in irregular clumps and strands—the so-called 'spaghetti and meatball' appearance. The abnormal connective tissue is also more basophilic than normal connective tissue and shows a similar staining pattern to elastic tissue when orcein-containing stains are used (Figure 2.3). The significance of this tinctorial similarity to elastic tissue is uncertain, but recent studies suggest that the abnormal elastic-staining tissue is indeed a form of elastic tissue.[7] The extent of this degenerative change varies with the dose of UVR received. In very severely

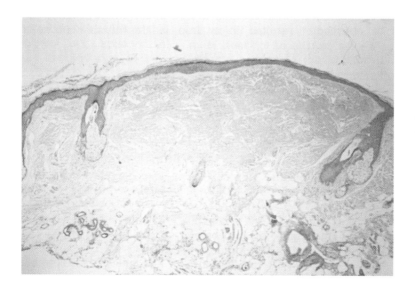

Figure 2.2

Severe solar elastotic degenerative change affecting the upper, mid and lower dermis. There is a band immediately beneath the epidermis that is not affected. The abnormal tissue is slightly more basophilic than usual and no longer possesses the fibrillar arrangement usually seen. The affected areas are more homogeneous looking than normal (H & E; ×25).

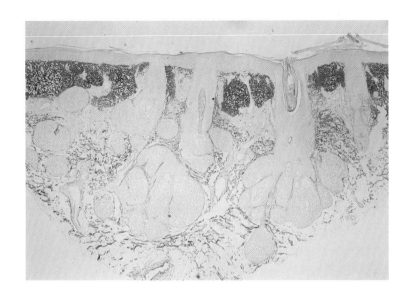

Figure 2.3

This photomicrograph shows a section stained specially to demonstrate abnormal solar elastotic tissue. Note the dark violet areas in the upper and mid dermis. The section was taken from a chronically sun exposed area of the face of an elderly man (elastic stain ×25).

affected areas virtually the whole of the upper and much of the mid dermis is replaced by the abnormal tissue. Curiously, the immediate subepidermal connective tissue stays free of elastotic change. The reason for this so-called Grenz zone is uncertain, but it is consistently present and seems likely to have a fundamental pathogenetic significance.

Sometimes the change is so profound that the interfollicular epidermis appears distended from the deposition of an abnormal homogenous basophilic material beneath, causing papules to appear clinically. This situation is known as 'colloid milium'[7] and is found in predisposed fair-skinned individuals who have had very heavy sun exposure.

Clearly there are mechanical consequences to chronic solar damage resulting from this alteration in the dermal connective tissue—evident in part by the droopiness and wrinkling of the skin. This has been difficult to document because of the impossibility of clearly distinguishing the effects of intrinsic ageing from those due to solar damage. It should be noted, however, that Pierard et al[8] have identified mechanical changes in the dermis due to psoralen UVA (PUVA) (see page 69), and presumably changes due to natural UVR are similar but less intense.

UV-induced epidermal damage and photocarcinogenesis

There can be no doubt that solar UVR is the major cause of solar keratoses and squamous cell carcinoma and is an important influence in the development of keratoacanthoma, Bowen's disease, basal cell carcinoma and melanoma. The strongest evidence is everyday clinical experience that these lesions are much more common in parts of the world that receive a large amount of sunshine and in pale-skinned individuals without strong protective melanin pigmentation. In addition there seems to be a dose–effect relationship as there is a much greater likelihood of skin cancer in people who work outdoors or who enjoy outdoor recreation. Further clinical evidence comes from patients with the disorder known as xeroderma pigmentosum, who develop large numbers of skin cancers on light-exposed skin while young. These individuals have an abnormality of DNA repair following damage by UVR.[9] Even more persuasive is the fact that psoriatic patients treated with photochemotherapy with UVA (PUVA) have a much higher incidence of skin cancers than expected.[10]

There is also a large amount of experimental evidence, mostly derived from the irradiation of mice, that UVR is carcinogenic.[11,12] The subject of photocarcinogenesis has become of considerable practical importance in recent years as well as of great theoretical interest, and the interested reader should consult recent reviews on the subject (eg, Epstein,[13] Marks,[14] van der Leun[15]).

The details of how UVR causes skin cancer are not known at present but there are several important clues. Langerhans cells seem particularly susceptible to damage by UVR.[16] As these cells appear to be vital for the development of delayed hypersensitivity, it has been suggested that sun-damaged epidermis is less able to eliminate rogue epidermal cells that may become neoplastic. It has also been demonstrated that UVR-induced tumours in mice can be transplanted into and not rejected by other UVR-irradiated mice, although non-irradiated mice will reject them.[17] This has suggested that UVR induces an antigen-specific series of T suppressor cells that allow the tumour to develop. Another observation that underlines the importance of the immune status in relation to the development of sun-induced skin cancer is the high prevalence of this group of disorders in immunosuppressed renal transplant patients.[18–20]

In addition to the changes mentioned above, alterations take place in UVR exposed epidermal cells that set off the whole process. Nuclear DNA seems to be a prime target. Abnormal crosslinks are produced which in normal individuals are enzymically excised and the base sequence repaired—a process that is inherently faulty in patients with xeroderma pigmentosum.[9] Presumably the repair process is not always adequate and other nuclear alterations occur, allowing the survival and growth of cells with abnormal nuclear DNA. Much work has appeared to show that solar UVR causes mutations in the important anti-tumour gene—P53. Recently it has been reported that mutations in this gene in mice after irradiation can be prevented by the use of sunscreens.[21] In addition, chronically UVR-stimulated skin shows epidermal hyperplasia and hyperproliferation as well as abnormal metabolic activity.[22] In particular there is enhanced glucose-6–phosphate dehydrogenase enzyme activity in the upper epidermis (Figure 2.2). This is observed as an increased width and intensity of the formazan reaction deposit seen in the enzyme cytochemical tests. It is also clear that all chronically UVR-damaged epidermis is abnormal, and cytological abnormalities are common even in skin that appears to be clinically normal.[23] Attempts have been made to quantify the degree of cytological atypia (dysplasia) using stereological, cell cycle analytic and biochemical techniques.[24] Although none of these methods are ideal, progress is being made in this area. It is not known which, if any, of the above changes are central to the development of neoplasia.

Clinical signs of solar elastotic degeneration

The most obvious changes in persistently sun-exposed skin are due to solar elastotic degeneration. Affected skin usually appears slightly thicker than normal and may have a sallow somewhat orangey-yellow or pale lemon-yellow hue (Figure 2.4). The surface is often, but not always, wrinkled or deeply furrowed, depending on the exact anatomical site.

The back of the neck shows deep furrows in individuals who have spent much time working outdoors in sunny climates (sailor's skin; see Figure 2.5). Sometimes there is a reddish background with the furrowing, especially in people with an auburn or gingery complexion, giving rise to the not very complimentary term 'rednecks' for Caucasian outdoor workers in the southern United States. Solar elastosis also causes small wrinkle lines radiating laterally from the external angle of the eye, referred to as crow's feet. These are almost inevitably present in white-skinned individuals after the age of 40 and are more evident during smiling or laughter. Small wrinkles also develop beneath the eye parallel to the lower lid, later progressing so that the skin of this area sags, giving rise to the familiar 'bags' beneath the eyes. The skin of this area is naturally lax and this change may develop because of other disorders besides solar elastotic degeneration. As elastotic degeneration becomes more severe, the number of wrinkle lines increases and they encroach on other facial areas including the cheeks (Figure 2.6).

How solar elastosis causes wrinkling is not entirely clear. Wrinkles do not develop over the

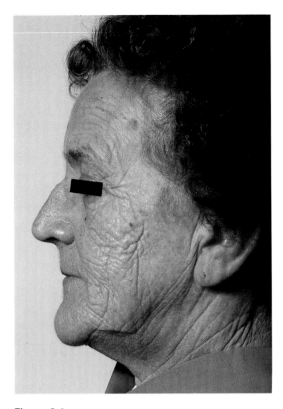

Figure 2.4a

Solar elastotic degenerative change showing wrinkling and yellowish appearance of the skin.

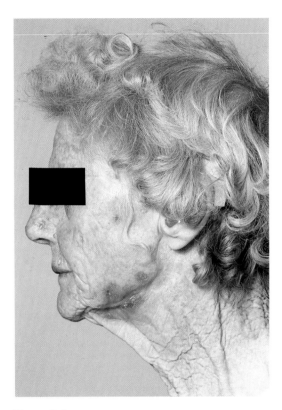

Figure 2.4b

Severe solar elastosis affecting the neck of an elderly Welsh lady. Note the 'chicken-neck skin' appearance. The reddened areas are solar keratoses.

nose, ears or forearms, which are histologically affected by solar elastosis, where considerable mobility of the skin is normally not required. It may be that the presence of wrinkle lines is a result of a change in the mechanical properties of the elastotic dermis in skin, which is normally extensile (see page 000). It is plain, however, that not all wrinkling is due to solar damage—wrinkle lines on the forehead, for example, seem to be partially genetically determined. The deep nasolabial furrows are also not due to solar damage and probably represent the ageing of subcutaneous tissue. Some wrinkle lines may also be due to the ageing process *per se*. Sagging of the skin of the trunk or upper arms is mostly due to obesity and intrinsic ageing and is irreversible (Figure 2.6c).

Telangiectasia and purpura

The lack of support for the vasculature of the subpapillary venous plexus allows these channels to dilate and to rupture after minor injury. The telangiectasia that results is particularly obvious over the cheeks (Figure 2.7). Senile purpura is the term used for crimson or purple patches developing over the forearms and the backs of the hands and sometimes elsewhere (Figure 2.8). The extravasated blood takes longer than usual to disappear and the normal colour changes of a bruise are muted. It seems that in the elderly this is partly due to depressed macrophage activity.[25] Similar clinical signs are caused by attrition of dermal connective tissue due to the action of glucocorticoids either from

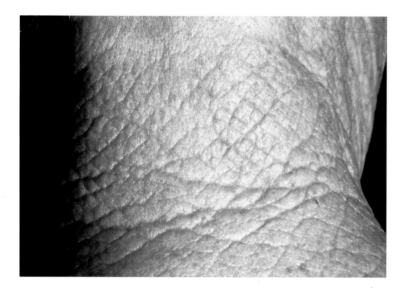

Figure 2.5a

Skin of back of neck of an elderly man showing deep furrowing and slight reddish background colour. This appearance gave rise to the term 'rednecks' to describe a particular group of individuals.

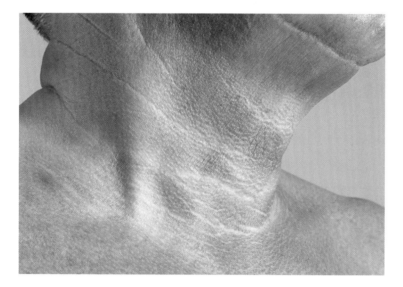

Figure 2.5b

Reddened appearance of skin of neck in man of 62 who persistently sunbathed. Note the comparative sparing of the areas that are not exposed because they are at the bottom of folds of skin.

the administration of these drugs or because of Cushing's syndrome.

Triradiate scars

If the skin of sun-battered individuals is examined closely, odd, irregularly shaped scars are sometimes found on the backs of the hands and forearms. These are linear, triradiate, stellate or angulate (Figure 2.9) and are usually 1–2 cm long. If questioned, their owners often attribute the existence of these scars to some former injury or activity. They seem, however, to arise either spontaneously or in response to quite minor traumata, and to occur specifically in sun-damaged skin. Their origins are mysterious, but they may reflect inefficient repair mechanisms in dermal

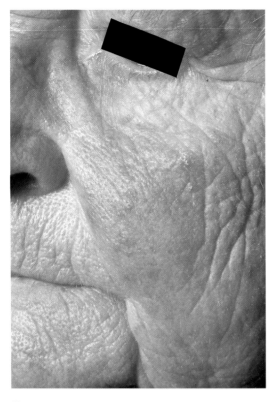

Figure 2.6a

Solar elastosis affecting an elderly lady, showing numerous wrinkles by the mouth and on the cheek. There is also redness of the cheeks due to persistent vasodilatation and telangiectasia.

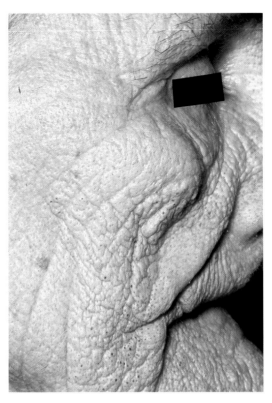

Figure 2.6b

Severe elastotic degeneration affecting the side of the face in a woman of 84.

Figure 2.6c

The droopy, saggy appearance of this elderly woman's upper arm is not due to solar elastosis but results from changes in her connective tissue due to senility and obesity.

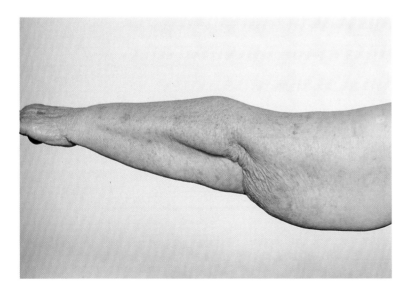

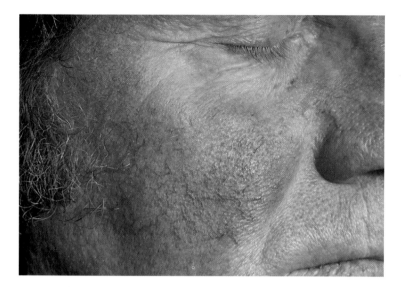

Figure 2.7

Intense erythema and telangiectasia of the cheeks due to solar elastosis and weathering in a farmer.

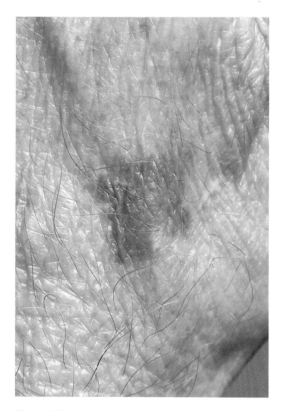

Figure 2.8

Senile purpura on back of hand.

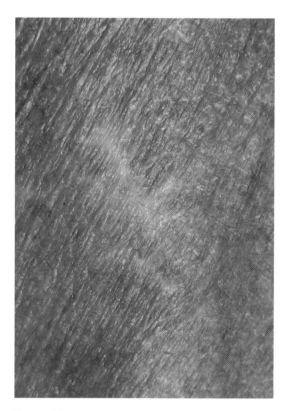

Figure 2.9

Triradiate scars. These are probably best called 'angulate' scars because, as seen in this example, the white scar marks are not often three-pronged but are irregular and angulated.

connective tissue affected by solar elastotic degenerative change.

Less common signs of solar damage

There are several other uncommon manifestations of solar elastosis (see Calderone and Fenske[26] for a recent review). Annular elastolytic granuloma, also known as actinic granuloma, is seen mostly on the dorsa of the forearms and the upper back, but it also occurs over the head and neck. Pink translucent papules develop and enlarge into ring-shaped lesions 1–3 cm in diameter. Histologically there is a focal marked granulomatous area of inflammation with evidence of the destruction of elastic tissue. Pseudocolloid milium is another uncommon lesion due to severe solar elastosis, typical signs are translucent papules and plaques on the upper face or the back of the hands and wrists.

Senile comedones and other pilosebaceous abnormalities

Dilated follicular orifices with comedonal plugging are not uncommonly found on the back and/or facial skin of the elderly. On the face these lesions occur around the eyes and on the upper cheeks, and they are reputed to be specifically associated with elastotic degenerative change. There may be just one or two such lesions or they may occur in large numbers (Figure 2.10a) and be the cause of some cosmetic distress. They can be removed quite easily: the skin is carefully pierced over each lesion and the follicular contents expressed. Unfortunately the comedone tends to reform after a few weeks. Our own epidemiological observations throw some doubt as to the relationship of these lesions to solar damage,[27] and histologically they are not always surrounded by dense elastosis.

Senile sebaceous gland hyperplasia is very common in elderly men (see also Chapters 1 and 9). Small yellowish papules (Figure 2.10b) are found, some with central puncta, over the cheeks and nose. They occur in areas of solar elastosis but the exact relationship is not clear. Occasionally giant comedones are found over the back in the elderly (Figure 2.10c), but again their significance is not clear.

The treatment and prognosis of solar elastosis and wrinkling

It has been tacitly accepted that once solar elastotic degenerative change has occurred it will be carried to the grave with its owner. However, the critical experiment of preventing further solar damage to skin affected by solar elastosis, with detailed and controlled observations over the ensuing years, has not, to my knowledge, been performed. From the recent results of studies in humans it now appears beyond doubt that the application of preparations containing all-trans retinoic acid or isotretinoin can improve the appearance of photoaged skin, at least while it is being used. The exact role of this agent is unknown, but the fact that it is at least possible to reverse some of the clinical sequelae of chronic solar irradiation has caused enormous interest.

Topical tretinoin has been shown in numerous well-controlled studies to improve the clinical appearance of photodamaged skin (eg, see Kligman et al,[28] Olsen et al[29] and Griffiths et al[30]). After 3–6 months use of topical preparations containing 0.025–0.1% tretinoin, there is a marked reduction in fine lines and some more prominent wrinkles, the sallow, yellowish appearance and the focal pigmented senile lentigines. Long-term use also reduces the number of solar keratoses. Individuals who have 'mild–moderate' changes of photodamage and who apply the preparations regularly as instructed show the best responses. The topical retinoid preparations may cause some skin irritation and skin dryness but this diminishes with time and is tolerable. One study showed that 0.025% tretinoin produced the same benefit with less irritation; the skin is also more sensitive to the sun during use.[15] After some 6–9 months maximum benefit is achieved and to maintain this, twice weekly applications of the

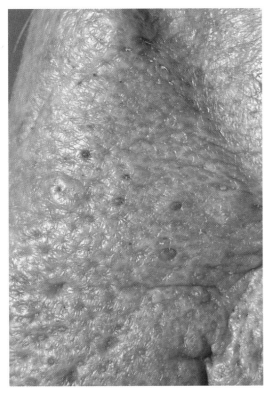

Figure 2.10a

Senile comedones.

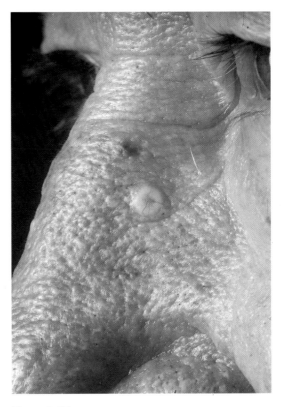

Figure 2.10b

Sebaceous gland hyperplasia in an elderly man. Note the central punctum in this yellowish nodule.

tretinoin preparation are sufficient. Patients who start on this treatment should feel committed to an altered lifestyle which includes decreased sun exposure and the use of sunscreens and emollients. Research studies in both mice and humans indicate that the topical tretinoin stimulates the synthesis of new dermal connective tissue that pushes down the solar elastotic degenerative dermis.[31,32] Tretinoin also accelerates epidermal cell production and modulates differentiation reducing the degree of epidermal dysplasia. In addition, these retinoids appear to stimulate neoangiogenesis and to 'normalize' melanin pigment distribution. Not unexpectedly topical isotretinoin has also been shown to have similar beneficial effects.

As mentioned previously, sunscreens have been shown to reduce the amount of solar elastosis present. Hydroxyacids are more recent additions to the anti-photodamage drug armamentarium[28] but as yet the evidence for their efficacy is less than overwhelming. Emollient creams and lotions may temporarily decrease the appearance of wrinkling by a flattening effect on the skin surface, but there is no evidence of any more fundamental change. 'Chemical peeling' has also been advocated. Detailed discussion of this procedure would be inappropriate here as the technique has not gained general acceptance and is potentially hazardous in the hands of the inexperienced and unskilled. Those experienced in the procedures claim that peels with 70% glycolic acid or

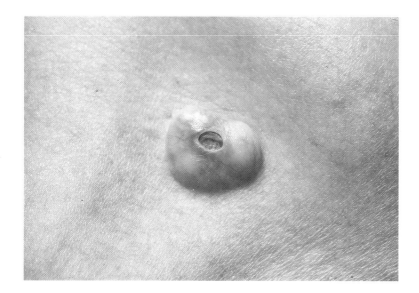

Figure 2.10c

Giant comedome on back of elderly woman. Why these lesions occur is a complete mystery.

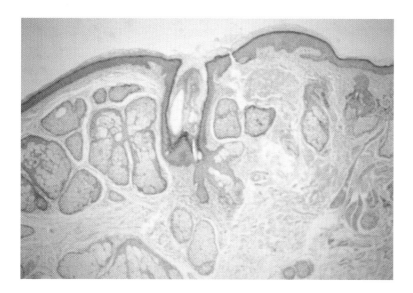

Figure 2.10d

Photomicrograph of sebaceous gland hyperplasia. Note large number of sebaceous glands in upper dermis (H & C).

trichloracetic acid can produce dramatic improvements in photodamaged skin. Plastic surgery is popular among the older, more affluent sections of the community—particularly in the USA. Undoubtedly the skin is made tauter and smoother by these techniques (details of the techniques may be found in Epstein and Epstein[33]).

Clinical signs of chronic solar damage to the epidermis

The clinical features of basal cell carcinoma, solar keratoses, Bowen's disease, keratoacanthoma, melanoma and squamous cell carcinoma are outlined in Chapter 9. Apart from the

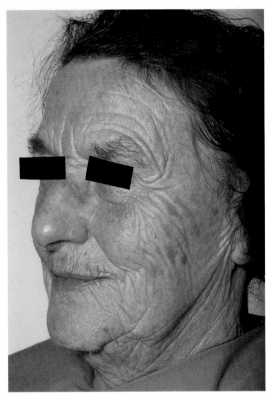

Figure 2.11a

Severe solar elastotic degenerative change and senile lentigos on the side of the face.

neoplastic lesions mentioned above, there are no established clinical sequelae from chronic solar exposure of the epidermis. However, chronically sun-exposed skin looks rough and coarse and has a dull mahogany discoloration. I believe these are the clinical counterparts of the minor histological abnormalities present in exposed but apparently normal skin.

Large, discrete light-brown patches over the temple, forehead or elsewhere on the face are known as senile lentigines (Figure 2.11). Smaller but similar lesions occur on the backs of the hands and are known colourfully by the French as *les medallions de cimitière*. Many of these are flat, seborrhoeic warts (see page 183); others are true lentigines with melanocyte hyperplasia and slight epidermal thickening. Yet others are large and lightly pigmented solar keratoses. Some seem to feature several abnormalities. They arise in sun-exposed skin and it seems likely that chronic solar exposure also has much to do with their aetiopathogenesis. The larger lesions must be carefully distinguished from lentigo maligna.

Chronic heat injury

The elderly often complain of feeling the cold more than they did in their youth, and where

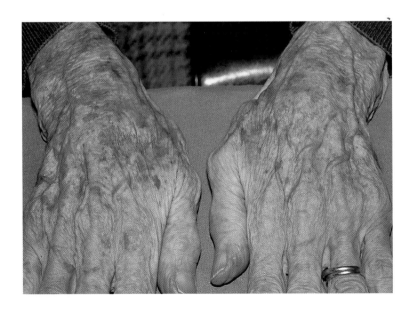

Figure 2.11b

Senile lentigos on back of hands.

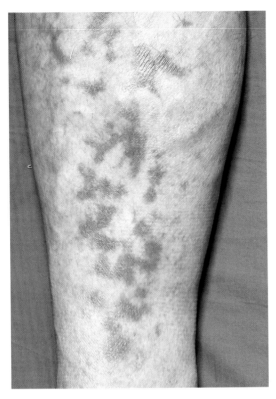

Figure 2.12

Typical reticulate pigmented appearance of erythema ab igne.

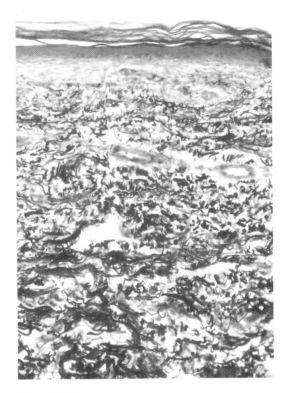

Figure 2.13

Elastotic tissue dispersed throughout the dermis in erythema ab igne (elastic stain ×25).

there is no central heating, they often warm themselves in front of focal sources of heat. This produces a characteristic reticulate, red-brown pigmentation over the front of the shins (Figure 2.12) or elsewhere and a series of other more unpleasant changes in the tissue, which are known as erythema ab igne. The reticulate pigmentation seems to be due primarily to deposition of haemosiderin, though why this should be in a reticulate pattern is unclear. The presence of pigment is confirmed histologically by the Prussian blue staining reaction; on biopsy material from patients with erythema ab igne this reaction reveals that most of the pigment is in the macrophages. The most striking alteration morphologically is the marked abnormality in the dermal fibrous tissue. Elastic tissue stains show that the abnormal degenerate material is

similar to that found in solar elastosis but differs in that it is evenly dispersed throughout the dermis (Figure 2.13) rather than clumped in the papillary and upper dermis. The dermal vasculature is also affected. The vessels are thickened and dilated.

In the more severely affected patients, small warty lesions appear on the involved skin. These are premalignant keratoses exactly analogous to solar keratoses.[34] Rarely, frank squamous cell carcinomas occur, completing the analogy to solar-induced skin damage.

Erythema ab igne is also seen occasionally over the trunk or in other areas subject to chronic heating. These may be found over the back or abdomen after the use of hot water bottles to relieve pain. Skin cancer has also been noted in individuals who carry containers of hot embers for heating.[35] It is interesting to speculate what role solar heating plays in the development of chronic solar damage. Recent studies show that when the skin is recurrently heated experimentally, the epidermis shows cell kinetic and enzyme cytochemical changes very similar to those that occur after UVR injury.

Cold injury

Repeated exposure to low temperatures can also damage the skin, but the effects of cold are in general less well documented than those of heat. As with any type of stimulus, the effects of cold on the skin depend on its strength and its rate of delivery. Clinical experience also suggests that the relative humidity, the presence of wind, and rapid warming after cold exposure modulate the type and severity of the injury produced. Chilblains are primarily a problem of north-west Europeans, and this has been explained by the cold, damp climate (and lack of central heating) in this area. Chilblains mostly affect the feet but they may be seen on the fingers and even on the face as well as other sites, particularly if these are well lined by subcutaneous fat and are either exposed to the cold or are usually flimsily clad. Chilblains have been described on the thighs, upper arms and buttocks and also on the flanks, though they are rarely found at these sites in the elderly.

Chilblains are easily recognized as mauve or bluish swollen areas which give rise to throbbing pain and itch—particularly when the affected areas are warmed. Histologically there is vascular dilatation, oedema and slight haemorrhage. Treatment of established lesions is not very effective, though advice on warm clothing and the use of rubefacients may give some relief.

Ordinary chilblains must be distinguished from the chilblain-like lesions seen in lupus erythematosus (see page 000), sarcoidosis and a preleukaemic disorder.[36] In all of these the lesions tend to be larger and more persistent.

Some dermatologists have suggested that continued exposure to the cold wind may contribute to the cause of rosacea but there is little evidence to substantiate this.

Low relative humidity

Low relative humidity tends to dry out the horny layer of the skin, causing chapping, xerosis and itchiness; this tendency is accentuated in the cold and also when there is an accompanying wind. It is particularly a problem in the elderly, especially in areas such as the northeastern United States. When the environmental conditions are compounded by unaccustomed frequent washing a form of eczema results. This is marked on the lower legs and is known as eczema craquelé because of the crazy paving appearance (see page 38).

Chronic mechanical injury

The chiropodists' waiting rooms are filled with elderly patients (mainly women) who in their youth crammed their feet into fashionable footwear. The corns and callosities that this bizarre societal behaviour produces are the cause of considerable discomfort and in some cases real disability (Figure 2.14). It is not clear whether all people are equally susceptible to these lesions, nor whether minor orthopaedic abnormalities of the feet are an essential feature of the problem.

Both types of lesions are painful (sometimes exquisitely so) but are clinically distinguishable. A corn (clavus) is a well-delineated hyperkeratotic area with a central area of even denser horn, which histologically appears to be largely 'subsurface'. A callosity is a more diffuse lesion marked by massive hyperkeratosis and epidermal hyperplasia.[37] Once they are established, it is difficult to rid the feet permanently of these annoying excrescences. They are usually treated by combinations of paring to remove the hard skin, salicylic acid dressings to assist in the same purpose and pads and other dressings to prevent weight bearing directly on the affected site. Advice on the choice of comfortable footwear is also essential. The paring down of the hyperkeratotic areas is not a job for amateurs—this should be done by chiropodists.

The hard horn over corns and callosities is inelastic and may crack with movement of the feet, allowing infection to develop. Such infected areas need urgent attention to prevent serious

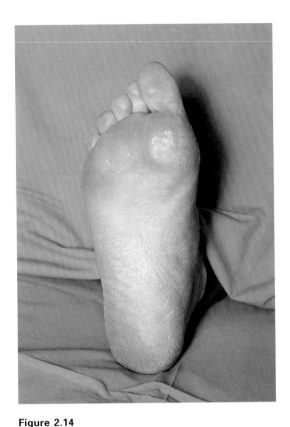

Figure 2.14

Corn and callosity on foot.

damage to the foot and often require systemic antibiotics.

Corns and callosities have to be distinguished from viral warts which, although uncommon in the elderly, do sometimes occur in this age group. Sometimes the distinction between a viral wart and a callosity can be made only by paring down the area and finding, in a viral wart, the characteristic hard white horn at the centre with punctate bleeding points. Squamous cell carcinoma may occasionally masquerade as a corn or callosity but the history of increasing size, atypical sites and warty irregularity of the surface should help differentiate this lesion.

Soft corns are macerated painful penetrating lesions found between closely apposed toes. Their exact aetiology is unknown but the constant friction between the abnormally close

toes probably plays the major role. Separation of the affected toes is the main component in their treatment and this can be accomplished using Sorbo rubber or some other soft resilient material.

General foot care is extremely important in the elderly as the additional disability of painful feet can cause total immobility in someone already troubled by osteoarthritis or chronic cardiorespiratory disorders. Foot care should include attention to the hyperkeratotic lesions discussed earlier as well as advice on hygiene and footwear.

Callosities are also found on the hands, knees, elbows and at other sites subject to repeated pressure and friction. Activities as varied as golf, housework and praying to Mecca can all cause callosities. Generally these lesions are not a problem for the elderly. However, continual mechanical trauma can contribute to the development of hand eczema and can localize various disorders including psoriasis (see page 56) and lichen planus (see page 70).

Chronic chemical trauma

The ability of alkalis, acids, detergents, oxidizing agents and other materials to irritate the skin and cause a primary irritant contact dermatitis is well known (see page 46). The ability of such irritants to cause other disorders after continuous or repeated long-term contact is less certain. Some substances (carcinogens) initiate skin cancer and others promote it,[38] but usually these substances are strictly regulated and are not ordinarily in contact with the skin. Chimney sweeps' cancer of the scrotum is a historically interesting example of a skin cancer once caused by chronic occupational exposure to a material (soot, in this instance) containing carcinogens. Pitch warts used to be seen in those who worked with pitch, and are another example of skin cancer from chronic exposure to chemical carcinogens. There is no firm evidence that other everyday materials currently in use contribute significantly to the development of skin cancer.

It would not be surprising if persistent chemical irritancy caused permanent changes in the skin. There is certainly evidence that the skin is not completely physiologically normal in individuals who have had an irritant dermatitis some time previously.[39]

References

1   Magnus I A. Sunlight. In: *Dermatological Photobiology*, (Blackwell: Oxford, 1976).

2   Davis S, Capjack L, Kerr N, Fedosejevs R. Clothing as protection from ultraviolet radiation: which fabric is most effective. *Int J Dermatol* (1997) **36:**374–9.

3   Klein K. Formulating sunscreen products. In: Lowe NJ, Sheath NA, eds. *Sunscreens*, (Marcel Dekker, 1990).

4   Kligman L K, Akin F J, Kligman A M. The contributions of UVA and UVB to connective tissue damage in hairless mice. *J Invest Dermatol* (1985) **84:**272–6.

5   Willis I, Menter J M, Whyte H J. The rapid induction of cancers in the hairless mouse utilising the principle of photoaugmentation. *J Invest Dermatol* (1981) **76:**404–8.

6   Beadle P C, Leach J F. Holidays, ozone and skin cancer. Skin cancer in Bristol—a comparison of theory with observation. *Arch Dermatol Res* (1982) **274:**47–56.

7   Bernstein E F, Chen Y Q, Kopp J B et al. Long-term sun exposure alters the collagen of the papillary dermis. Comparison of sun-protected and photoaged skin by northern analysis, immunohistochemical staining, and confocal laser scanning microscopy. *J Am Acad Dermatol* (1996) **34:**209–18.

8   Pierard G E, Franchimont C, de la Brassinne M et al. Photosclerosis induced by long wavelength ultraviolet light and psoralens. In: Marks R, Payne P, eds *Bioengineering and the Skin*. (MTP Press: Lancaster, 1981) 71–8.

9   Kraemer K H. Xeroderma pigmentosum. In: Demis D J, Dobson R L, McGuire J, eds *Clinical Dermatology*, Vol 4, (Harper and Row: London, 1980).

10 Stern R S, Laird N, Melski J et al. Cutaneous squamous cell carcinoma in patients treated with PUVA. *New Engl J Med* (1984) **310:**1156–61.

11 Blum H F. *Carcinogenesis by Ultraviolet Light* (University Press, Princeton: New Jersey, 1959).

12 Freeman R G. Action spectrum for ultraviolet carcinogenesis. *Natl Cancer Inst Monogr* (1978) **50:**27–9.

13 Epstein J H. Photocarcinogenesis, skin cancer and aging. *J Am Acad Dermatol* (1983) **9:**487–502.

14 Marks R. Premalignant disease of the epidermis— some light on neoplasia. *J R Coll Phys Lond* (1986) **20:**116–21.

15 van der Leun J C. UV carcinogenesis. *Photochem Photobiol* (1984) **39:**861–8.

16 Aberer W, Schuler G, Stingle G et al. Ultraviolet light depletes surface markers of Langerhans cells. *J Invest Dermatol* (1981) **76:**202–10.

17 Kripke M L. Immunologic mechanisms in UV radiation carcinogenesis. *Adv Cancer Res* (1981) **34:**69–106.

18 Shuttleworth D, Marks R, Griffin P J A, Salaman J R. Dysplastic epidermal change in immunosuppressed patients with renal transplants. *Q J Med* (1987) **243:**609–16.

19 Hardie I R, Strong R W, Hartley L C J et al. Skin cancer in Caucasian renal allograft recipients living in a subtropical climate. *Surgery* (1980) **87:**177–83.

20 Blohme I, Larkö O. Skin lesions in renal transplant patients after 10–23 years of immunosuppressive therapy. *Acta Derm Venereol* (Stockh) (1990) **70:**491–4.

21 Anathaswamy H N, Loughlin S M, Cox P et al. Sunlight and skin cancer: Inhibition of p53 mutations in UV irradiated mouse skin by sunscreens. *Nature Med* (1997) **3:**510–14.

22 Pearse A D, Marks R. Quantitative changes in respiratory enzyme activity in premalignant lesions and experimentally irradiated skin. *Bull Cancer* (1978) **65:**351–6.

23 Pearse A D, Marks R. Actinic keratosis and the epidermis on which they arise. *Br J Dermatol* (1977) **96:**45–50.

24 Barton S P, Pearse A D, Marks R. Derivation of a dysplasia index for epidermal neoplasia. *Dermatology* (1992) **185:**190–5.

25 Shuster S, Scarborough H. Senile purpura. *Q J Med* (1961) **30:**33–40.

26 Calderone D C, Fenske N A. The clinical spectrum of actinic elastosis. *J Am Acad Dermatol* (1995) **32:**1016–24.

27 Kumar R, Marks R. Sebaceous gland hyperplasia and senile comedones: a prevalence study in elderly hospitalised patients. *Br J Dermatol* **117:**231–6.

28 Kligman L H, Due C H, Kligman A M. Topical retinoic acid enhances the repair of ultraviolet damaged dermal connective tissue. *Connect Tissue Res* (1984) **12:**139–50.

29 Olsen E A, Katz I, Levine et al. Tretinoin emollient cream: a new therapy for photodamaged skin. *J Am Acad Dermatol* (1992) **26:**215–24.

30 Griffiths C E M, Kang S, Ellis C N et al. Two concentrations of topical tretinoin (retinoic acid) cause similar improvement of photoaging but different degrees of irritation. *Arch Dermatol* (1995) **131:**518–22.

31 Schwarz E, Kligman L H. Topical tretinoin increases the tropoelastin and fibronectin content of photoaged hairless mouse skin. *J Invest Dermatol* (1995) **104:**518–22.

32 Schwarz E, Cruickshank F A, Mezick J A et al. Topical all-trans retinoic acid stimulates collagen synthesis in vivo. *J Invest Dermatol* (1991) **96:**975–8.

33 Epstein E, Epstein E, Jr. *Techniques in Skin Surgery* (Lea & Febiger: Philadelphia, 1979).

34 Shahrad P, Marks R. The wages of warmth: changes in erythema ab igne. *Br J Dermatol* (1977) **97:**179–86.

35 Svindland H B. Kangri cancer in the brick industry. *Contact Dermatitis* (1980) **6:**24–6.

36 Marks R, Lim C C, Barrie P F. A perniotic syndrome with monocytosis and neutropenia. *Br J Dermatol* (1969) **81:**327–31.

37 Thomas S E, Dykes P J, Marks R. Plantar hyperkeratosis. A study of callosities and normal plantar skin. *J Invest Dermatol* (1985) **85:**394–7.

38 Boutwell R K. The biochemistry of preneoplasia in mouse skin. *Cancer Res* (1976) **36:**2631–5.

39 Al Jaberi H, Marks R. Studies of the clinically uninvolved skin in patients wiht dermatitis. *Br J Dermatol* (1984) **111:**437–43.

3
The inflammatory scaling dermatoses

The eczematous dermatoses and psoriasis have much in common and, despite their different causes, their similarities seem to be exaggerated in the elderly. For this reason it was decided to describe eczematous dermatoses and psoriasis, together with a few rarer dermatoses, in the same section of this book.

The eczematous dermatoses

Introduction

This group of disorders is characterized by a particular variety of epidermal inflammation in which the predominant pathological feature is intercellular oedema (spongiosis). The oedema collects to form vesicles which erupt to 'weep' at the surface if the eczema develops acutely. Epidermal thickening is seen in all varieties of eczema after the acute phase has passed.

The terms eczema and dermatitis are regarded as synonymous and are used interchangeably in this chapter.

The commoner varieties of eczema in the elderly are set out in Table 3.1. The pattern of eczema differs markedly between age groups. Atopic dermatitis is quite uncommon in the elderly but other types of eczema, such as asteatotic eczema and discoid eczema, are virtually restricted to this age group. The reason for this changing pattern across the lifespan is unclear, but it should be noted that the intensity and timing of experimentally produced inflammation of the skin differs markedly in the older age group. For example, the time taken for suction blisters to appear is greater in the elderly[1] and ammonium hydroxide blistering is similarly prolonged in this age group.[2] Similarly,

the reaction to a battery of irritants appears to be muted in the elderly.[3] The elderly also show a reduced erythema response to UV irradiation.[4] The various structural and functional differences in the skin of the elderly may dictate that the elderly epidermis is less capable of reacting to an injurious stimulus with an eczematous reaction. In addition the inflammatory process itself appears to be modified in the aged.[5]

As pointed out in the previous chapter there is a reduction in Langerhans cells in the skin of the elderly. This is one component of the reduced capacity to mount a delayed hypersensitivity response in the elderly, but the other elements are less well characterized. This diminished immune responsiveness must also influence the pattern of eczema in the elderly.

Seborrhoeic dermatitis

Definition

Seborrhoeic dermatitis is a common, persistent eczematous disorder of unknown origin which typically results in a reddened, scaling eruption that affects the scalp, facial flexures, the central parts of the upper trunk and the major body flexures.

Aetiopathogenesis

There is increasing evidence that most forms of the disease (particularly pityriasis simplex—or dandruff) are due to a disturbance of the skin microflora.[6] In particular, the disorder has been ascribed to overgrowth of *Pityrosporon ovale*

Table 3.1 Common eczematous conditions in the elderly

Clinical varieties of eczema	Major features
Seborrhoeic dermatitis	Involvement of scalp and face are frequent; in more severe varieties the disorder spreads to involve the central part of the trunk and limbs; major flexural areas are also affected; men are more frequently affected
Asteototic eczema (syn. eczema cracquelée)	Typically the lateral aspects of the lower legs are affected by a cracked 'crazy-paving' type of scaling; may spread to other extensor aspects of the limbs and trunk
Gravitational eczema (syn. venous eczema)	This occurs as part of the gravitational syndrome most often around ulcerated areas but can spread to affect other areas; must be distinguished from allergic contact dermatitis due to applied medicaments
Allergic contact dermatitis	Occurs as a result of sensitization to an applied or contacted chemical agent; is at first restricted to the sites of contact but may spread to other areas later; often due to applied medicaments in the elderly
Primary irritant dermatitis	This is due to exposure to chemical irritants and usually presents as 'hand eczema'
Hand and foot eczema	Typical vesicular eczema of these sites (pompholyx) is uncommon in the elderly but more persistent and disabling
Infectious eczematoid dermatitis and intertriginous eczema	This occurs as an exudative dermatosis in the major body folds; it is more common in the obese and may be a major problem in elderly obese women in the retromammary areas; may involve the ears and surrounding skin
Discoid eczema	Coin-sized or larger areas of eczema appear on the limbs and trunk
Lichen simplex chronicus	Well-defined, thickened scaling plaques over certain sites such as the back of the scalp, around the wrists, elbows and knees and the dorsum of the foot characterize this disorder; it tends to be persistent and resistant to treatment
Photodermatitis	A dermatitis affecting the light-exposed sites and often due to a drug or a material applied to the skin previously

and an altered skin response to this. Seborrhoeic dermatitis of a specially persistent and severe type is a well-known complication of AIDS complex, presumably reflecting the reduced cellular immunity in this disease.[7] The disorder also occurs in other diseases in which there is a chronic deficiency of T-helper lymphocytes.[8]

Clinical features

The disorder is seen at all ages and in both sexes but seems quite common in the late middle-aged and the elderly. It usually starts in the scalp and may be mistaken for severe dandruff. Later the rash progressively involves the frontal scalp margin, the eyebrows, the eyelids, the paranasal areas, the external ears, the retroauricular regions, the remainder of the face (Figure 3.1), the sides of the neck, the front of the chest, the central part of the upper back and the major body flexures. In the most severely affected individuals

the disorder becomes generalized and is one cause of an erythroderma (Figure 3.2). The rash itself is pink or red with marked scaling, and macular or very slightly raised. Affected areas are usually quite well defined but not so sharply as in psoriasis (see page 56). As with most eczematous conditions, seborrhoeic dermatitis causes itching. Untreated, the disorder is persistent, and even when treated successfully it tends to recur.

Differential diagnosis

Sebhorroeic dermatitis may be difficult to distinguish from psoriasis in some patients, and even the histological appearance may not supply a definitive answer. Flexural psoriasis and facial psoriasis can be especially difficult to distinguish from seborrhoeic dermatitis. In fact, the frequent clinical confusion has been epitomized by a spoof name for the condition—'seborrhiasis'. Virtually the only ways of differentiating between

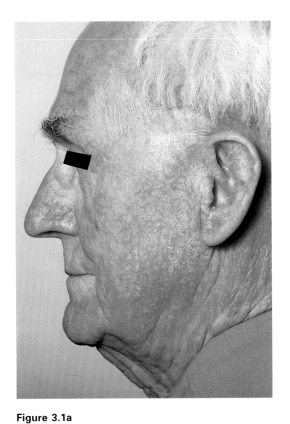

Figure 3.1a

Seborrhoeic dermatitis affecting the face.

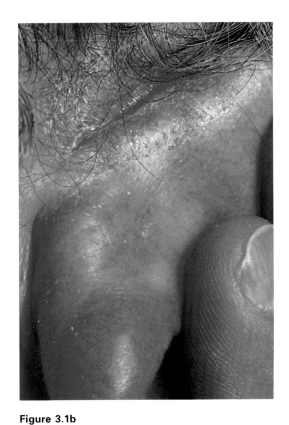

Figure 3.1b

Presternal scaly patch of seborrhoeic dermatitis.

Figure 3.1c

Scaling, redness and cracking behind the ears in an elderly woman with seborrhoeic dermatitis.

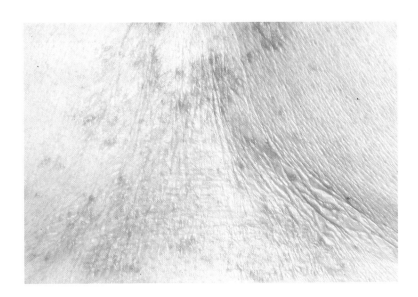

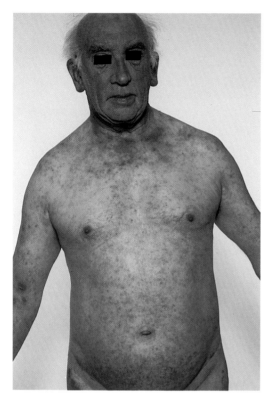

Figure 3.2

Widespread seborrhoeic dermatitis affecting the face, trunk, arms and legs.

these two conditions to establish a diagnosis are from the patient's history and the evolution of the disorder.

The other major differential conditions are allergic contact dermatitis and photodermatitis. The eruption of allergic contact dermatitis rarely involves the scalp, but does usually involve the fingers in addition to other areas. Patch testing with the standard battery, as well as with any suspected medicament or toiletries, should be performed (see page 000). The distribution of photodermatitis usually differs from that of seborrhoeic dermatitis in that light-induced eruptions do not affect the hairy scalp (but may involve a bald pate) and are most pronounced on the convexities, unlike seborrhoeic dermatitis, which is found in the creases. The backs of the hands and the V of the neck are also frequently affected in a rash due to light exposure.

The condition may occasionally resemble rosacea superficially but the predominance of scaling rather than erythema, and the accentuation of the rash in the folds and creases, usually easily distinguishes seborrhoeic dermatitis.

Treatment

When the condition is merely an embarrassment and is confined to the scalp, ears and eyebrows, traditional treatments may be tried. Shampooing with a detergent-based shampoo (with or without antimicrobial compounds), use of an emollient cleanser such as unguentum emulsificans aquosum (BNF). Hydrocortisone preparations may be all that is required. More potent agents (eg, betamethasone-17–valerate) may be needed when the condition is resistant to all else.

As mentioned earlier, there is a view that seborrhoeic dermatitis is the result of a disturbance to the cutaneous microflora, suggesting that antimicrobial measures may be helpful in its treatment. The addition of antimicrobial agents to corticosteroids may be more helpful than preparations containing corticosteroid alone for treating some varieties of eczema, and many dermatologists also find this to be the case for seborrhoeic dermatitis. A combination of miconazole or econazole and hydrocortisone seems useful if it is decided to adopt this approach.

Some patients respond well to a preparation containing 8% lithium succinate and 0.05% zinc sulphate (Efalith20®)The mode of action of this topical agent is uncertain.

In the uncommon situation that the condition spreads relentlessly to become erythrodermic, it may be necessary to administer systemic steroids.

Asteatotic eczema (eczema craquelée)

Definition

Asteatotic eczema is an eczematous disorder of the elderly which typically has a crazy-paving appearance. It is prone to occur on the extensor aspects of the limbs and trunk in debilitated individuals in conditions of low relative humidity—usually while hospital inpatients.

Clinical features

The disorder is often seen after admission to hospital during the course of some other illness. It is virtually restricted to those in their late 60s and older. It seems to be more common in the winter months and in air conditioned environments. The rash consistently appears over the lateral aspects and shins of the lower legs but may spread to involve the thighs, the back and rarely even the upper arms. There is a characteristic cracked or crazy paving appearance in the affected areas (Figure 3.3), which merge imperceptibly into the surrounding normal skin. The condition is pruritic but often there is a complaint of soreness that troubles the patient more than the itch. Asteatotic eczema does not generally persist for long and is often a transient disorder lasting only while the patient's general debility or the ambient conditions of low humidity persist. It mostly responds quite readily to treatment.

Treatment

The mainstays of treatment for this disorder are the increase in the ambient humidity if at all possible and the application of emollients. The best is the one the patient finds most helpful and pleasant to use (see Chapter 12) but the greasier the better. Preparations based on white soft paraffin tend to be more occlusive and more efficient at hydration of the stratum corneum. Avoidance of hot baths, vigorous washing with ordinary soaps and rubbing with rough towelling will also help. Bathing in lukewarm water containing a bath oil, using an emollient soap and gentle patting dry is acceptable. If this simple treatment is insufficient to clear the disorder, applications of weak corticosteroids may be used.

Figure 3.3

Eczema craquelée. There is a reticulate, crazy-paving type of pattern typical of this condition.

Gravitational eczema

The term gravitational eczema or even venous eczema is much better than the older one of 'stasis dermatitis' as it has been shown on several occasions that there is an increased rate of total blood supply to skin, rather than the reverse, as stasis would imply[9] (see also Chapter 11).

Definition

Gravitational eczema is a form of eczema occurring as part of the gravitational syndrome on the lower legs of individuals suffering from venous hypertension.

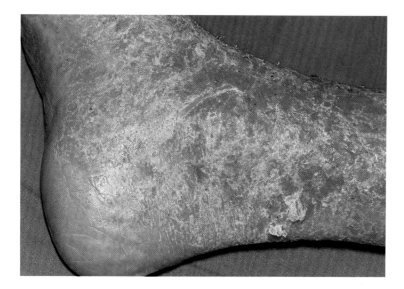

Figure 3.4

Gravitational eczema.

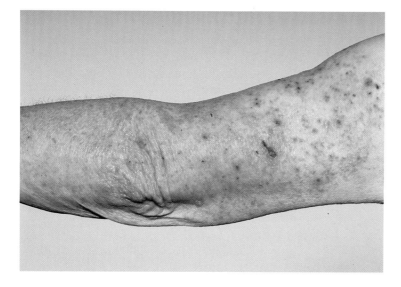

Figure 3.5

Dissemination of eczematous rash in gravitational eczema. The outer aspect of the upper arm is a typical site.

Clinical features

The disorder typically occurs on the lower halves of the lower legs in patients with severe or moderately severe venous hypertension and the gravitational syndrome. Gravitational ulceration, superficial varices, ankle oedema, lipodermatosclerosis and pigmentation are frequent accompaniments of the eczematous rash. It usually starts insidiously and may progress to involve most of the affected lower leg (Figure 3.4). Later the other lower leg may become affected, even though there may be little in the way of venous incompetence in this limb. For reasons that are as yet unclear the eczematous process disseminates in a small proportion of affected individuals to involve the fronts and sides of the thighs, the upper arms, the flanks, the back and elsewhere (Figure 3.5). At one time this was dubbed autosensitization eczema, and was believed to be due to sensitization to tissue breakdown products in the patient's originally affected skin. The finding of cytotoxic antibodies in a small number of such individuals gives some support to this hypothesis.[10]

Gravitational eczema tends to be persistent and it frequently relapses after what appears to be successful treatment.

Differential diagnosis

The major differential diagnosis is allergic contact dermatitis to a medicament used to treat a gravitational ulcer (see later). It appears that patients with the gravitational syndrome are particularly easily sensitized, though why this should be so is unclear.[11] All patients with gravitational eczema should be patch tested and a set of patches containing medicaments should be included.

Treatment

Treatment of the gravitational syndrome is dealt with in Chapter 11. Treatment directed to the underlying venous hypertension should be instituted. The treatment of the eczematous component of the gravitational syndrome is similar to the treatment of other types of eczema. The use of emollients is recommended as a first-line measure and then, if required, weak (or if necessary moderately potent or potent) corticosteroids are indicated. Because of the danger of dermatitis medicamentosa in this group of patients, applications containing lanolin, neomycin and gentamicin and other sensitizers should be avoided.

Allergic contact dermatitis

Definition

Allergic contact dermatitis is an eczematous reaction that occurs at the site of contact with an agent to which the individual has developed a specific acquired hypersensitivity of the delayed hypersensitivity type (type 4 reaction).

Clinical features

The eruption appears a variable period after secondary contact with the specific allergen. Typically the latent interval is about a day, but it can range from a few hours to 4 days or, rarely, even longer. However, the interval between primary contact with the allergen and the subsequent secondary contact which elicits the eczematous reaction is obligatorily at least 10 days. The sites involved in allergic contact dermatitis are the sites of secondary contact with the sensitizing agent. The diagnosis is by no means always straightforward, and an extremely detailed and painstaking history-taking session is often needed before an apparent mystery is solved. This in itself may be difficult in the elderly, whose memory may be poor (Figure 3.6).

If contact with the sensitizer is not prevented after the reaction has been produced, the eczematous rash may spread to involve areas of skin that have not been in contact with the allergen, making clinical diagnosis even more difficult. The appearance of the eruption itself is variable and dependent on the sites involved, the extent of the exposure and the degree of sensitization. Typically the affected area will first appear as an itchy swollen pink area on which vesicles, exudation and crusting may arise in quick succession (Figure 3.7). Thickening, scaling—and in some normally mobile sites, fissuring—occur subsequently (Figure 3.8). The disorder resolves after the responsible allergen has been identified and further contact prevented.

The commoner contact sensitizers are set out in Table 3.2. Nickel, rubber additives, dyes, lanolin, plants and antibiotics are among the most frequent offenders, but sensitization is possible to an enormous range of substances. For comprehensive descriptions of the allergens and materials containing them the reader should consult monographs on this topic (eg, Rycroft et al,[12] Nater and de Groot[13]). Once the sensitivity has developed it persists for many years and may be permanent. Unexpectedly some recent

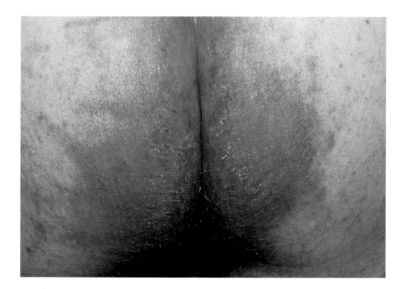

Figure 3.6

Allergic contact dermatitis in an elderly man who had pruritus ani. He had at first forgotten that he had used an antipruritic cream containing a local anaesthetic.

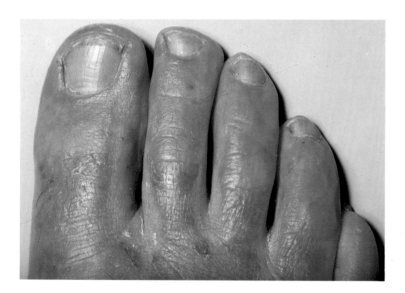

Figure 3.7

Allergic contact dermatitis on the dorsa of the toes and feet in a man who became sensitive to one of the constituents of his shoes.

studies suggest that in some cases the hypersensitivity actually diminishes over the years. Allergic contact dermatitis may be slightly less common in the elderly than in younger adults; however, there are limited data to support this and the apparent lesser frequency may be due to a combination of lesser opportunity for exposure to sensitizers in the elderly and a depressed skin reactivity to any insult—immunological or irritant. Some studies have suggested that positivity to common allergens actually increases with age,[14] although the ability to become sensitized, is actually decreased in the elderly (see Chapter 8).

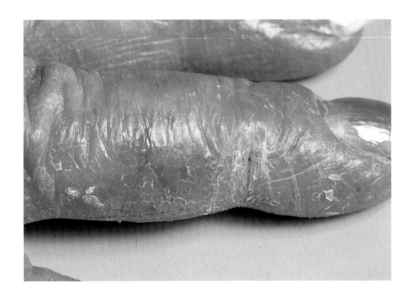

Figure 3.8a

Dermatitis affecting the fingers. This was thought to be due to handling irritant cleansing agents.

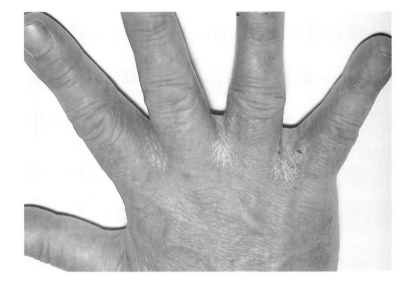

Figure 3.8b

Hand dermatitis. The main areas involved are between the fingers. The cause was never found in this patient.

Mechanisms

In recent years our views on the pathogenesis of allergic contact dermatitis have been greatly modified. Sensitizers are not themselves complete antigens and there is good evidence that the chemical agent (hapten) conjugates with some unidentified protein component of the epidermis before it becomes able to spark off a hypersensitivity reaction. However, it is unknown at which stage this conjugation occurs. It appears that after penetration of the stratum corneum the molecules of antigen are sequestered in Langerhans cells[15,16] which then carry and present

Table 3.2 Some common contact sensitizing substances

Substance	Where found	Comment
Metals		
Nickel	Steels, alloys, precious metals,	Extremely common (c. 5% in female
Chromates	'plated' metals,	population)
Dyes		
Paraphenylene diamine	Blue, black dyes	Many black hair dyes contain this
Paratoluenediamine	Red dyes	All the dyes may cause clothing or shoe
Azo dyes	Orange, yellow, red dyes	dermatitis
Rubber additives		
Mercaptobenzothiazole	Natural and synthetic rubbers	There are many substances in rubbers that
Thiouram		can cause allergic contact dermatitis
Paratertiarybutylphenol		
Resins, plastics, adhesives		
Colphony 'plaster'	Contact adhesives	Common cause of dermatitis
Epoxy resin adhesives	Adhesives	A not infrequent cause of industrial dermatitis
Formalin resins	Waterproofing in fabrics	A cause of clothing dermatitis
Cosmetics and topical medicaments		
Wool alcohols (lanolin)	Many ointments and creams	Common (but less sommon than previously)
Parabenz esters	Preservatives in many creams	causes of dermatitis due to cosmetics and
Chloroxylenol	Antiseptic	topical preparations
Cetavlon	Antiseptic	
'Caine' local anaesthetic	In 'anti-itch' preparations	
Neomycin	Antibiotic used in topical treatments	
Diphenhydramine	Antihistamine used in topical treatments	
Plants		
Primula		May cause dermatitis of face and hands
Chrysanthemums		resembling photodermatitis
Tulip bulbs		
Poison Ivy (USA)		Extremely common seasonal dermatitis in parts of USA

the antigen to immunocompetent T lymphocytes. Clones of lymphocytes that are specifically sensitized to the particular antigen are then produced by a rapid series of cell divisions. The site of production of 'sensitized' lymphocytes appears to be in the regional lymph nodes. It is unclear how the committed lymphocyte actually causes the eczematous reaction. So far as the final manifestation of this sequence is concerned (ie, epidermal spongiosis and vesiculation), it seems that several mediators are involved and that prostaglandins of the E series are among these.[17] For a more complete account of the mechanisms responsible for allergic contact dermatitis the reader should consult Hanifin.[18]

Diagnosis

A high degree of clinical suspicion is required for accurate diagnosis of allergic contact dermatitis.

When the suspicion has been roused (as, for example, in a patient with a dermatitis of the face and hands) the real sleuthing begins, and a detailed social and occupational history should be obtained. Confirmation is obtained by patch testing. The suspected allergen is placed in contact with the skin and held there in occlusive contact for 48 hours. After a further 48 hours the site is scrutinized for the presence of a positive eczematous-type reaction. Elderly subjects may take longer to develop a positive patch-test reaction than younger patients. It is customary to use a battery of commonly incriminated antigens (or groups of antigens) as a screen initially and then, if this does not give the answer, to employ other series of substances appropriate to the history and pattern of dermatitis of the particular patient. For example, a woman with a predominantly facial dermatitis should be tested with a series of agents that are found in cosmetics and that occasionally cause allergic contact dermatitis.

Patch testing is not a technique for the amateur. It is an expert's province, as much misinformation can be generated if the pitfalls are not recognized; the details of the technique are important. The International Contact Dermatitis Research Group (ICDRG) has performed a great service by recommending a standard practice, and most dermatology clinics now adhere to this. Either aluminium chambers ('finn' chambers) or aluminium-backed strip dressings are used to apply the materials occlusively to the skin of the back. The concentrations of the allergens in the test materials and the vehicles in which they are contained are of vital importance and the advice given by the ICDRG should be heeded.[19] Care must be taken to distinguish true positive from false positive reactions, which may be due to primary irritation. A series of false positive reactions can also be caused by patch testing the subject too soon after the original attack of dermatitis has subsided. This has been termed the 'angry back syndrome', which adequately describes the propensity of the skin to break out at this time at the slightest stimulus.

If a particular article (eg, clothing, toiletry or cosmetic) is suspected but the full list of constituents is not known or cannot be obtained, then it is permissible to perform an 'as is' or a 'use' test. In these tests the material is applied to the skin in its complete state ('as is') or is used as it would normally be used and the sites of application inspected as described previously.

Reactions are usually graded according to their severity, using a scoring system. The more vigorous the reaction the more likely is the test to be relevant to the individual's problem although this is by no means invariable. It also gives some indication as to the degree of sensitivity present and the likely outcome of further exposures.

Treatment

The most important component of treatment is identification of the material containing the contact allergen responsible and prevention of further contact with it. Other articles in which it may be or materials that contain similar substances to which the patient may cross-react

must also be avoided. The rash should then gradually subside. To speed it on its way, emollients and topical corticosteroids may be used as for other varieties of eczema.

Primary irritant contact dermatitis

Definition

Primary irritant contact dermatitis is an eczematous response of the skin at the site of toxic chemical and/or mechanical trauma.

Clinical features

This type of dermatitis tends to be significantly less common in the elderly as for the most part they are no longer exposed to the potentially injurious substances encountered occupationally. In addition, and as pointed out previously, the skin of the older subject reacts much less vigorously than that of younger folk. Typically the hands are affected by scaling, fissuring and erythema with involvement of the fingers (see Figure 3.8). Both the palms and dorsal surfaces may be involved. Vesiculation is uncommon though may be seen if the condition is aggravated by sudden and vigorous exposure to an injurious agent.

The condition tends to be more common and more severe in the winter time when the low temperature and humidity induce chapping. A form of irritant dermatitis may also develop in the groins, around the genitalia and on the buttocks of incontinent elderly patients—in reality a form of napkin dermatitis.

Treatment

Removal of the substance causing the irritation will usually promote healing. Resolution may, however, be a slow process and it is best to aid it by supplying emollient soaps and applications. These help to stop fissuring (which in itself perpetuates the eczematous process) and may have a mild anti-inflammatory effect. If these measures are not sufficient, weak corticosteroids may be used.

Hand and foot eczema

Definition

This eczematous disorder occurs on the hands and/or feet and defies further definition. It may in fact be several disorders.

Clinical features

Scaling, reddened patches make their appearance primarily on the palms and/or soles, although other areas may also be affected. The condition is usually symmetrical although one hand may be much more severely affected than the other (Figure 3.9). Vesiculation is sometimes seen when the condition flares, but this is less frequent than its counterpart in young adults. More often, fissuring and hyperkeratosis are observed. Sometimes the hyperkeratosis is the major manifestation so that patients present with thickened fissured and disabling gloves and sandals of hyperkeratosis. Central palmar regions and the instep and sole are the areas mostly affected—sites not conspicuously involved in allergic contact or primary irritant contact dermatitis. The disorder tends to be persistent or subject to remission and relapse for some months.

In diagnosis it is important not only to exclude any sort of contact dermatitis but also psoriasis and ringworm. The latter tinea infection can be excluded by examination of scales microscopically and by culture (see page 168). It is much more difficult to distinguish psoriasis if there are no other signs of the latter disease. One feature that favours psoriasis is the existence of a well defined and curved upper margin to the rash on the palm.

The cause of this disorder is unknown but it has been suggested, with very little evidence, that it is a manifestation of atopy in the adult.

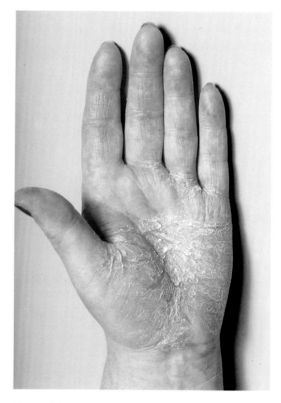

Figure 3.9

Hand dermatitis. Both of the patient's hands were involved and he also had a similar problem on one foot. Constitutional factors were probably involved.

Treatment

Avoidance of unnecessary skin irritation is one aspect of the treatment and the use of emollient soaps and emollient creams and lotions is to be encouraged. Topical corticosteroids sometimes give relief—but not as much as may be thought—and some of their success may well be due to the elegant bases with which they are formulated. If this disorder is improved by one particular topical corticosteroid the improvement is rarely maintained for long periods as tachyphylaxis seems to occur[20] and it is then necessary to change to another preparation. Preparations containing tar are occasionally useful, but are messy and are not popular with patients. As compliance is less good in the elderly anyway this problem has to be kept in mind if tar preparations are prescribed. Tars contain carcinogenic substances. Concerns over this have been answered by large scale surveys of patients who have used tar preparations over long periods which have not shown any excess occurrence of neoplastic disease due to this form of treatment.[21,22] Recently use of tar containing shampoos has been shown to result in tar absorption and the excretion of carcinogenic polyaromatic hydrocarbons in the urine.[23] It is clear that this is a problem that won't 'go away', but the data available to date does not indicate any appreciable risk from the use of tar preparations. They are quite well tolerated if it suggested that the preparation is used at night together with cotton gloves.

Infectious eczematoid dermatitis and intertriginous dermatitis

Definition

The term infectious eczematoid dermatitis has been applied to an acute exudative eczematous dermatosis that affects ears or other cavities harbouring a bacterial infection. Intertriginous dermatitis (or just 'intertrigo' when mild) is in all probability the same or a similar disease involving the major body flexures.

Clinical features

The major feature is the presence of an acutely inflamed eczematous dermatosis involving either the skin around a cavity (eg, ear, umbilicus, nostril) or the flexures symmetrically. Affected skin is often red and swollen and bears vesicles, pustules and crusts (Figures 3.10 and 3.11). The disorder is quite common in the elderly and seems more frequent in the warm summer months and in obese patients with dubious hygiene. Minor degrees of erythema develop in the creases of the deep flexures due to the trauma of movement between skin surfaces. Sweating increases the friction between the skin

surfaces and promotes microbial growth on the skin surface. When there are large pendulous folds of skin in the very obese these effects are exaggerated and intertriginous dermatitis beneath the breasts and in the groins of elderly fat ladies is often seen in summer months. If bacterial swabs are taken from the inflamed areas a wide variety of micro-organisms may be cultivated including Gram-negative rods and *Candida albicans*. A frequent story is that minor soreness and irritation has been present in these flexures for several weeks before the acute inflammation starts quite explosively within 2 or 3 days. When severe, the disorder causes great discomfort with soreness and tenderness of the skin and even slight fever and malaise. In these patients the rash can spread to involve large areas of skin.

Treatment

When acute and severe, bed rest is needed—if only to minimize the chafing between areas of sore skin in the flexures. If there is exudation the areas should be treated by packs kept moist with normal saline or 1:10 000 potassium permanganate solution and by bathing. If swabs indicate that bacterial infection is a significant factor, the appropriate antimicrobial compound should be given systemically. When *Candida* appears to be important in the aetiology, systemic treatment is not needed in the first instance, as topical measures usually suffice. As the condition subsides, weak topical corticosteroid preparations or corticosteroid antimicrobial combinations may be used, eg, hydrocortisone with miconazole. Most patients respond rapidly unless there is underlying disease such as diabetes. However, recurrences are common, especially in the obese, who should be encouraged to reduce weight.

Discoid eczema (nummular eczema)

Definition

Discoid eczema is a common eczematous dermatosis of unknown cause characterized by

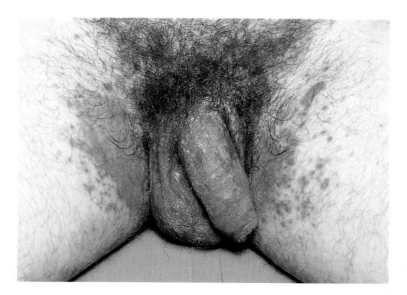

Figure 3.10

Infectious eczematoid dermatitis. The axillae were also involved.

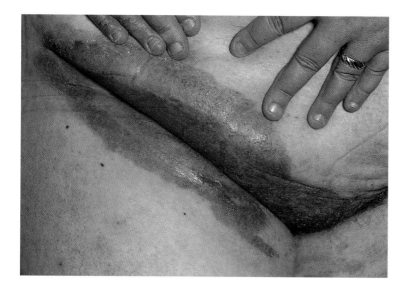

Figure 3.11

Intertriginous dermatitis.

the presence of rounded (discoid) scaling red areas of skin.

Clinical features

Typically the disease affects individuals over the age of 40 and seems to be more common in men. The disorder may start abruptly with severe itching, swelling, bright erythema and vesiculation in the rounded involved areas. Usually, however, it is less vigorous and the discoid patches are scaly (Figure 3.12) rather than oozing and crusted. The limbs, especially the legs, are mainly involved, though patches sometimes appear on the lower trunk. Often there are only three or four patches, each 1–3 cm in diameter, but the disorder is capricious and may be much more extensive. Discoid eczema often lasts for some months before remitting and it relapses quite frequently.

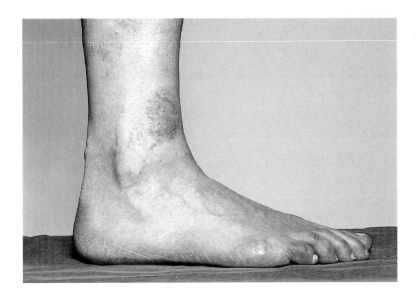

Figure 3.12a

Discoid eczema. Similar round, scaling irritant patches were also evident on this patient's thighs and arms.

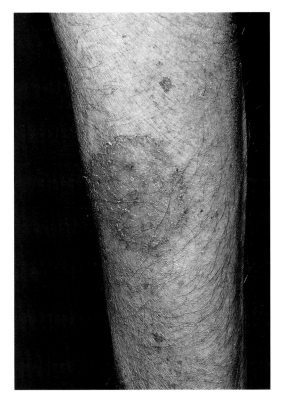

Figure 3.12b

Patch of discoid eczema.

Differential diagnosis

The differential diagnosis is set out in Table 3.3. It is most important to distinguish the disorder from psoriasis, where there are often lesions on the trunk and scalp and in which the scaling tends to be more prominent, from ringworm, in which the edge tends to be raised, and from Bowen's disease and superficial basal cell carcinoma (see pages 197 and 203).

Treatment

Treatment with emollients may give some symptomatic relief, as may applications containing corticosteroids or tars, but the condition tends to resist most therapeutic efforts and remits spontaneously after some weeks or months.

Sulzberger–Garbe disease (oid–oid disease)

Opinion seems divided as to whether this rare disease really exists or not.[24] It was originally described as occurring in late-middle-aged and elderly Jewish businessmen in New York, but has occasionally been described in others as

Table 3.3   Differential diagnosis of round, red, scaling patches

Disease features	Clinical features	Differentiating
Discoid eczema	Multiple coin-sized, red, round, scaling areas on limbs	History of oozing and crusting
Psoriasis	Multiple rounded or polycyclic, raised, dull-red, thickly scaling areas, discrete margins	Family history
Lichen simplex chronicus	One or several scaling, lichenified red patches in characteristic sites	Persistence and extreme itchiness
Ringworm	One or several rapidly expanding scaling pink areas with a ring-line configuration	Microscopy and culture of scales
Bowen's disease	Usually solitary scaling patch on legs	
Superficial basal cell carcinoma	One or several slightly scaling, discrete patches on trunk or limbs, edge often raised, thin and 'hair like'	The histopathology of these lesions is quite distinctive
Mycosis fungoides	Multiple red, irregularly thickened scaling areas which persist	

well. Its distinctive features include the appearance of inflamed exudative patches over the legs, genitalia and trunk. From the descriptions it appears to represent a very vigorous type of discoid eczema.

Lichen simplex chronicus (circumscribed neurodermatitis)

Definition

Lichen simplex chronicus (LSC) is an extremely itchy localized chronic eczematous disorder which shows clinical and histological signs of epidermal hypertrophy.

Clinical features

LSC can occur at any age in adults, but may be more frequent in those over the age of 60. The disease has a curious predilection for certain areas of the skin including the occipital region of the scalp and adjoining part of the upper neck, the dorsum of the foot, the ulnar border of the upper part of the forearm, the front of the wrist

and around the knees (Figures 3.13 and 3.14). Affected sites vary greatly in size from 3–4 cm^2 to 30–40 cm^2. Each patch is well defined and raised. The reddened surface tends to be slightly scaly and there is exaggeration of skin surface markings—a sign known as lichenification. There may be only one affected area but commonly there are several such patches. The disorder is extremely itchy and the thickening is the result of the persistent rubbing and scratching. Many patients with this disorder seem to have an atopic background.

Differential diagnosis

The well defined edge, the redness and the scaling surface may make differentiation from psoriasis difficult. When the lesion occurs on the back of the scalp, confusion with psoriasis is the rule rather than the exception. Close inspection will generally reveal the lichenification of the skin surface, which makes psoriasis unlikely. The disorder can also be confused with hypertrophic lichen planus, especially when the lesions are on the lower legs. Generally, hypertrophic lichen planus lesions are mauvish and the surface is warty rather than scaly and lichenified. In addition, in lichen planus there is often a characteristic white lacework tracery

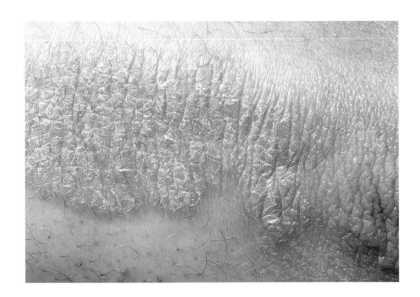

Figure 3.13

Lichen simplex chronicus. There is a raised lichenified scaling patch typical of this condition.

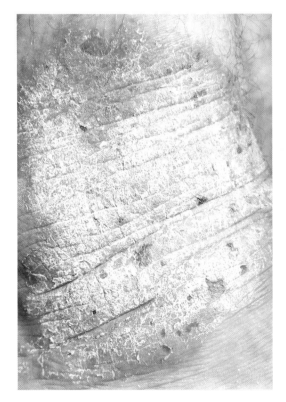

Figure 3.14

Lichen simplex chronicus. This patch shows more obvious signs of scratching than Figure 3.13.

(Wickham's striae) over the surface (see page 000). Discoid eczema is not thickened and is not lichenified.

Histopathology

The correct diagnosis should be reached clinically but can be confirmed histologically, although there may be a superficial similarity in the histopathology to psoriasis. However, in lichen simplex chronicus the epidermal hypertrophy is very marked and irregular and there are very few or no inflammatory cells in the epidermis and stratum corneum. There may be parakeratosis but this is not invariable, and when present it is not as marked as with psoriasis. There is usually a marked inflammatory cell infiltrate in the dermis. Interestingly, there is a similarly high rate of epidermal cell production in lichen simplex as in psoriasis (Figure 3.15).[25]

Treatment

This disease is notoriously resistant to treatment. Indeed, it has been suggested that it is probably best not to treat it but to allow patients to

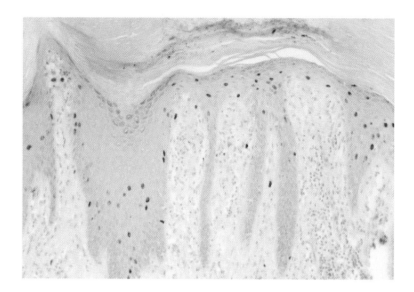

Figure 3.15

Photomicrograph from biopsy of lichen simplex chronicus showing irregular thickening of the epidermis, parakeratosis and a dermal inflammatory cell infiltrate. Two days prior to biopsy the site had been injected with a small quantity of tritiated thymidine. There are many cells within the epidermis that have become labelled (visible as black dots) indicating a high rate of epidermal cell production and migration through the eidermis (H & E; ×45).

continue to use it as an outlet for their tensions and aggressions for fear that something worse will happen if treatment is successful. Topical corticosteroids—even the most potent ones—rarely shift the patches. The best form of local treatment is with strong tar preparations. Painting with crude coal tar has even been tried by some. One regimen that is sometimes successful is to prescribe a simple but pleasing emollient and to request the patient that they use this instead of scratching or rubbing.

Photodermatitis

Definition

This is a group of eczematous disorders that are wholly or partly caused by exposure to solar radiation.

Aetiological factors

In almost all instances it is the long-wave segment of solar ultraviolet radiation that is responsible. In many patients with this type of disorder it is possible to incriminate a prior exposure to a photosensitizing chemical or drug which may have been contacted topically (photocontact dermatitis) or given systemically. Sometimes there is a phototoxic reaction and in other patients it seems that a photoallergic mechanism is responsible. In a phototoxic reaction it is thought that the UVR excites the molecule involved, making it much more reactive and toxic to the skin.

In a photoallergic reaction the UVR changes the chemical involved via a photochemical reaction so that the drug or chemical becomes a sensitizer and elicits an immunological reaction. Examples of substances that elicit phototoxic and photoallergic reactions are given in Table 3.4. Photosensitizing chemicals can produce an eczematous reaction after either systemic administration or topical application, and in practice it can be difficult to sort out the mechanism responsible. A particular difficulty is that some individuals continue to react to UVR long after the chemical or drug responsible has been removed from the patient's environment.[26] This is seen particularly frequently in elderly men.

Paradoxically many sunscreen filter chemicals are now known to be photosensitizers.[27] A photosensitivity dermatitis may also occur

Table 3.4 Examples of phototoxic and photoallergic reactions

Materials responsible	Comment
Psoralens (eg methoxypsoralens in oil of bergamot)	Photodermatisis from plants and fruit or their extracts; this photochemical reaction is the basis of PUVA treatment
The Compositae and Umbelliferae flowers	These are suspected of containing substances responsible for the persistent light reaction
Halogenated salicylanilides	These compounds were often added to toiletry products and were the cause of acute and persistent light reactions
The phenothiazine drugs (eg chlorpromazine)	Responsible for pigmentary abnormalities in light-exposed sites
Amiodarone	Responsible for pigmentary abnormalities in light-exposed sites
Sulphonamides	Can cause acute photodermatitis
Tetracylines (particularly demethylchlortetracycline)	Can cause acute photodermatitis and photo-onycholysis
Benoxyprofen notorious	Now withdrawn; was a cause of photodermatitis and photo-onycholysis
Nalidixic acid	Light-induced blistering reactions have been recorded
Frusemide	Can cause blistering and erosions stimulating porphyria in light-exposed sites
Naproxen	As with Frusemide
Hydralazine erythematosus	May produce a lupus erythematosus like condition especially in slow acetylators of HLA B-8 DR3 haplotype

without exposure to an identifiable photosensitizing chemical. As with so many 'idiopathic' disorders, 'idiopathic' photosensitive eczema becomes rarer as more causes for it are found. None the less, at the time of writing there is still a small hard core of patients for whom this designation is most appropriate. If their eruption is basically eczematous, but at times nodular and/or plaque type, the term polymorphic light eruption is used. This is mainly a disorder of young and middle-aged women. Photosensitive eczema with no identifiable cause is occasionally seen in the elderly.

These specific light-induced disorders should be distinguished from non-specific 'light-aggravated' dermatitis, in which dermatitis from a wide variety of causes is made worse through the general irritative effects of UVR. This is most common in young people with atopic dermatitis, but it is also seen in facial seborrhoeic dermatitis of the elderly.

Clinical features

The eruption appears in the light-exposed sites of the face and neck (Figure 3.16), on the backs of the hands and elsewhere depending on the prevailing fashion in clothes. The bald pate is often badly affected—standing out in marked contrast to the white skin of the hair-covered scalp. The forehead, nose, chin, ears, cheeks and neck receive the most UVR and are worse affected in contrast to the comparatively shaded paranasal area, the upper lip and the cleft of the chin. The V of the neck and the lower legs are often involved in women. Clothing may only partially protect against UVR. Figure 3.17 shows the effect of wearing shoes with small holes in a highly photosensitive elderly man who was passionately fond of gardening. Thin shirts and blouses may not prove much of a light barrier and the development of a rash after sun exposure through this type of clothing is not particularly unusual (see page 17).

Photosensitive eczematous rashes may appear at any time when there is enough incident UVR energy, but in patients with long-standing photosensitivity the rash usually remits in late September or October, to reappear in March or even in late February. The time between exposure to the sun and the development of the eczematous rash is variable, but is usually about a day or two. It may start off as a very vigorous affair (Figure 3.18) with swelling of the affected areas—particularly around the eyes. In most people the rash eventually subsides after avoidance of sun

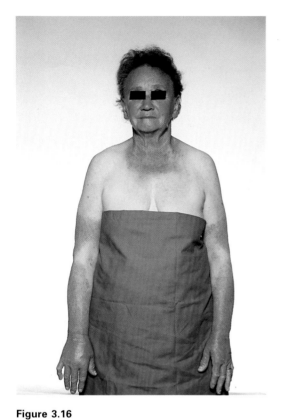

Figure 3.16

Photodermatitis. All the exposed sites show evidence of an eczematous rash.

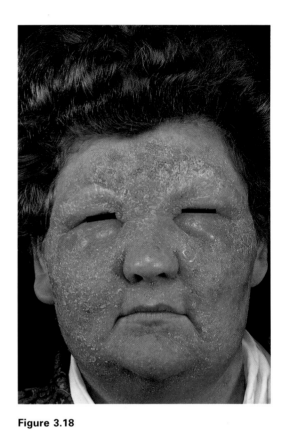

Figure 3.18

Patient with severe exudative eczematous rash on the face, showing swelling around the eyes due to light sensitivity.

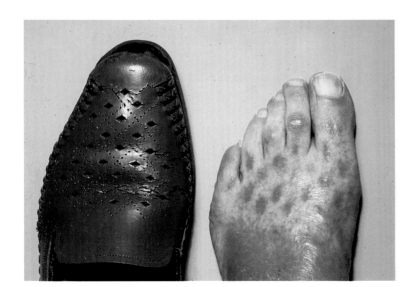

Figure 3.17

Photodermatitis. The odd pattern on this man's foot is due to the holes in his shoe where light has been able to shine through.

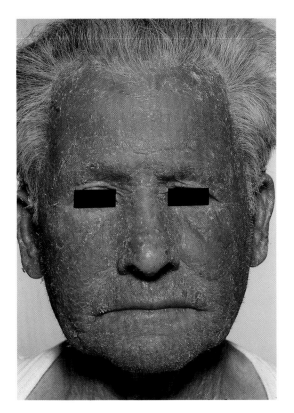

Figure 3.19

Actinic reticuloid in elderly man. The affected areas are thickened and scaling and some areas appear hyperpigmented.

intense inflammatory cell infiltrate in the subepidermal region, with some of the appearances of a reticulosis, which is found in biopsies of affected sites in such patients. However, not all patients show this change and the condition does not appear to be due to a lymphoma. Many of this group have been shown to have positive photopatch tests to fragrance materials.[28]

Diagnosis

The characteristic distribution of the eruption in the light-exposed skin and the history of aggravation after exposure should allow diagnosis of a light provoked or aggravated dermatitis. Patch tests, photopatch tests, other light tests and biopsy may then all be necessary to pinpoint the aetiological type. Photopatch tests are similar to ordinary patch tests save that two sets of test substances are applied to the skin. One is kept covered after the initial exposure while the other is irradiated with UVR containing long wavelength UV. The exact times of irradiation and the energy of the radiation source are of great importance and for details the reader should consult an excellent review by the British Photodermatology Group.[29] Some plants (eg, Compositae and Umbelliferae) contain substances responsible for persistent photosensitivity.[30]

Determining the degree of sensitivity to UVR is helpful in confirming that UVR is important aetiologically and in giving advice as to management. It may also assist in diagnosis by evoking a small area of rash under controlled conditions. In order to pinpoint the wavelengths responsible it is necessary to irradiate test sites with single wavelengths or narrow bands of wavelengths with a monochromator.

Differential diagnosis

The major issue in differential diagnosis is whether the disorder is provoked by or aggravated by light energy or whether the eruption merely simulates a photodermatosis. Seborrhoeic dermatitis and allergic contact dermatitis may occur in the distribution of a photodermatosis. The former eruption also involves the hairy scalp

exposure, though there are some very sensitive individuals whose rash persists despite this strategy (persistent light reactors). A proportion of these are still, unintentionally, exposed to the unidentified photoallergic compound and are receiving enough UVR energy to make their rash persist.

In one unfortunate group of individuals the eruption takes on particular clinical signs. The skin thickens—particularly over the back of the neck and the forehead (Figure 3.19)—and it becomes darker red or mauve, and there may also be irregular areas of hyperpigmentation. This condition has come to be known as 'actinic reticuloid'. Characteristically the affected individuals are exquisitely sensitive to UVR; not only to long-wave UVR, but sometimes also to visible light. The term 'reticuloid' is derived from the and the light-protected flexural areas and the latter usually involves the hands and fingers as well. It is not usually as symmetrical as a photo-dermatosis. Rosacea may also simulate a photo-dermatosis but occurs only over the face. Close inspection will demonstrate that it is not in fact eczematous but marked by erythema, telangiecta-sia and papules. Systemic lupus erythematosus may be more difficult to distinguish and indeed is a light-provoked dermatosis. However, complaints and signs relating to other systems, as well as the presence of abnormal laboratory findings, should allow its identification.

Treatment

Nowhere in dermatology is it more correct to say that the key to proper management is in the understanding of the causative factors in each patient. The provoking drug, topical application or inadvertently encountered substances responsible must be eliminated from the environment. During the process of identification and while the individ-ual is still sun sensitive, all steps must be taken to avoid exposure to UVR. In extremely sensitive individuals this may even involve replacement of fluorescent lamps by tungsten filament bulbs, as the former emit some UVR. Some patients may even require nursing in the dark for a short time. Sun screens (see page 17) are not generally helpful as they are not very efficient at blocking out longer UV wavelengths. Some patients are helped by administration of beta-carotene, the substance in vegetables converted to retinol in the gut, as some is deposited in the skin and absorbs the damaging UVA.

When the rash is present its treatment is exactly the same as for other types of eczema-tous dermatoses. Emollients and topical corti-costeroids should be used as required (see page 268).

Psoriasis

Definition

Psoriasis is a common persistent inflammatory dermatosis of the skin of unknown cause with a prominent hereditary component characterized by the appearance of well-defined plaques of scaling and erythema.

Introduction

Psoriasis is one of the most common skin disor-ders. It affects some 1–2% of the population of most parts of the world surveyed.[31] However, it may be less common in the Japanese and black African ethnic groups.[32] It may also be more common in some areas such as Scandinavia.[33] Because of its persistence and the disabilities that it causes, psoriasis is of great importance economically and socially. For example, it has been computed that the disease cost the United States $248 000 000 in 1977.[34] The unhappiness and disability that it causes are more difficult to quantify but are none the less evident even to the casual observer.

The disease may begin at any age but commonly first makes its appearance in the latter part of the second decade. It is the author's impression that there is another peak of incidence in the seventh decade and a recent study has confirmed this. Evidence was presented that whereas the group presenting in early life were likely to have a family history of the disease and a high prevalence of histocompatibility leukocyte antigen (HLA) type CW6, this was not the case in the late onset group.[35] Whether or not this is true, the disorder is common in the older age groups and they are often more disabled by it than are younger people. Some surveys have shown that it is more common in men, sometimes by up to one and a half to two times more frequent.

Clinical features

Common plaque type psoriasis

Sites that are frequently involved include the extensor aspects of the knees and elbows, the sacral region and the scalp. As the disorder progresses no area of skin surface is immune. Indeed, it may spread to involve the whole of the skin in psoriatic erythroderma. It is quite common for psoriatic patches to develop at the

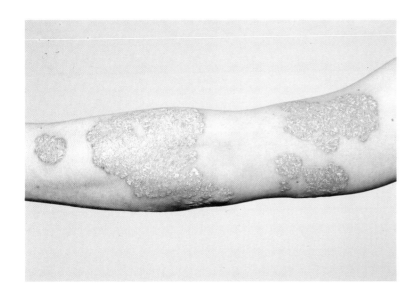

Figure 3.20

Typical plaques of psoriasis on the arm.

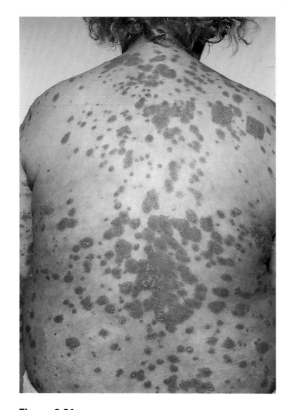

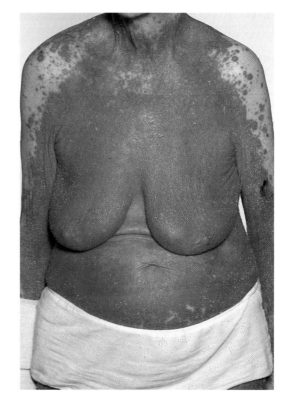

Figure 3.21a

There are many small plaques of psoriasis affecting the back.

Figure 3.21b

Severe widespread psoriasis which has almost become erythrodermic.

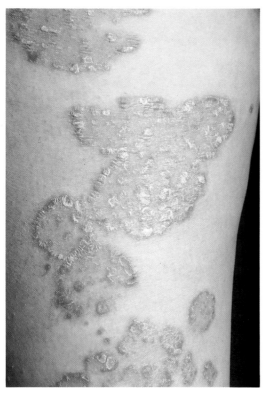

Figure 3.22

Psoriatic plaques in which there has been clearance at the centre and expansion at the periphery, giving an annular appearance.

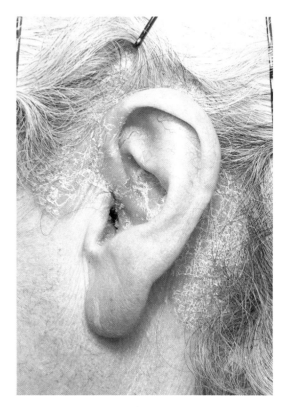

Figure 3.23

Psoriasis affecting the scalp margin and ears.

sites of injury. This is known as the Koebner phenomenon or the isomorphic response. The appearance of new lesions at the site of injury is not specific to psoriasis and is also seen in lichen planus and discoid lupus erythematous.

The typical psoriatic plaque is oval, rounded or polycyclic and has a sharply demarcated border (Figures 3.20 and 3.21). The colour of psoriatic lesions is variable but is frequently a striking homogenous darkish red. The scale has been described as silvery, and indeed so it often is, but as with the colour, it varies considerably between patients. Many lesions tend to heal spontaneously at the centre but spread peripherally (Figure 3.22), sometimes causing annular lesions.

The scalp and the scalp margin are frequently affected and this is often very disabling in the elderly (Figure 3.23).

Only the inexperienced attempt to predict the course of an attack of psoriasis. While it is true that there is a general tendency to resolution, some patients' disease seems doggedly to stay put. In others the disease appears to melt away. Some patients appear to relapse at the same time (or times) each year but without this information from the patients themselves, there is no special way of predicting the development of a further attack or time to remission.

Flexural psoriasis

This pattern of psoriasis is more frequently seen in those past the age of 60 but is by no means restricted to this age group. The obese seem to

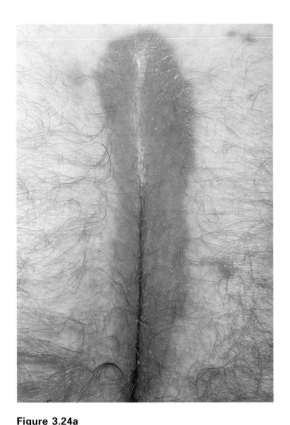

Figure 3.24a

Flexural psoriasis affecting the natal cleft.

be especially prone to flexural psoriasis or are at least particularly troubled by the disorder when it makes an appearance.

The psoriatic patches appear in the groins and on the genitalia, in the axillae, in the umbilicus and in the folds of fat around the abdomen (Figure 3.24). The facial flexures are also affected—particularly perinasally and retroauricularly. Scaling is not generally as prominent as in ordinary psoriasis and the surfaces tend to have a glazed, moist look to them. In other respects the affected areas resemble plaque type psoriasis of the usual kind.

Pustular psoriasis

Pustular psoriasis of the palms and soles

Palmoplantar pustular psoriasis is the most common form of pustular psoriasis and is not uncommon in the elderly. In 1985 it was reported that this disorder is strongly associated with cigarette smoking.[36] Some 95% of patients with pustular psoriasis were found to be smokers! Despite the strong association in the author's experience, there is a poor response to giving up

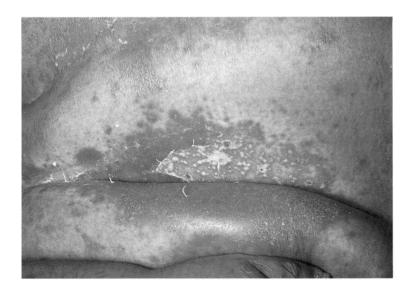

Figure 3.24b

Submammary psoriasis in an overweight elderly woman.

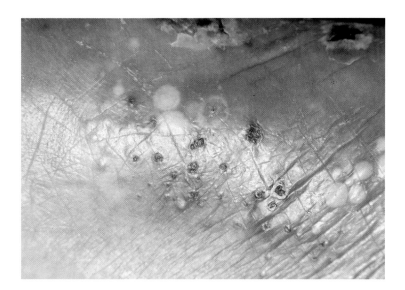

Figure 3.25

Pustular psoriasis affecting the soles. Note the presence of typical yellow pustules.

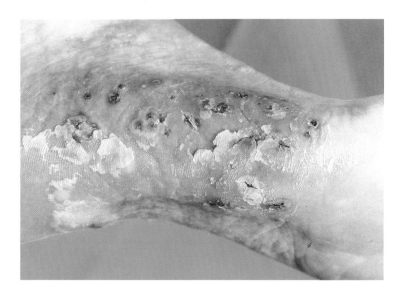

Figure 3.26

Pustular psoriasis affecting the sole of the foot. There are many brownish lesions resulting from old pustules.

the habit. Although it is not particularly uncommon to find patches of ordinary psoriasis elsewhere, most patients with this type have pustular lesions restricted to the palms and soles. The pustules appear deep-set on a reddened background and are often confined to one or two areas of the palmar and plantar skin. Newer pustules tend to be a lemon yellow. Older pustules are brownish and then become scaly (Figures 3.25 and 3.26). The disorder may affect palms and soles symmetrically but it is more usual for one palm or one sole to be worse. Pustular psoriasis can be quite disabling as it causes pain and soreness. In addition, because the pliability and resilience of the palmar and plantar skin is affected by the inflammatory process, it fissures causing even more pain and discomfort.

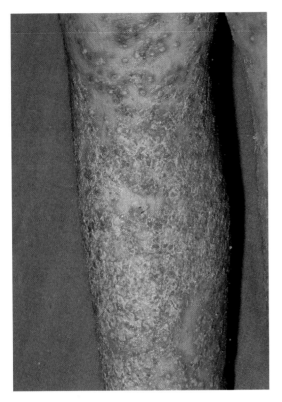

Figure 3.27

Acute generalized pustular psoriasis. This patient was affected by showers of pustules which later became scaly and crusted.

Generalized pustular psoriasis (von Zumbusch's disease)

This disorder may be seen at all ages but is particularly devastating in the elderly. It is relatively rare. The disorder may start spontaneously in a previously perfectly fit individual or may affect someone who has had ordinary plaque type psoriasis for some time. There is a sudden and generalized intense erythema superimposed on which crops of small yellowish-white superficial pustules appear (Figure 3.27). Often the pustules seem to coalesce so that lakes of pus develop. Sometimes the process is so vigorous that the pustules do not have time to form and all that can be seen is sheeted desquamation. The crops of pustules are accompanied by malaise, pyrexia, arthralgia and leukocytosis. The generalized erythema there also causes considerable heat loss and a danger of hypothermia. In addition, there is massive loss of fluid via the diseased skin because of the disturbed barrier function so that patients are usually considerably dehydrated. The erythema may also result in ankle oedema, raised jugulovenous pressure and high volume pulse, due to the increased blood supply to the skin acting as a 'shunt'. Although there are signs of high output failure, genuine cardiac decompensation does not generally occur unless there is accompanying myocardial disease. Patients with generalized pustular psoriasis are usually extremely ill, and unless carefully nursed and given the appropriate treatment, they may die.

Erythrodermic psoriasis

Patients with severe plaque-type psoriasis may develop universal erythema without pustules for no apparent reason. It may then be difficult to distinguish their disorder from other causes of an erythroderma (see Chapter 5). Although, like pustular psoriasis, plaque-type psoriasis may be abrupt in onset, it may also start insidiously in some patients. The generalized erythema causes dehydration and heat loss similar to that seen in patients with pustular psoriasis. There are also the signs of a high output state.

Psoriasis and arthritis

Patients with psoriasis have an increased incidence of arthritis. The pattern in most patients is similar to that of rheumatoid arthritis in that it is the metacarpophalangeal joints and proximal interphalangeal joints that are mainly involved. Some 5 or 6% of patients with psoriasis have this form of arthritis.[37,38] Very much less common is a pattern of joint disease commonly referred to as 'psoriatic arthropathy'. The relationship of this disorder to the other rheumatoid type arthropathy is unclear—some regard them as essentially the same disease. Whether they represent the same underlying disease

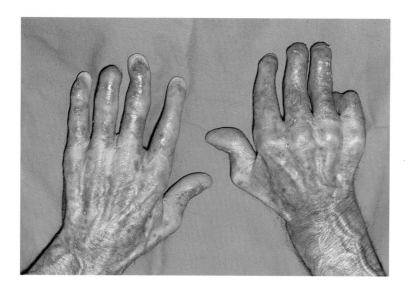

Figure 3.28

Psoriatic arthropathy with severe deformity of the terminal interphalangeal joints.

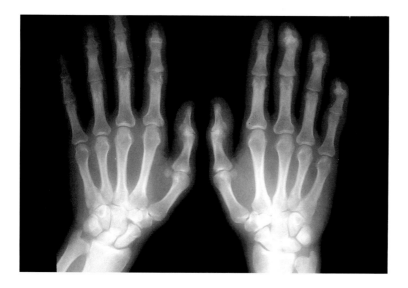

Figure 3.29

X-ray from psoriatic arthropathy showing destruction of the terminal interphalangeal joints with bony arthrosis in places.

process or not, the clinical features of psoriatic arthropathy are quite different. The distal interphalangeal joints bear the brunt of the disease rather than the proximal interphalangeal and metacarpophalangeal joints (Figure 3.28). Other joints typically affected include the temporomandibular, posterior zygohypophysial and the sacroiliac; other joints are occasionally involved. The inflammatory process seems more aggressive in psoriatic arthropathy and bone erosion, destruction and eventual ankylosis are fairly common findings (Figure 3.29). Oddly enough, despite the massive destruction and the resulting disability little pain seems to result. As an end result of this unpleasant destructive process the fingers may be 'telescopic' and virtually ablated (arthritis mutilans) (Figure 3.30). The elderly are more often affected by disabling arthritis in psoriasis and it is an additional burden for them to bear.

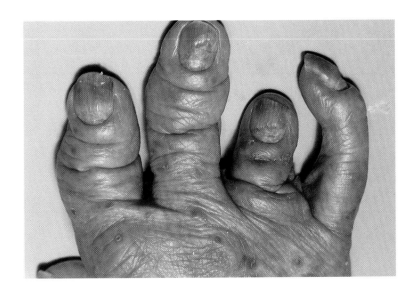

Figure 3.30

Arthritis mutilans showing severe deformity of the hand in a patient with longstanding psoriatic arthropathy.

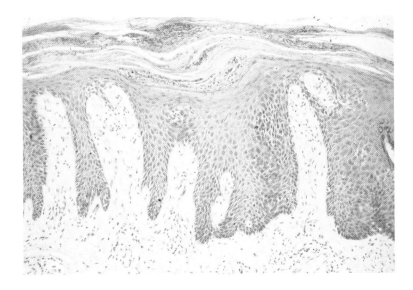

Figure 3.31

Histology of psoriasis. Note the regular epidermal hyperplasia and marked parakeratosis. (H & E; ×90).

Pathology and pathophysiology

The histological hallmark of plaque-type psoriasis is regular epidermal hypertrophy. The rete pattern is greatly exaggerated so that the rete pegs may be thickened to five or six times their usual thickness (Figure 3.31). The epidermis overlying the expanded dermal papillae, however, may be relatively thinned. The affected epidermis is surmounted by layers of parakeratotic horn, amongst which may be found small collections of desiccated polymorphs—the so-called Munro microabscesses. Epidermal oedema and inflammatory cells are often scattered throughout the epidermis (Figure 3.32). The dermal papillae are expanded by dilated tortuous papillary capillaries. There is a variably dense infiltrate of lymphocytes, predominantly in the upper dermis.

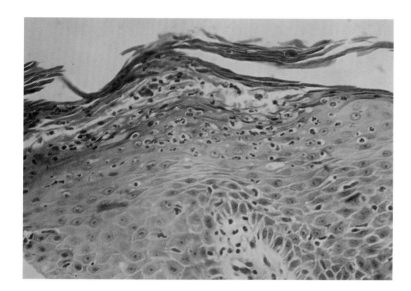

Figure 3.32

There are collections of polymorphs in and just below the stratum corneum in this photomicrograph from a biopsy of a patch of psoriasis (H & E; ×150).

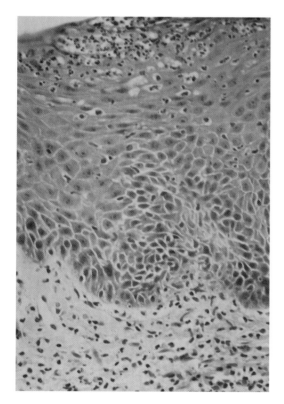

Figure 3.33

Diffuse infiltration of polymorphs in pustular psoriasis (H & E; ×150).

In pustular psoriasis there is much less epidermal hypertrophy, but instead there is exaggeration of the inflammatory component. There are collections of polymorphs within the epidermis and marked spongiosis (Kogoj spongiosis) (Figure 3.33).

The epidermal hypertrophy is caused by an increase in the rate of epidermal cell production to some four to seven times normal. It is not known whether this increase is due to an increase in the rate of cell division by the existing germinative population, or to an increase in the germinative cell population, or whether both types of change occur. Autoradiograph studies using the DNA precursor tritiated thymidine readily demonstrate that there is an increased number of 'labelled cells'—the labelling index being in the region of 25% as compared with the normal 4 or 5% (Figure 3.34). The rate of travel of epidermal cells from the basal germinative compartment of the epidermis to the surface is increased, so that the transit time within the epidermis is decreased. Normally it takes some 28 days for new cells produced in the basal layer to reach the surface of the stratum corneum. In psoriasis this process takes only four or five days; the cells have less time to differentiate properly, resulting in a stratum corneum that is structurally, biochemically and functionally very different from normal. In particular, the abnormal

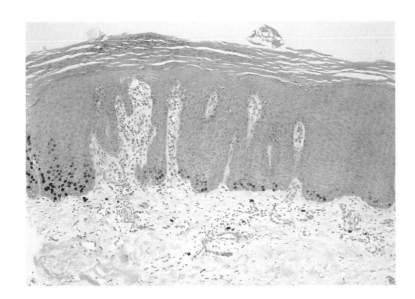

Figure 3.34

Autoradiograph after intracutaneous injection of a small quantity of tritiated thymidine showing large numbers of labelled cells indicating a high rate of epidermal cell production (H & E; ×45).

stratum corneum has a disturbed barrier function, resulting in the loss of 12 to 13 times more water than normal from the skin's surface. If large body areas are affected, dehydration can result. Absorption of substances applied to the skin is also enhanced—and this must be remembered in relation to the topical treatment of the disease.

The blood vessels in the affected skin are widely dilated and the rate of blood supply to the skin is greatly increased. This can result in a significant loss of heat from the skin and, despite the skin feeling hot, the patient may be hypothermic. This can be a particular problem in the elderly, especially if their homes are poorly heated. Additionally there are haemodynamic changes from a 'shunting' effect in the skin. If large areas of skin are affected there will be a high volume pulse and even a raised jugulovenous pressure from a compensatory increased plasma volume. This is not a problem for a healthy cardiovascular system, but in elderly patients, whose myocardium is often compromised by atherosclerosis, cardiac failure can result.

The papillary capillaries are not only dilated; they are also tortuously convoluted. The endothelium of these oddly prominent capillaries has a disproportionately increased volume,[39] although the endothelial cells do not appear structurally abnormal.

Aetiopathogenesis

The cause of psoriasis remains an enigma. It is clear that there is a genetic component to the disease.[40] Some 30% of psoriatic parents will have a child with psoriasis; however, if both parents are affected there is a 60% chance of an offspring with the disease. From various studies it has been estimated that the heritability is 90% overall. It has been found that possession of certain HLA groupings is associated with an increased likelihood of having the disease. Thus B13, B17, B37, Cw6 and Dr7 are particularly associated with ordinary adult onset type I (see later) plaque-type psoriasis but none is particularly associated with pustular psoriasis of the palms and soles. Cw6 is found in some 85% of patients with early onset disease.[41] Using sequence specific amplification primers it was confirmed that CW602 is especially prevalent in type I psoriatics.[42] In summary, the evidence points to there being an inherited predisposition to psoriasis but no straightforward inheritance pattern. Many researchers believe that it is the susceptibility that is inherited, and the chase is on to identify a susceptibility gene or genes for psoriasis.

Many biochemical alterations have been recorded in affected skin but for the most part they appear to be either a consequence of the altered pattern of epidermal cell production or the consequent deficient epidermal differentiation. For example, an altered profile of keratin polypeptides in the epidermis has been found[43] and proposed as an indicator of an underlying basic fault in the keratinization process, although as pointed out earlier, this seems unlikely. In particular, keratins 6 and 16 are found in psoriasis, but they do not seem to be specific to the disease as they are also found in other hyperproliferative states.[44]

Although no bacterium or virus has been consistently identified in the lesions and there are no epidemiological features to suggest that psoriasis is an infection, there have been some interesting findings. Research workers have identified viral-like particles in the lesions and urine of psoriatics.[45] It certainly seems possible that viral infection could play some role in the disorder, perhaps in a similar way to viragenes in cancer, and these findings should not be dismissed lightly.

There has been much research on the cause of the increase in epidermal cell production that characterizes psoriasis. Abnormalities in cyclic nucleotide metabolism with deficient adenyl cyclase activity and increased cyclic GMP (guanosine monophosphate) concentration,[46] increased ornithine decarboxylase and polyamine concentrations[47] and increased concentrations of arachidonate metabolites, and in particular lipoxygenase products,[48] have all been identified in psoriasis and considered as possible reasons for the increased rate of epidermopoiesis. It has also been suggested that growth hormone may be responsible for the increased rate of cell production.[49]

The inflammatory reaction has also been considered of central importance in the disease. Some workers have reported enhanced neutrophil migratory activity[50] and others have found that factors are present in the blood of psoriatics that stimulate neutrophil migration activity.[51] In addition there may well be an important immunopathogenetic component to psoriasis. We all possess antibodies to stratum corneum in the blood, and in psoriasis these are deposited in the stratum corneum.[52] It has also been suggested that the basal keratinocytes in psoriasis are leaky and stimulate an autoantibody response. In addition, there have been

several reports of abnormalities in the numbers and ratios of T-lymphocyte subsets, but it is difficult to evaluate their significance.

The fact that cyclosporin is such an effective remedy (see later) would also suggest that T-lymphocytes play an important role in the disease.[53] Patients with AIDS are sometimes afflicted with a particularly aggressive form of psoriasis.[54] A major component of HIV infection is disturbance in T-cell function and deficiency in T-helper cell numbers, and this may be another indication of the importance of lymphocytes in the pathogenesis of the disease. Further and persuasive evidence of the intimate involvement of T lymphocytes comes from work in which these cells have been injected intracutaneously into mice with severe combined immunodeficiency; lesions reminiscent of psoriasis resulted.[55,56]

As yet there is no reasonable unitary hypothesis that can account for all the manifestations of psoriasis. Intensive research activity has unravelled much of the cell kinetics and biochemical alterations in psoriasis, but there have been few pointers to the initiating causative events.

It has not even been decided whether psoriasis is one disease or several and the clinical manifestations are merely the final common pathway for a number of aetiological agencies.

Treatment

General issues concerning advice and topical treatments for the elderly are covered in Chapter 12. In particular it must be remembered that scaling, hyperkeratotic skin is not well tolerated by the elderly and that cosmetic concern may be as great as that in younger people.[53] It is not known for certain how any of the remedies for psoriasis exert their effects. Many of the treatments (eg, antimitotic agents, corticosteroids) have an antimitotic effect and certainly it would appear reasonable to suppose that this is their main mode of action. However, this may not be the case with the vitamin D analogues and the retinoids, which may work by promoting epidermal differentiation. The way that tar or dithranol works is also very much a mystery. They certainly have an antimitotic effect but they also have marked effects on intermediary metabolism and on the release of mediators. Anti-inflammatory and immunosuppressive effects are clearly also important for a therapeutic effect in psoriasis as for example with cyclosporin or tacrolimus.

Topical treatments

Emollient creams and baths may be all that is required when a few patches of psoriasis are present. Topical preparations containing tar (1–6%) and salicylic acid are quite useful for isolated plaques. If they are prescribed, the patient and relatives must be warned of their smell, appearance and potential for staining clothes and bedclothes. If tars are prescribed, the patient should be informed that tars have fallen under suspicion as potential carcinogens even though it has never been confirmed that the therapeutic use of tars has been responsible for human cancer. They can be applied at night under gauze bandages or early in the morning for 2 or 3 hours before being washed off. Tar ointment, tar paste and tar and salicylic acid are old favourite generic prescriptions. Cosmetically more acceptable tar preparations are now available either as creams or gels.

One of the most effective topical preparations for psoriasis is dithranol. This compound is used in concentrations matched to the patients' tolerance. Dithranol is a powerful oxidizing agent and acts as an irritant to the skin. Maximal therapeutic benefit is obtained by using the substance in concentrations just below that which causes irritation. The initial concentration used is 0.1%. Tolerance to it is extremely variable; some patients (perhaps 10–15%) cannot tolerate any concentration while others may eventually use a 5% (or even higher) concentration. Apart from irritating, it always stains the skin a brown-purple colour. It also stains clothes and bedclothes the same colour. If patients are treated intensively in hospital, dithranol clears some 80% in approximately 4 weeks. It used to be said that dithranol treatment was suitable only for hospital use, but this is no longer the case. The older preparations in a stiff paste (Lassar's paste) are gradually being replaced with more elegant and acceptable proprietary preparations which are quite suitable for use at home. In recent years it has been demonstrated that relatively short periods of skin contact with dithranol are required for a therapeutic effect.[54] In this short contact type of treatment the dithranol is applied in the mornings for 30–60 minutes and then washed off and there is no further treatment that day. Clearly this has tremendous advantages for outpatient treatment and, understandably, this form of treatment has become very popular.

Preparations containing dithranol are not suitable for use on the face, scalp and flexures. Owing to their irritant and staining properties they are rarely tolerated at these sites.

There has been an intensive search for more 'patient friendly' analogues of dithranol, but unfortunately none have emerged that are non-staining, non-irritating, stable and clinically effective.

There is considerable controversy concerning the use of topical corticosteroids (see page 268) in psoriasis. They are extensively used for treatment of the disorder in the USA but much less prescribed for this purpose in the UK. The more potent varieties do have a suppressive effect on psoriatic plaques, but the patches recur with renewed vigour almost immediately the treatment is withdrawn—which is not the case with dithranol or the vitamin D_3 analogues. In addition, their use seems to be associated with the development of pustular psoriasis.[55] Weak or moderately potent topical corticosteroids may be used on the scalp, the genitalia or flexures. If the face is affected, hydrocortisone preparations can be quite useful. Surprisingly, this is often adequate and the facial lesions rarely persist for long. Analogues of vitamin D_3 have been introduced for the topical treatment of psoriasis in the past decade. Calcipotriol was the first of these followed by tacalcitol, but others are developed and awaiting licensing. Calcipotriol was reported as more effective than betamethasone-17–valerate[56] and equally effective as dithranol.[57] Although topical calcipotriol (50 µg/g) causes some skin irritation in up to 15% of patients, it does not stain and is well accepted by patients. The theoretical hypercalcaemia that could result from excessive percutaneous penetration of the compound is excessively rare, and there are reports of psoriasis being well controlled by the use of calcipotriol for a year.[58]

Topical retinoids have always appeared to hold potential for use in psoriasis, but it was not until the mid-1990s that receptor-selective retinoid compounds had been shown to exploit that potential. Tazarotene is an acetylenic retinoid which binds particularly with nuclear receptors of type RAR (Retinoic Acid Receptor) alpha and beta that has been found to have good therapeutic activity in plaque-type psoriasis.[59] A once daily application of the 0.1% gel appears to be effective in some 65% of patients,[60] and its activity is enhanced by concurrent use of a medium potency corticosteroid.[61] Early onset of action and prolonged remission are other claimed attributes. As with other topical retinoids it can cause local irritation and burning in 15–20% of patients.

Systemic treatments

Some form of systemic medication is usually required for patients with severe widespread and persistent plaque-type psoriasis, erythrodermic or generalized pustular psoriasis. Because some of the elderly cannot cope with complex regimens of topical treatment, it may be appropriate to treat them with drugs given systemically even though the extent of the psoriasis would not warrant this in a younger individual. Methotrexate, the folate reductase inhibitor antimetabolite which functions as a cytostatic agent, has been found useful for psoriasis since the mid-1950s. Unfortunately its use is associated with a number of toxic side-effects, which limit its more widespread use. In particular, prolonged methotrexate use is associated with hepatocellular damage and fibrosis; the longer it is used and the larger the dose, the greater the risk of serious hepatotoxicity. It also causes marrow suppression, resulting in leukopaenia, thrombocytopaenia and anaemia in some patients. Nausea, vomiting and diarrhoea are other side-effects. Nevertheless, used with caution by an experienced clinician, the drug does provide much-needed relief in some patients.

Generally the use of methotrexate is restricted to those over 40 years old, and checks are made on the blood for haematological status and liver function at regular intervals. Liver biopsy every year (or less, if indicated) is also recommended by some practitioners to monitor the effects on the liver. The higher the cumulated dosage, the greater the incidence of hepatic fibrosis and serious functional hepatic disorder.[62] Weekly administration (oral or intramuscular) is said to be associated with a lesser incidence of serious toxic side-effects. Doses of 5–30 mg are given weekly, depending on the response. An alternative regimen which has found favour in some quarters is the administration of methotrexate 12 hourly over 36 hours each week. The rationale behind this administration at intervals is that the drug is likely to 'hit' more dividing epidermal cells over the shortened cell cycle. Generally, elderly patients tolerate methotrexate well, although there may be more gastrointestinal disturbance in this group.

Other antimitotic agents and antimetabolites are not as effective as methotrexate in psoriasis. Hydroxyurea has been found helpful by some clinicians but has not gained general acceptance. Razoxane appears to be as effective[63] but unfortunately, although its short-term marrow toxicity is manageable, its longer term toxicity may include leukaemia[64] so that its use has become unacceptable.

Although of considerable use for patients with severe psoriasis (particularly those patients who are erythrodermic or who have generalized or intractable localized pustular psoriasis), the older oral aromatic retinoid drug, etretinate, has been replaced by its more water-soluble metabolite—acitretin. Acitretin only starts to be effective after 2 weeks of treatment and maximal effects are seen after some 6 weeks. The recommended dose of acitretin is 0.3–0.6 mg/kg body weight daily. Virtually all patients who take the drug experience dryness and scaling of the lips. Other side-effects are less frequent and include transient and slight loss of scalp hair, dryness of the nasal, oral, anal and genital mucosae, and generalized itchiness. These side-effects may be more frequent in the elderly and can be irksome, but they are generally tolerable and do not usually result in the treatment having to be abandoned. More recently some cases of hyperostosis and ligamentous ossification have been reported in patients taking etretinate for several years. It is still too early to evaluate the clinical significance of these findings particularly with regard to the use of acitretin.

A potentially more hazardous side-effect is the hyperlipidaemia that occurs in some 25–35% of patients taking retinoids. For this reason the drug should not be given to patients with atherosclerotic arterial disease or those with pre-existing hyperlipidaemia. Etretinate and acitretin are teratogenic and even the oldest of patients treated with these retinoids should be informed of this lest they give the drug to their young relatives 'to try', as sometimes happens. Some authors have suggested that the oral retinoids are of particular value given in conjunction either with UV treatments (see below)[65] or with dithranol.[66] These reports are very encouraging and these forms of combination therapy seem worth considering in those who are resistant to more established treatments.

The fungal metabolite cyclosporin A is a potent immunosuppressive agent that was first used to prevent immune rejection in patients who had received organ transplants. It was later found to be very effective in the treatment of severe intractable plaque-type psoriasis[67,68] and is now often the treatment of choice for elderly patients. It is prescribed in 3–5 mg/kg body weight doses per day and usually the psoriatic lesions begin to remit after a few days. Unfortunately the lesions also rapidly reappear after treatment has been withdrawn. Side-effects that limit its use include a nephrotoxic effect and the development of hypertension. While cyclosporin is being given the patient should be regularly monitored for blood creatinine and blood pressure. If either of these parameters show significant rises the dose of cyclosporin must be reduced by 1 mg/kg daily for 2–3 weeks; if the levels of creatinine and/or blood pressure do not recover, the cyclosporin should be stopped. Other side-effects include nausea, paraesthesia and hirsuties.

Phototherapy

Treatment with various forms of UV irradiation is often a successful, if somewhat inconvenient, form of treatment. Ordinary artificial UV radiation (using lamps emitting primarily in the UVB range, see page 270) was frequently used as a treatment adjunct in patients using tar or dithranol. It does speed clearance of psoriatic plaques, but fell out of fashion when PUVA (see below) was introduced. It is now being used

again in many departments. If given, it must be administered by experienced staff who are aware of its potential for causing severe sunburn in the short term and chronic photodamage in the long term.

Exposure to the sun can be helpful for some patients, but the elderly are often too bashful to expose themselves in public and there is inadequate effective sunshine in Europe. However, treatment at the Dead Sea in Israel in spa conditions is remarkably successful for many patients.[69]

Since the early 1970s a new form of phototherapy has been available. This is photochemotherapy with ultraviolet radiation in the long-wave (A) part of the spectrum—so called PUVA therapy.[70] This form of treatment depends on the photosensitizing effect of a group of drugs known as the psoralens. The most frequently used is 8–methoxypsoralen, which is given (usually starting at a dose of 0.2 mg/kg) 2 hours before irradiation. The long-wave UV (UVA) is given in specially constructed apparatus (either cabinets or beds) so that the whole body can be treated at the same time. Smaller units are available for treatment of limited areas of the body such as the hands, feet and scalp. It is usual to start off with a short irradiation time to determine the patient's tolerance. Irradiation is gradually increased to 15–20 minutes per treatment and is given up to three or four times per week until clearance of the psoriasis has been achieved. PUVA is a clean treatment and the absence of messy ointments is much appreciated by patients; it is also popular with patients because of the tan that accompanies the clinical improvement.

Before patients start PUVA treatment they should be counselled and the risks and precautions carefully reviewed. Patients who cannot tolerate sun exposure and who burn easily are clearly unsuitable. Usually all type I subjects and many type II subjects are excluded. Male subjects should have their genitalia shielded as genital skin seems particularly at risk for PUVA-induced skin cancer (see later). To minimize the risk of UVA-induced ocular damage (including cataracts), UVA-blocking sunglasses must be worn both during treatment and for 12 hours after treatment. There are some patients who cannot tolerate being enclosed in a PUVA cabinet because of claustrophobia. The elderly sometimes find difficulty in standing for the required period. An important practical problem is that a course of treatment requires either inpatient treatment or frequent visits to a hospital centre offering this facility. The latter may be difficult for someone of advanced years with decreased mobility, and, of course, is also costly. PUVA can produce unpleasant burns if the treatment is advanced too rapidly. It also causes generalized pruritus and a dryness and scaliness of the skin, to which the elderly patient is prone anyway. Emollients are often needed for this side-effect. In the longer term, PUVA treatment damages dermal connective tissue and causes elastotic degenerative change.[71] A change termed photosclerosis also occurs in which specific alterations in the collagenous structure and mechanical properties have been noted.[72] In addition, there are now many reports documenting the rapid development of preneoplastic and neoplastic lesions of irradiated skin.[73,74] This may be a particular risk for fair-skinned patients and those who have previously had some other mutagenic treatment such as X-irradiation or systemic treatment with arsenic. Researchers in Boston suggest that the risk of developing a squamous cell carcinoma is some 12 times greater in those receiving PUVA treatment compared to those psoriatics who do not. The recorded risk seems specifically increased for the development of squamous cell carcinomas and not for basal cell carcinomas or melanomata. This does not mean that there is not an increased risk for these latter two lesions, merely that it has been more difficult to incriminate PUVA in these disorders.[75] The development of PUVA lentigines[75] suggest that pigment cells are indeed disturbed by the PUVA rays.

Lichen planus

Definition

Lichen planus is a common inflammatory disorder of the skin and mucosae of unknown cause, characterized pathologically by basal cell degenerative change, and clinically by the appearance of itchy, small, mauvish, flat-topped papules.

Clinical features

The disorder is uncommon in children but is seen in most other age groups, being most common between the ages of 30 and 60. It occurs equally frequently in men and women, and seems to affect most racial groups. A familial occurrence has been reported, though this is not usual. The antigens HLA 5, HLA 7 and B8 appear to be more common in patients with lichen planus. It is reputedly more common in some Asiatic communities. It accounts for 0.14–1.2% of all dermatological consultations. The typical lesions are small, shiny, flat-topped, polygonal papules, which vary in colour though characteristically have a mauve tint. Older lesions tend to be brownish, while new lesions are pink. On larger lesions a feathery white patterning may be seen over the surface—the so-called Wickham's striae.

The flexor creases of the wrists and the dorsa of the feet are typical involved sites (Figure 3.35) but anywhere on the limbs or trunk may be affected. When the palms and soles are involved, diagnosis may be quite difficult (Figure 3.36). Most patients with the disorder develop some 20–100 papules quite rapidly, which last for some months before remitting. However, lichen planus is notoriously variable in its expression. Buccal mucosal lesions are seen in 30–50% of patients. They are recognized as a feathery white lacework, or less commonly as a white punctate rash. When the lesions persist they may become thicker and less lacework-like (Figure 3.37). It is in this variety that squamous cell carcinomatous change may occur. The tongue, palate and lips may also be affected by lichen planus. Rarely other mucosae are involved—particularly the vulvovaginal and rectal mucosae. Lichen planus papules may appear at the site of skin trauma (the Koebner phenomenon, or isomorphic response).

Rarely the disorder has a dramatic onset and presents as an acute widespread scaling erythema. In other patients the trunk and limbs are densely covered by tiny but none the less typical lichen planus lesions (Figure 3.38). At the other end of the spectrum there may be just a few large, thickened lesions—the hypertrophic variety. This hypertrophic type is most frequently seen on the lower legs and forearms and tends to be persistent and very itchy (Figure 3.39). It

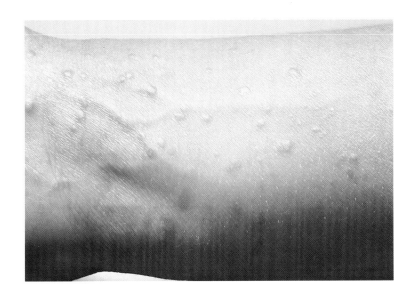

Figure 3.35a

Many typical papules of lichen planus affecting the wrist.

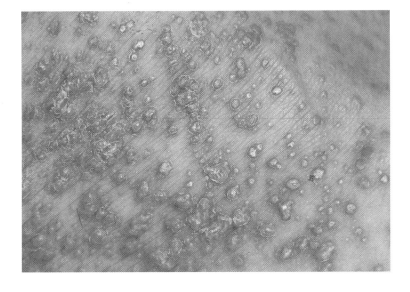

Figure 3.35b

Many typical papules of lichen planus. Some have typical white marking of Wickham's striae; others have a small amount of scale on their surface.

may be more frequent in the elderly. A very rare complication of the hypertrophic variant is squamous cell carcinoma. Two such patients have recently been seen in Cardiff in the UK. Yet another clinical variant is the annular form in which thin shiny rings, 0.5–2 cm in diameter, with atrophic centres form on the trunk and genitalia in particular (Figure 3.40).

Lichen planopilaris is a variant in which the brunt of the disease process is borne by the follicular epithelium. Aggregates of follicular horny plugs or horny pink papules are characteristic of the disorder. When lichen planus affects the scalp, scarring occurs after the inflammation subsides, and the resulting bald patches cannot be distinguished clinically from those due to lupus erythematosus.

In micropapular lichen planus and lichen nitidus there are a myriad of minute pink shiny papules. Lichen nitidus has been thought by

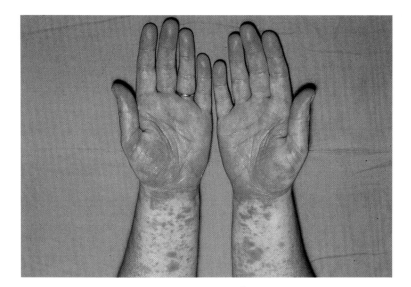

Figure 3.36

Lichen planus affecting the palms.

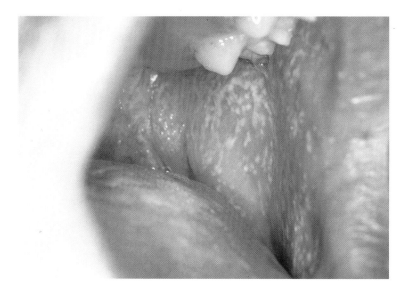

Figure 3.37

Buccal lichen planus.

some practitioners to represent a separate disorder,[54] and it certainly has a distinctive histopathological picture (see later).

Rarely bullous lesions appear—lichen planus pemphigoides. This complication may occur alongside severe destruction of the nail tissues, resulting ultimately in loss of nails. The bullous and destructive forms seem more common in the elderly, affecting the feet and the periungual tissues in particular.[76]

The nails are involved in some 10% of patients. The most frequently seen nail change is a rather characteristic longitudinal ridging, but more severe types with a destructive pterygium formation, nail deformity and even total permanent nail loss are not uncommon (Figure 3.41).

Lichen planus is a self-limiting disorder and approximately 50% of patients are free of the disease after 6 months; most patients are clear after 2 years. When the papules disappear,

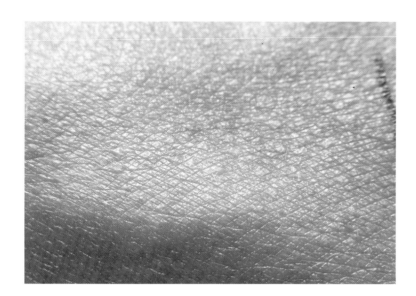

Figure 3.38

There are myriads of tiny papules of lichen nitidus on the skin.

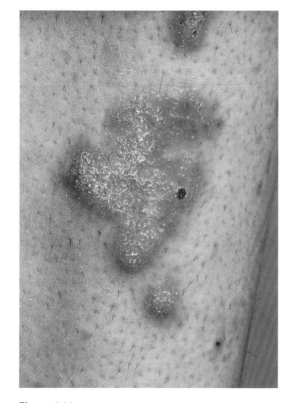

Figure 3.39

Thickened patch of hypertrophic lichen planus.

brown patches remain for some time afterwards; recurrences are quite common.

Pathology and pathophysiology

The most characteristic histopathological finding is a focal liquefactive degenerative change of the basal layer of the epidermis. At some sites pink, globular, homogeneous bodies known as cytoid bodies (or Civatte bodies or colloid bodies) (Figure 3.42) are found. These have been thought to represent dead epidermal cells on which immunoprotein has been deposited.[77] Ultrastructurally they have a fibrillar structure despite their homogeneous appearance in the light microscope, but the fibrils are more like those of amyloid than keratinous tonofilaments.[78] It was thought that the disordered basal layer precluded generative activity but labelling studies employing the DNA synthesis marker tritiated thymidine and an autoradiographic technique have shown that this is not the case. Rather than there being a reduction in the rate of cell production, an increase was found.[79] It seems most likely that the increase represents reparative activity to make good the damage produced by the disease.

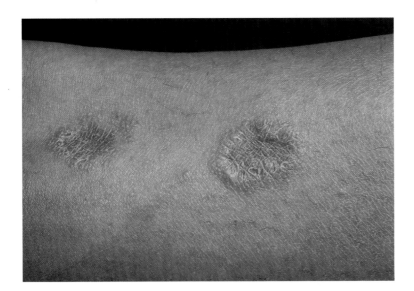

Figure 3.40

Annular lesions of lichen planus.

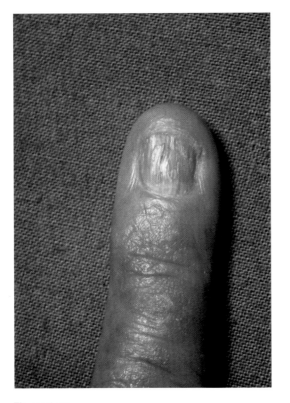

Figure 3.41

Longitudinal ridging and partial destruction of the nail in lichen planus.

Smaller, spindle-shaped epidermal cells are also found at the base of the epidermis (Figure 3.43). These seem to be another sign of repair as they resemble migrating epidermal cells seen in other wounded sites. The erosion of the basal layer causes a characteristic saw-tooth type of profile (Figure 3.44). Epidermal thickening is also a feature of the inflamed area. In addition, the epidermal cells in the mid and upper epidermis seem larger than usual and there is hypergranulosis. This upper epidermal hypertrophy seems paradoxical in the face of epidermal destruction at the base of the epidermis, but may be the result of simultaneous attempts at healing and repeated episodes of epidermal damage.

Immediately below the epidermis there is an infiltrate of lymphocytes and histiocytes of variable relative proportions. This so-called lichenoid band may be prominent or quite inconspicuous. Some of the cells occasionally cross into the epidermis. Amidst the infiltrate, pigment particles are seen—the result of epidermal melanin being released from damaged epidermal cells to be engulfed by histiocytes of the infiltrate (melanophages). Occasionally clefts appear subepidermally at the sites of pronounced basal cell damage; when clefting is pronounced, bullae arise.

In hypertrophic lichen planus the epidermal hypertrophy is very marked and may reach

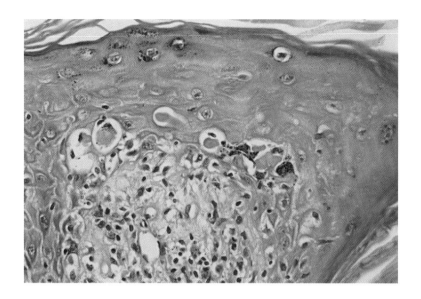

Figure 3.42

Basal cell damage in lichen planus. Note the formation of pink globular colloid bodies at the base of the epidermis (H & E; ×150).

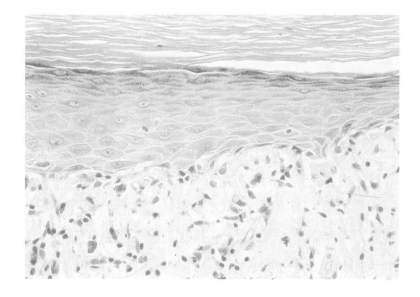

Figure 3.43

Spindle shaped cells at the base of the damaged epidermis beginning to repopulate the damaged areas (H & E; ×150).

pseudo-epitheliomatous proportions. In atrophic lichen planus there is no hypertrophy; instead there is marked atrophy of the epidermis. In lichen nitidus the cellular infiltrate is tucked up high in the papillae and there is suprapillary thinning of the epidermis. The infiltrate is sometimes frankly granulomatous.

Immunopathogenesis and associated immunological findings

There is strong circumstantial evidence that immunological mechanisms are involved in the production of the lesions of lichen planus. This

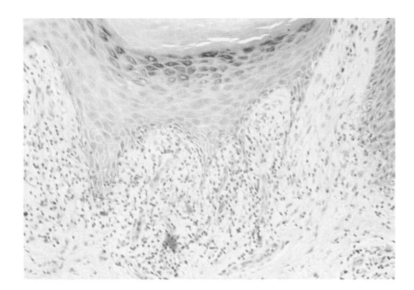

Figure 3.44

Saw-toothed profile in lichen planus. Note the relatively dense inflammatory cell infiltrate in the upper epidermis and the marked thickening of the granular cell layer (H & E; ×45).

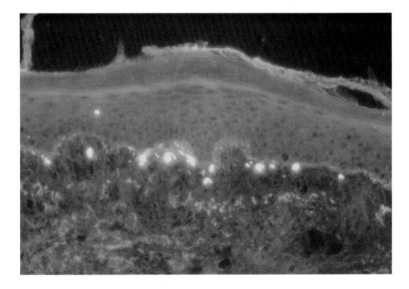

Figure 3.45

Immunofluorescence photomicrograph of lichen planus to show cytoid bodies staining with anti-human IgM reagent. (×90).

does not necessarily imply that the ultimate cause of the disease is an immunological disturbance but it does imply that immunological pathways are in some way responsible for the manifestations of this disease. The evidence for immune involvement may be summarized as follows;

1. The inflammatory cell infiltrate contains a large number of T-lymphocytes[80] and these are in close contact with the site of epidermal damage at the base of the epidermis.

2. Characteristically there are deposits of IgM and fibrin at the dermo-epidermal junction.[81] These can be detected using immunofluorescent techniques (Figure 3.45) or some other immunolocalization procedure. The IgM is mainly located in globules the size of epidermal cells or a little larger, which are thought to represent deposits of this immunoglobulin

47 Lowe N J, Breeding J, Russell D H. Cutaneous polyamines in psoriasis. *Br J Dermatol* (1982) **107:**21–6.

48 Greaves M W. Prostaglandins and dermatology. *Proc R Coll Physicians Lond* (1982) **16:**219–25.

49 Weber G, Neidhardt M, Schmidt A et al. Korrelation von Wachstumshormon und klinischem Bild der Psoriasis. *Arch Dermatol Res* (1981) **270:**129–40.

50 Dubertret L, Le Breton C, Touraine R. Neutrophil studies in psoriasis: in vitro migration, phagocytosis and bacterial killing. *J Invest Dermatol* (1982) **79:**74–8.

51 Kohwohl G, Szperalski B, Schroder J M et al. Polymorphonuclear leukocyte chemotaxis in psoriasis: enhancement by self activated serum. *Br J Dermatol* (1980) **103:**527–33.

52 Jablonska S, Beutner E H. Stratum corneum antibodies. In: Roenigk H H Jr, Maibach H I, eds, *Psoriasis*, (Marcel Dekker Inc: New York, 1985).

53 Graham J A, Kligman A M. Physical attractiveness. Cosmetic use and self perception in the elderly. *Int J Cosmet Sci* (1985) **7:**85–97.

54 Jones S K, Campbell W C, MacKie R M. Outpatient treatment of psoriasis: short contact and overnight dithranol therapy compared. *Br J Dermatol* (1985) **113:**331–7.

55 Baker H. Generalised pustular psoriasis. In: Roenigk H H Jr, Maibach H I, eds, *Psoriasis*, (Marcel Dekker: New York, 1985).

56 Cunliffe W J, Berth-Jones J, Claudy A et al. Comparative study of calcipotriol (MC903) ointment and betamethasone-17-valerate in patients with psoriasis vulgaris. *J Am Acad Dermatol* (1993) **26:**736–43.

57 Berth-Jones J, Chu A C, Dodd W AH et al. A multicentre parallel group comparison of calcipotriol ointment and short contact dithranol therapy in chronic plaque psoriasis. *Br J Dermatol* (1992) **127:**266–71.

58 Ramsay C A, Berth-Jones J, Brundin G et al. Long term use of topical calcipotriol in chronic plaque patients. *Dermatology* (1994) **189:**260–4.

59 Lew Kaya D A, Sefton J, Krueger J J et al. Safety and efficacy of a new retinoid gel in the treatment of psoriasis [abstract]. *J Invest Dermatol* (1992) **98:**600.

60 Weinstein G D, Krueger G G, Lowe N J et al. Tazarotene gel, a new safety retinoid for topical therapy of psoriasis: vehicle controlled study of safety, efficacy and duration of therapeutic effect. *J Am Acad Dermatol* (1997) **37:**85–92.

61 Tazarotene Clinical Study Group. Poster at European Academy of Dermatology and Venereology. October 1996, Lisbon.

62 Roenigk H H Jr, Maibach H I. Methotrexate. In: Roenigk H H Jr, Maibach H I, eds, *Psoriasis*, (Marcel Dekker Inc: New York, 1985).

63 Horton J J, Atherton D J. 'Razoxan'. In: Roenigk H H Jr, Maibach H I, eds, *Psoriasis* (Marcel Dekker: New York, 1985).

64 Horton J J, Caffrey E A, Clarke K G A et al. Leukaemia in psoriatic patients treated with razoxane. (Letter). *Br J Dermatol* (1984) **110:**633–4.

65 Lauharanta J, Juvakoski T, Kanerva K et al. Combination of etretinate and PUVA. A new effective way to treat psoriasis. In: Farber E M, Cox A J, eds, *Psoriasis: Proceedings of the 3rd International Symposium*, (Grune & Stratton: New York, 1982). 499–500.

66 Grupper C, Berretti B. Retinoid combinations. In: Roenigk H H Jr, Maibach H I, eds, *Psoriasis* (Marcel Dekker: New York, 1985).

67 Bos J D, Meinardi M M H M, Joost Th van et al. Use of cyclosporin in psoriasis. *Lancet* (1989) **ii:**1500–2.

68 Laburte C R, Grossman J, Abi-Rahed J. Efficacy and safety of oral cyclosporin A (CyA; Sandimmune®) for long term treatment of chronic severe plaque psoriasis. *Br J Dermatol* (1994) **130:**366–75.

69 Avrach W W. Climatography at the Dead Sea. In: Farber E M, Cox A J, eds, *Psoriasis: Proceedings of the 3rd International Symposium*, (Grune & Stratton: New York, 1982).

70 Stern R H, Hönigsmann N H, Parrish J A et al. Oral psoralen photochemotherapy. In: Roenigk H H Jr, Maibach H I, eds, *Psoriasis*, (Marcel Dekker: New York, 1985).

71 Zelickson A S, Mottaz H, Zelickson B D et al. Elastic tissue changes in skin following PUVA therapy. *J Am Acad Dermatol* (1980) **3:**186–92.

72 Pierard G E, Franchimont C, Cawvenberge T et al. PUVA and specific changes in the dermis. In: Farber E M, Cox A J, eds, *Psoriasis: Proceedings of the 3rd International Symposium*, (Grune & Stratton: New York, 1982). 459–60.

73 Stern R S, Laird N, Melski J et al. Cutaneous squamous cell carcinoma in patients treated with PUVA. *New Engl J Med* (1984) **310:**1156–61.

74 Stern R S, Nichols K T, Valeka L H. Malignant melanoma in patients treated for psoriasis with Methoxsalen (psoralen) and ultraviolet A radiation (PUVA). *New Engl J Med* (1997) **336:** 1041–5.

75 Lever L, Farr P M. Skin cancers and premalignant lesions occur in half of high dose PUVA patients. *Br J Dermatol* (1994) **131:**215–19.

76 Black MM. Lichen planus and lichenoid disorders. In: Champion RH, Burton JL, Ebling FJG, eds, *Rook/Wilkinson/Ebling Textbook of Dermatology*, (Blackwell Scientific: Oxford, 1982) 1684–98.

77 Ueki H. Hyaline bodies in subepidermal papillae. *Arch Dermatol* (1969) **100:**610–17.

78 Clausen J, Kjaergaard J, Bierring F. The ultrastructure of the dermo-epidermal junction in

lichen planus. *Acta Derm Venereol* (Stockh) (1981) **61**:101–6.

79   Marks R, Black M M, Wilson-Jones F. Epidermal cell kinetics in lichen planus. *Br J Dermatol* (1973) **88**:37–45.

80   Schmitt D, Thivolet J. Use of monoclonal antibodies specific for T-cells subsets in cutaneous disorders. II. Immunomorphological studies in blood and skin lesions. *J Clin Immunol* (1982) **2**:111–19.

81   Baart de la Faille-Kuyper E H, Baart de la Faille H. An immunofluorescence study of lichen planus. *Br J Dermatol* (1974) **90**:365–71.

82   James W D, Odom R B. Graft v host disease. *Arch Dermatol* (1983) **119**:683–9.

83   Davies M G, Gorkiewicz A, Knight A, Marks R. Is there a relationship between lupus erythematosus and lichen planus? *Br J Dermatol* (1977) **96**:145–54.

84   Graham-Brown R A C, Sarkany I, Sherlock S. Lichen planus and primary biliary cirrhosis. *Br J Dermatol* (1982) **106**:699–703.

85   Van Den Haute V, Antoine J L, Lachapelle J M. Histopathological discriminant criteria between lichenoid drug eruption and idiopathic lichen planus: retrospective study on selected sample. *Dermatology* (1989) **179**:10–13.

86   Swanbeck G, Thyresson N. Electron microscopy of intranuclear particles in lichen planus: a preliminary report. *Acta Derm Venereol* (1964) **44**:105–6.

87   Maidhof R. Zur systemischen Behandlung des oralen lichen planus mit einem aramatischen Retinoid [Ro 10-9359]. *Z Hautkr* (1979) **54**: 873–6.

88   Kersle K, Mobacken H, Sloberg K et al. Several oral lichen planus: treatment with an aromatic retinoid (etretinate). *Br J Dermatol* (1982) **106**:77–80.

4
Itching and other dry skin disorders

As mentioned elsewhere in this book, apparent dryness of the skin surface and itchiness is a major problem in the elderly. It is a component of many skin disorders in the elderly, including psoriasis and the eczematous dermatoses (see Chapter 3). It should be taken into account when prescribing for these diseases.

Senile pruritus (senile xerosis)

This is the term for persistent itchiness of the skin in the elderly accompanied by apparent dryness of the skin, but without other obvious cause. Generally it is a problem found in those over 70 years old. The skin looks and feels dry although until recently there have been precious little data to confirm that there is less water in the stratum corneum than in other age groups. Using a dynamic mechanical method to study the propagation and attenuation of low frequency shear waves in skin, Potts and coworkers[1] found that the major part of the response came from the stratum corneum and that the results depended on the water content of the stratum corneum. Changes were recorded in older subjects, suggesting that there was less moisture in the horny layers of their skin. The skin surface in senile xerosis has a dull matt appearance and there is often a fine scale, but examination is otherwise unrewarding (Figure 4.1). Patients complain bitterly of the persistent itch despite the lack of physical signs. The pruritus is worse at night and temporarily aggravated by hot baths. At the moment there is no rational explanation for this unpleasant and often disabling symptom.[2]

Figure 4.1

Close-up of 'dry' skin with some scaling on upper leg of man of 83.

Other causes of generalized itching should be excluded before a diagnosis is attempted. It has to be remembered that the elderly are not immune from scabies and it is embarrassing for all concerned for this common infestation to be missed. It is also prudent to exclude systemic causes of pruritus, including obstructive jaundice, renal failure, hyperthyroidism, the reticuloses and polycythaemia rubra vera. Curiously, excoriations are not prominent in senile pruritus and this may be helpful in the differential diagnosis.

Treatment should begin with general advice. The condition often seems worse in winter time and in a centrally heated environment when the relative humidity is at its lowest. This is particularly a problem in the north eastern USA, but winter may even aggravate the condition in our damp northern islands. Humidifiers improve the situation so far as central heating is concerned and wrapping up well in warm clothes when outside in a cold wind may be of some assistance. Soaking in hot baths should be avoided. Showering is best, although quick tepid baths will have to suffice if, as is often the case, showers are not available. Vigorous towelling after bathing can also aggravate itching, and so the skin should be patted dry.

Special emollient soaps designed to provide only a mild detergent effect should be used instead of ordinary toilet soap. Bath oils are sometimes helpful as they leave a thin emollient film of oil on the skin surface. The application of emollient preparations gives slight temporary relief and should be prescribed. The most appropriate product is the one that the patient finds most soothing and pleasant to use. Several may have to be tried before the one that is most acceptable and gives the most relief is found. Unfortunately there are no topical preparations that specifically attack the problem of itch. There is a fortune waiting for the pharmaceutical company that introduces an effective and safe antipruritic. Topical doxepin does appear to give some relief from pruritus, but mainly in atopic dermatitis, and its effect in other pruritic conditions is uncertain. Mentholated preparations may give slight transient relief and should be tried. Oily calamine lotion with 0.5% menthol is helpful for some individuals. Weak topical corticosteroids are sometimes used, but I do not think that these are any more effective than emollients for most patients.

Drugs used systemically rarely give assistance. The antihistamines only relieve itch when histamine release is the cause of the symptom and there is no evidence that this is the case in senile pruritus. The sedative effect of older antihistamine preparations may be helpful, but can also cause confusion in the elderly. If a sedative effect is thought necessary then it is probably better to prescribe one of the benzodiazepines.

As can be gathered from the above, the treatment of itch in the elderly is not easy. It requires experience, patience, sympathy and perseverance.

Psychiatric disorder and pruritus

Severe persistent and generalized itch causes sleeplessness and general debility and can result in a depressive reaction. This must be watched for and treated if present.

Persistent itch is very occasionally the primary presenting complaint of a delusional psychotic disorder. Parasitosis is a rare disease of this type sometimes seen in the elderly in which there is an unshakeable belief that the skin is inhabited or attacked by some form of parasite.[3] It is not uncommon for these patients to bring to the clinic (carefully wrapped up in tissue paper or in a matchbox) various bits of detritus that they have scraped off the surface of their skin and which they proudly present as the parasite. Such patients often have severe excoriations and even deep gouge marks on the skin where they have attempted to dig the parasites out. Despite explanation and reassurance and their apparent normality in other respects, they hold steadfastly to the belief that they are infested. Patients with parasitosis need to be referred for psychiatric assessment, although psychiatrists find this condition as tough to manage as do dermatologists. However, the drug pimozide has proved helpful to many patients with this complaint.[4]

Another disorder that is almost as difficult to manage as parasitosis is the condition known (unjustifiably) as neurotic excoriations. This is mainly seen in late-middle-aged women, but is sometimes seen in older individuals as well. It is characterized by persistent pruritus which

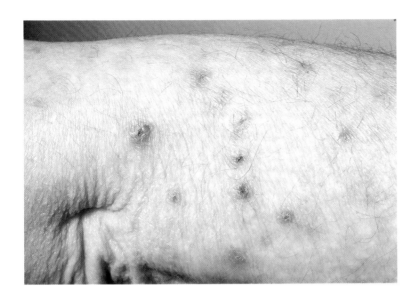

Figure 4.2a

Excoriations on side of arm in woman of 79.

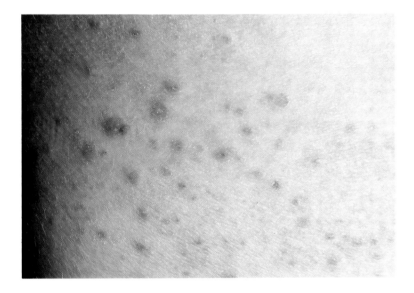

Figure 4.2b

Prurigo papules as a result of scratching, with neurotic excoriations.

may or may not be generalized. There is usually pronounced excoriation over the back and shoulders and possibly the forearms (Figure 4.2). Apart from mild anxiety these patients do not have an overt psychiatric disturbance and despite intensive investigation no cause is found for the symptom. Management should be along the lines indicated for senile pruritus.

Pruritus ani and vulvae

Irritation of the perianal, perineal and genital skin is extremely common and not confined to the elderly although it is certainly common in the older age groups. The sensitive areas are subjected to high humidity, irritating secretions, tight underclothing and a variety of toilet procedures apart from being the subject of a

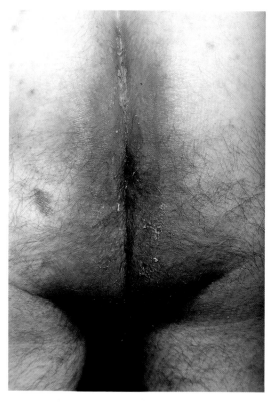

Figure 4.3

Perianal region and buttocks showing acute allergic contact dermatitis due to sensitization to one of the local anaesthetics in a proprietary preparation used for the relief of irritation due to piles.

Probably the commonest identifiable cause of pruritus ani is haemorrhoids, which should be considered for surgical treatment if they are severe. When, as is often the case, no cause for the pruritus can be found, especial care should be taken that self-medication is not aggravating or perpetuating the condition. Patch testing to determine whether there are contact hypersensitivities sometimes reveals sensitivity to a constituent of a topical application which the patients themselves have been using. Cinchocaine and amethocaine are included in some local preparations for haemorrhoids and may cause an allergic contact dermatitis (Figure 4.3). Benzocaine and procaine are less potent sensitizers, and preparations containing these substances are less frequently the cause of problems.

Symptomatic relief for such patients is often difficult to obtain despite employing the regimen described above for senile pruritus and advice concerning hygiene for the troublesome part. Regrettably such patients often end up as chronic outpatient attendees oscillating between dermatologist, gynaecologist, surgeon and psychiatrist.

variety of sexual fantasies and practices. It is hardly surprising that the skin of the area occasionally capitulates and causes intense itchiness.

Luckily the irritation is mostly transient and needs no special attention. When it is persistent, care must be taken to ensure that it is not the result of a disorder of either the skin or the anogenital mucosa. There can be no excuse for not examining the area in detail and performing rectal and vaginal examinations. Conditions such as carcinoma of the rectum or carcinoma of the cervix may rarely cause pruritus. Lichen sclerosis et atrophicus, leukoplakic vulvitis and atrophic vaginitis can also cause irritation and should be appropriately treated when present.

Disorders of keratinization

Congenital disorders of keratinization in which there is a genetically determined fault in the process of epidermal differentiation or desquamation are diseases that affect the whole lifespan and persist into old age. Complete descriptions of these may be found elsewhere.[5] However, it is appropriate to describe briefly here how they affect the older age groups.

The scaling of all the ichthyotic disorders, including autosomal dominant ichthyosis, sex-linked ichthyosis, non-bullous ichthyosiform erythroderma, bullous ichthyosiform erythroderma and lamellar ichthyosis, tends to become more pronounced in old age. Presumably this is due to the general tendency of the skin to be dry and scaly in the elderly anyway (Figure 4.4). Despite this, it is uncommon for patients with these diseases to seek attention for them in old age—presumably because they have learnt to live with them. They are usually discovered incidentally during the course of examination for another complaint.

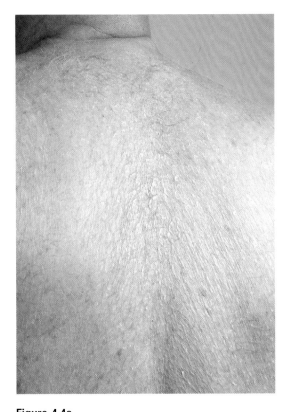

Figure 4.4a

Autosomal dominant ichthyosis in elderly man.

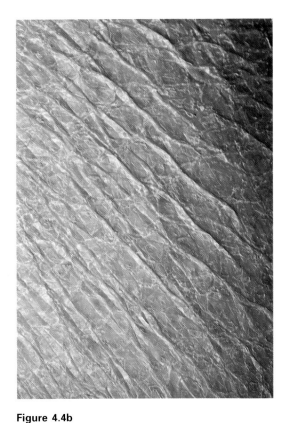

Figure 4.4b

Close-up of thigh of patient with autosomal dominant ichthyosis.

Patients with the rare dominantly inherited disease, bullous ichthyosiform erythroderma (also known as epidermolytic hyperkeratosis) lose the tendency to blister after early adult life and the redness becomes much less marked as well. The latter is also the case for patients with the similarly rare recessive non-bullous ichthyosiform erythroderma. However, the hyperkeratosis and severe scaling persists and in fact may worsen in old age (Figure 4.5). The rare lamellar ichthyosis is also inherited as a recessive feature, but has different clinical, histological and cell kinetic features.[6] This too worsens in old age (Figure 4.6).

Patients with severe palmoplantar hyperkeratosis as a result of one of the localized disorders of keratinization may experience worsening of the fissuring of the skin in old age. This may be quite disabling and need urgent attention. Often there is no option but to put the affected area to rest. Local treatment should include greasy emollients and if these are insufficient the addition of either 2% salicylic acid in white soft paraffin or bandaging at night should be considered.

Acquired ichthyosis is characterized by the onset of the ichthyotic disorder in later life and is dealt with in Chapter 10.

Nodular prurigo

This is an uncommon itching dermatosis of unknown cause which is characterized by the

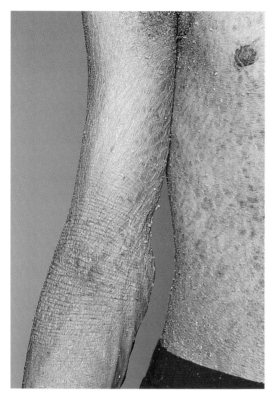

Figure 4.5a

Arm of patient with non-bullous ichthyosiform erythroderma. Note rippled appearance.

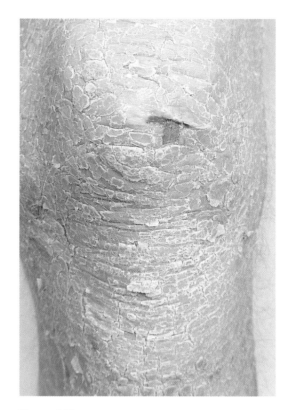

Figure 4.5b

Patient with bullous ichthyosiform erythroderma (epidermolytic hyperkeratosis). The remnants of one or two small blisters can be seen. Even though this man is middle aged, he is still suffering from blisters on occasion. Note the iregular dark hyperkeratotic areas.

appearance of variably sized excoriated papules and nodules. Small prurigo papules occur as part of atopic dermatitis and are also seen in scabies and occasionally in or near lesions of lichen simplex chronicus (see page 50). Why some individuals react in this odd and specific manner is quite mysterious, but a comprehensive study of the disorder found that a substantial proportion had a valid systemic cause for pruritus.[7] Histologically, there is a massive epidermal hypertrophy and considerable inflammation. Treatment with topical agents such as corticosteroids is not often successful, but topical tacalcitol has proved successful within 4 weeks in 9 of 11 cases treated with this agent.[8]

Oral thalidomide has also been claimed as helpful.

Pityriasis rubra pilaris

This disease is usually described as a disorder of keratinization, although there is no evidence to incriminate any particular pathophysiological mechanism. There are several forms of the disorder,[9] but the only one that need concern us here is the acquired adult form. This is an uncommon, but by no means rare, condition in the elderly. Usually the disorder has a fairly rapid onset in

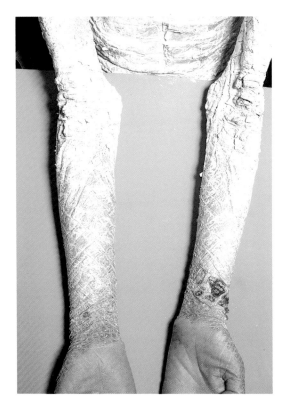

Figure 4.6a

Severe lamellar ichthyosis affecting the arms in a man agd 72.

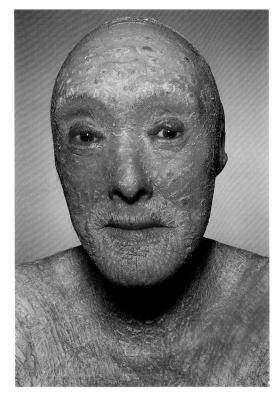

Figure 4.6b

Face of same patient as in Figure 4.6a. Note the severe ectropion and poor ear development. These are quite common in this disorder.

an individual without a previous history of skin disorder. The face and scalp are often the first sites to be affected and a little later the trunk and limbs are involved so that the condition may become erythrodermic. The rash itself often superficially resembles psoriasis and indeed it can be difficult to distinguish the two conditions. There is marked erythema and scaling but the redness has a distinct and characteristic orange tint unlike the plum red colour of psoriasis. Other points of distinction are the facial involvement which nearly always affects the entire face and scalp early in the disease and the presence of small islands of normal skin in pityriasis rubra pilaris. The hair follicle orifices of the backs of

the hands and the sides and fronts of the thighs and maybe elsewhere may have horny plugs—giving the disease its name (Figure 4.7). The palms and soles may also be thickly hyperkeratotic in pityriasis rubra pilaris.

Pityriasis rubra pilaris persists for a variable period but usually remits in 1–3 years or sometimes less. Occasionally there are relapses, but mostly the disorder is not a long-term problem.

Histologically the characteristic clubbing of the epidermal rete pegs and the suprapapillary plate thinning of psoriasis are not seen, although the overall appearance is that of 'psoriasiform hyperplasia'. The epidermis is

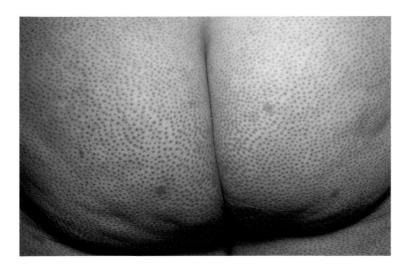

Figure 4.7a

Pityriasis rubra pilaris with marked follicular involvement of the buttocks.

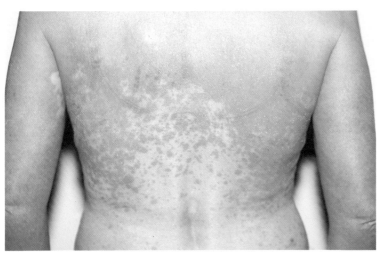

Figure 4.7b

Pityriasis rubra pilaris in a woman of 64. The disorder started suddenly on her face and scalp and spread to her trunk, looking very like psoriasis in places.

Figure 4.7c

Pityriasis rubra pilaris showing follicular accentuation.

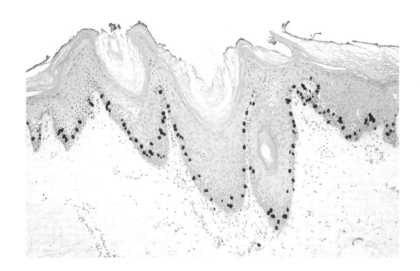

Figure 4.8

Autoradiograph from patch of pityriasis rubra pilaris. There are many autoradiographically labelled cells in the basal and suprabasal regions. There is little parakeratosis but considerable epidermal thickening in this section with follicular plugging. It is not the picture expected in psoriasis (H & E; ×90).

hyperproliferative in that there is an increased thymidine autoradiographic labelling index (Figure 4.8). Furthermore there are no Munro microabscesses and there is less inflammatory cell infiltrate than in psoriasis.

Treatment

As mentioned earlier, the condition spontaneously remits, so that it is easy to be convinced that a particular treatment has been effective if given just at the time of improvement. In general the topical treatments for psoriasis are not very effective. Treatment with oral retinoids is often helpful[10] but Clayton et al (1997) found that oral retinoids supplemented with low dose weekly methotrexate resulted "in 25–75% improvement in 17 of 24 patients after 16 weeks of therapy".[11]

References

1   Potts R O, Buras E M, Chrisman D A. Changes with age in the moisture content of human skin. *J Invest Dermatol* (1984) **82:**97–100.

2   Kligman A M. Perspectives and problems in cutaneous gerontology. *J Invest Dermatol* (1979) **73:**39–46.

3   Tullet G. Delusions of parasitosis. *Br J Dermatol* (1965) **77:**448–55.

4   Cotterill J A. Psychiatry and skin disease. In: Rook A J, Maibach H I, eds, *Recent Advances In Dermatology*, Vol 6. (Churchill Livingston: Edinburgh, 1983) 189–212.

5   Traupe H. *The Ichthyoses* (Springer Verlag: Heidelberg, 1989).

6   Hazell M, Marks R. Clinical, histological and cell kinetic discriminants between lamellar ichthyosis and non-bullous ichthyosiform erythroderma. *Arch Dermatol* (1985) **121:**489–93.

7   Rowland Payne C M E, Wilkinson J D, McKee P H, Jurecka W, Black M M. Nodular prurigo—a clinicopathological study of 46 patients. *Br J Dermatol* (1985) **113:**431–9.

8   Katayama I, Miyazaki Y, Nishioka K. Topical vitamin D_3 (tacalcitol) for steroid-resistant prurigo. *Br J Dermatol* (1996) **135:**237–40.

9   Griffiths A. Pityriasis rubra pilaris. Etiologic considerations. *J Am Acad Dermatol* (1984) **10:**1086–8.

10 Goldsmith L A, Weinrich A E, Shupack J. Pityriasis rubra pilaris response to 13-cis-retinoic acid (isotretinoin). *J Am Acad Dermatol* (1982) **6:**710–15.

11 Clayton B D, Jorizzo J L, Hitchcock M G et al. Adult pityriasis rubra pilaris: a 10 year case series. *J Am Acad Dermatol* (1997) **36:**959–64.

5
Drug eruptions and acute exanthematic disorders

The older one becomes, the more drugs are prescribed to keep you going! As long as 'more things go wrong' in old age and pharmacotherapy remains the main thrust of our therapeutic efforts, this tendency is irreversible. An inevitable consequence is that drug reactions of all types are more common in the elderly than in younger age groups.[1] Drug-induced rashes are no exception. Some of the acute generalized eruptions seen in the elderly which are due to the administration of a drug are identical to disorders for which no drug cause can be found. These will also be included in this chapter.

At the outset it has to be stated that we are still at a primitive stage of understanding with regard to drug-induced disease. Usually we have little idea as to the pathogenesis of the disorder and consequently have few diagnostic tests or specific treatments.

Some drugs are especially prone to cause drug eruptions. These include the non-steroidal anti-inflammatory agents, antibiotics and non-antibiotic antimicrobial agents (eg, the penicillins, the sulphonamides, metronidazole and clotrimazole), diuretics, such as the thiazides, some psychotropic agents, including the phenothiazines and drugs used in the control of epilepsy including phenytoin and Tegretol®. Recommended reviews on the topic include Wintroub and Stern[2] and Merk and Hertl[3]. The general principles and the problems only as they affect the elderly will be covered here. To avoid repetition and to obtain a broad overall view of the topic, the subjects of clinical signs and symptoms, pathogenesis, diagnosis and treatment are each considered for all drug eruptions.

Clinical signs and symptoms

Any part of the skin or mucosae may be involved in a drug reaction. In addition there is often a systemic component with slight fever and a feeling of being unwell. The time of onset of the rash after the drug has been started is very variable and it may indeed suddenly develop for no apparent reason in someone who has been taking a drug for some time. Generally, however, the rash starts some 7–21 days after the culprit drug was started.

Severe generalized eruptions

Erythema multiforme

This pattern of skin disorder may be evoked by a variety of stimuli (Table 5.1). Discoid or annular reddened swollen patches suddenly appear

Table 5.1 Main causes of erythema multiforme

Type	Agent
Infective	Herpes simplex
	Orf
	Vaccina
	Deep fungus infections (eg coccidioidomycosis, histoplasmosis)
	Streptococcal infection
Drug-induced	Sulphonamides (particularly long-acting sulphonamides)
	Non-steroidal anti-inflammatory agents
	Hydantoinates
	Sulphonylureas
	Trimethoprim
	Metronidazole
	Thiazides
Miscellaneous	Exposure to solar UVR
	X-irradiation of neoplastic disease

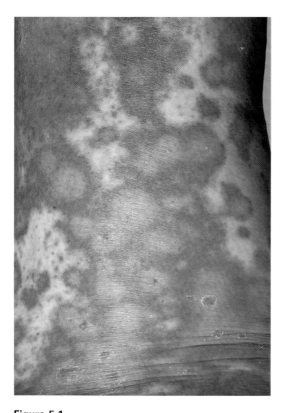

Figure 5.1

Many target lesions of erythema multiforme.

symmetrically over the limbs, particularly hands and forearms, although any area can be affected when the condition is severe. The lesions are often annular and sometimes target shaped with an area of necrosis centrally (Figure 5.1). There is frequently a bullous component with the blisters arising on the patterned, reddened lesions or sometimes independently on other reddened areas. In most patients the buccal mucosa is patchily eroded, and when the disorder is severe the nasal, conjunctival and even genital mucosae are also inflamed and eroded (Figure 5.2). The severe generalized form with marked mucosal involvement tends to be known eponymously as the Stevens–Johnson syndrome. When the mucosal lesions are prominent the patient is often severely ill with swollen, exudative and ragged areas over the lips, tongue, palate and genitalia. All such patients are ill, and when the disease occurs in the elderly it can be life-threatening (with a mortality of 20 or 30%). The worst of the disease is over in 7–10 days, but it usually takes 2 or 3 weeks before the lesions begin to disappear. The disease should be clearly differentiated from toxic epidermal necrolysis (Table 5.2). There are characteristic histological appearances in early lesions which assist the differentiation. Focal epidermal cell necrosis and a lymphocytic infiltrate are seen, and blisters form subepidermally (Figure 5.3).

Figure 5.2

Involvement of the lips in erythema multiforme. The buccal mucosa was also involved in this patient.

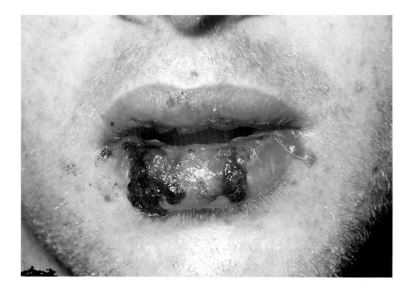

Table 5.2   Main points of differentiation between toxic epidermal necrolysis and erythema multiforme

	Toxic epidermal necrolysis	*Erythema multiforme*
Population affected	Rare disorder; any group, but appears to be predilection for elderly women	Not uncommon disease; any group
Clinical signs	Wide confluent areas of exudation and desquamation	Symmetrical round or annular or target-shaped lesions with central necrosis or blistering
Mucosal involvement	Muscosal involvement extensive and severe	Mucosal involvement common in severe forms
Morbidity and mortality	Always serious disease; mortality approaches 50%	Variable in severity; mortality perhaps 20% in elderly when severe
Pathology	Separation and necrosis of upper epidermis with marked inflammation and exocytosis	Inflammatory change in papillary dermis and necrosis at base of epidermis

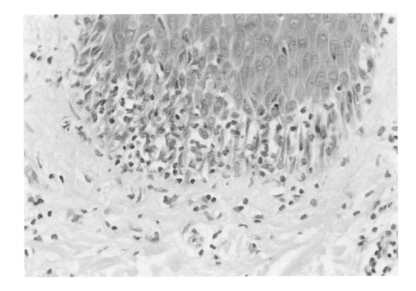

Figure 5.3

Pathology of erythema multiforme. There are many inflammatory cells invading the epidermis.

Toxic epidermal necrolysis

This condition has often been confused with a widespread exfoliative disorder in neonates caused by particular toxigenic strains of staphylococci and best known as the staphylococcal scalded skin syndrome. Toxic epidermal necrolysis mostly occurs in the middle-aged or elderly and is either due to a drug or has no identifiable cause.[4] The drugs with which the disorder has been associated include the non-steroidal anti-inflammatory agents, the hydantoinates and the oral hypoglycaemic agents. The disorder is rarer than erythema multiforme, which is just as well as it is more serious and has a higher mortality. Biopsies will reveal a dense mixed cellular infiltrate in the upper dermis which involves the epidermis as well. The upper part of the epidermis is necrotic (Figure 5.4).

The disease starts abruptly with fever, malaise and a widespread erythematous macular rash. It rapidly worsens as the mucosae become inflamed and eroded and the rash begins to desquamate over large areas (Figure 5.5). At this stage there is usually severe constitutional disturbance with fluid and electrolyte imbalance and heat loss from the erythroderma. In the most severely afflicted there may also be peripheral

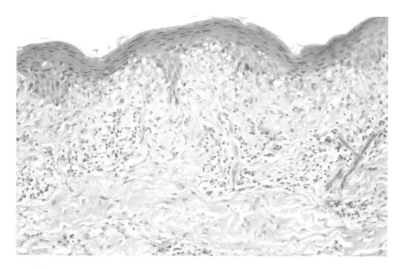

Figure 5.4

Pathology of toxic epidermal necrosis. There is intense upper dermal and sub-epidermal inflammatory cell infiltrate with involvement of the epidermis, which is necrotic in areas (H & E; ×90).

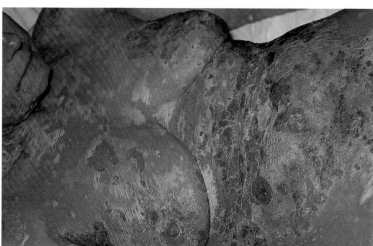

Figure 5.5a

Toxic epidermal necrosis in an elderly woman. This woman unfortunately died.

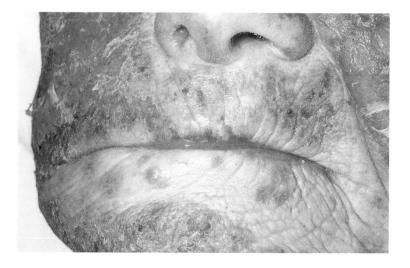

Figure 5.5b

Toxic epidermal necrosis in an elderly woman, showing the lower face.

vascular failure and finally central cardiorespiratory failure. No other skin disorder is such a challenge to management.

Erythema nodosum

This is an inflammatory nodular panniculitis affecting the front of the shins predominantly and provoked by many agencies, including tuberculosis, sarcoidosis, streptococcal infection, deep fungal infections, virus infections and drugs occasionally, including sulphonamides. Unfortunately the cause is identified in only about 30% of patients. It is uncommon in the elderly but certainly is seen at times, as in the patient shown in Figure 5.6. The nodules (1 to 3 cm in diameter) are tender and painful and develop bruise-like discoloration before disappearing within 2–4 weeks. Erythema nodosum may develop rapidly, with mild pyrexia and arthralgia—particularly in the ankles.

Erythematous and morbilliform eruptions

The sudden onset of a macular or morbilliform eruption starting at the periphery and spreading over the next 2 or 3 days is probably the commonest type of drug-induced skin problem (Figure 5.7). When more severe, the rash can

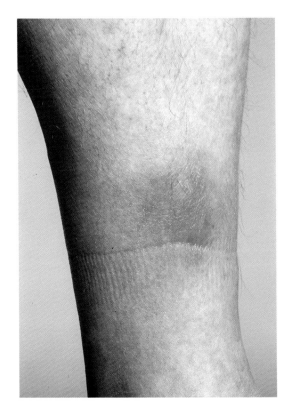

Figure 5.6

Erythema nodosum on the leg of an elderly man.

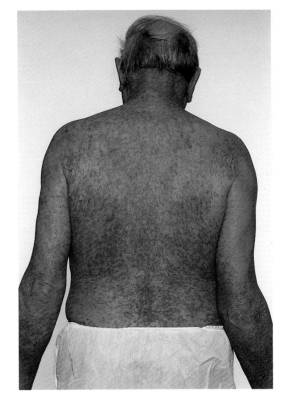

Figure 5.7a

Widespread diffuse erythematous eruption in an elderly man after he had taken a barbiturate drug.

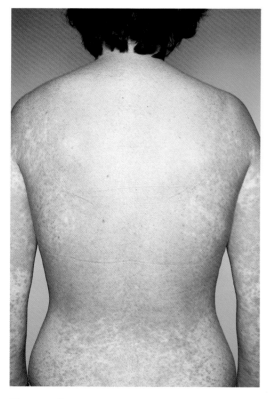

Figure 5.7b

Widespread morbilliform rash due to ampicillin.

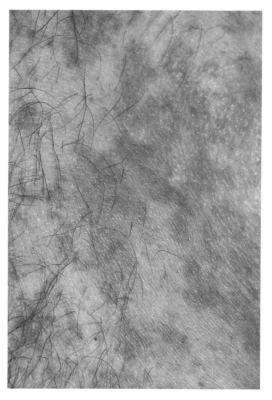

Figure 5.7c

Close-up of lesions due to a thiazide drug. There are papules as well as erythematous patches.

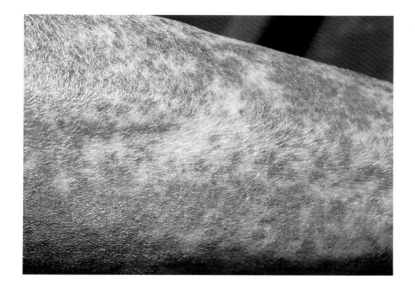

Figure 5.7d

Drug eruption with purpuric compo-nent to the rash.

Table 5.3 Causes of urticaria

Cause	Agents
Type I (immediate) hypersensitivity	Food allergy, eg, shellfish, eggs, milk Drug hypersensitivity, eg, penicillin Airborne allergens, eg, cat, dog, guinea pig dander, pollen Infestation with intestinal and other parasites
Direct chemical stimulus to mediator release	Aspirin, morphine alkaloids, food additives, eg tartrazine Cholinergic urticaria induced by exercise and hot baths
Physical stimuli to mediator release	Cold Solar ultraviolet radiation Heat Pressure Water
As component of other disorders	Dermatitis herpetiformis Vasculitis Henoch-Schoenlein purpura Lupus erythematosus

affect most of the skin surface and even provoke an erythroderma. When acute and severe there may be a purpuric element to the rash (Figure 5.7a). A wide variety of drugs may be responsible, including all those mentioned as causing erythema multiforme and toxic epidermal necrolysis as well as numerous others, including ampicillin and its analogues, the phenothiazines, thiazide, diuretic agents and hypotensive agents. Ampicillin is notorious for causing a widespread morbilliform rash in some 50% of patients who have glandular fever.[5]

In the large majority of patients who develop this type of complication of drug treatment there are no dire consequences, although there may be the added discomfort of an itch while the disorder persists. Bland emollients or at most, weak corticosteroids are all that is required for treatment—other than stopping the drug responsible. In a few, however, the rash progresses relentlessly to produce a persistent erythroderma, even though all drugs being administered are stopped. In this erythrodermic group it may be difficult to know what role the drug has played in the precipitation and persistence of the disorder, as it behaves similarly in patients in whom no drug cause has been identified.

It should be noted that in contrast to the frequency of these erythematous eruptions, drug-induced eczematous rashes are uncommon, although the once often used anticoagulant phenindione, the now withdrawn beta-blocker practolol, and gold injections, are all capable of causing this side-effect.

Urticarial rashes

This is one of the commonest of problems for the dermatologist. When urticarial lesions have persisted for more than a few weeks and no particular cause or pattern has been established, it is most unlikely that a cause will be found despite intensive investigation. The same is not true for severe urticaria of acute onset, in which a drug-related cause may account for perhaps 20 or 30% of those affected. The most notorious drug causing urticaria is penicillin and its various derivatives. However, numerous other drugs can cause an urticarial reaction, including aspirin, morphine and various morphine analogues. Some of the causes of urticaria are given in Table 5.3. The disorder is easily distinguished by the transient nature of the eruption and its

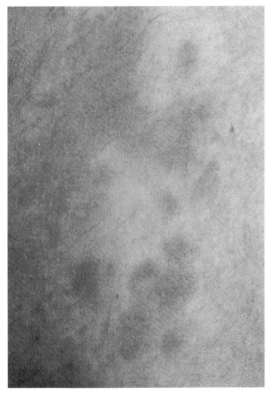

Figure 5.8a

Urticaria on the trunk in an elderly patient.

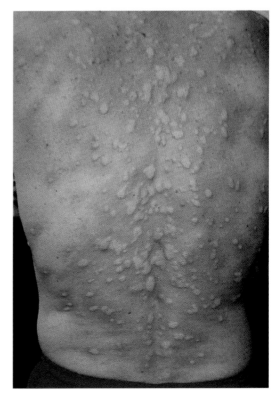

Figure 5.8b

Many urticarial lesions on back.

raised, wheal-like, oedematous appearance (Figure 5.8). Lesions last a few hours to a day before fading, usually to appear elsewhere some time later.

Generally this type of reaction (type I, immediate hypersensitivity reaction) is the cause of pruritus and embarrassment but little else. In a few patients this is not the case and acute penicillin hypersensitivity has an appreciable mortality.[6] In these patients there is immediate anaphylactic shock after a penicillin injection has been given, with severe bronchoconstriction, hypotension and shock. If the patient survives, areas of angio-oedema (large, deep oedematous swelling) and generalized urticarial wheals may appear. A serum sickness like illness can also result from penicillin hypersensitivity. This may not occur until 10 days to 3 weeks after the injection of penicillin, and is often accompanied by a glomerulonephritis, mild fever and arthralgia, as well as an urticarial eruption. These unpleasant urticarial reactions are rather less common in the elderly than in other groups, but whether this is a reflection of the different usage of drugs in this group rather than a different host-immune response, is unknown.

Some more distinctive patterns of drug reaction

Lichenoid drug reactions

A rash that looks clinically and histologically like lichen planus is described as a lichenoid eruption. Generally this indicates that the

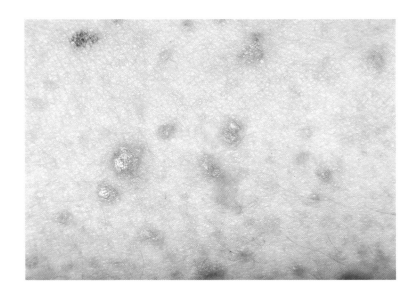

Figure 5.9

Lichenoid drug eruption.

eruption is mauve-red, itchy and papular. The antimalarial drugs (mepacrine in particular), gold injections, captopril, beta-blockers, carbamazepine and methyldopa are among the drugs that have been described as causing a lichenoid drug reaction (Figure 5.9) but many other drugs have been incriminated (see Halevy[7]: Table I). Often the rash can be distinguished from spontaneously occurring lichen planus by some atypical clinical or histological features though usually there is quite a close resemblance.

Photosensitivity eruptions

Drug-induced rashes may be localized to the light-exposed areas. These are the face and neck and backs of the hands in both sexes, and the lower legs and central parts of the upper chest and back in women alone (Figure 5.10). The sulphonamides, tetracyclines, amiodarone, nalidixic acid and phenothiazines can all cause this pattern of drug eruption. Many topically applied drugs can also produce a photosensitivity. The type of rash produced is variable but is often sunburn-like rather than eczematous. Most light-induced drug reactions are phototoxic rather than photoallergic,

although both are possible. It is the long-wave component of solar ultraviolet radiation (UVA, 310–400 nm) that provokes the skin problem in most cases. Artificial sources of light may contain sufficient UVA to spark off or perpetuate the problem. It should be noted that a pseudoporphyria-like picture with blisters occurring in light-exposed areas has been described in patients taking frusemide or naproxen (Figure 5.11).

Lupus erythematosus-like syndromes

Hydralazine, procainamide, captopril and beta-blockers can induce a lupus erythematosus-like picture. This interesting phenomenon has been most studied with hydralazine. The appearance of the condition is dose related and is most likely to occur in slow acetylators and those with HLA DRW 3 cell surface antigens.[7,8] Apart from its reversibility after the drug responsible has been stopped, and its comparatively benign nature, it behaves almost identically to spontaneously occurring lupus erythematosus. Drug-induced lupus is seen equally in men and women compared with the spontaneously occurring

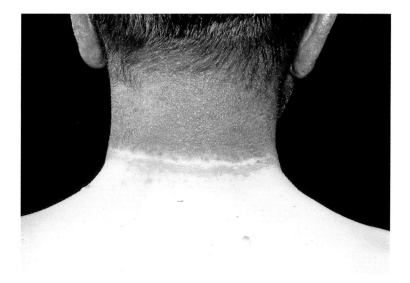

Figure 5.10a

Photosensitivity in a man due to a sulphonamide. Note the sparing where he was wearing a necklace.

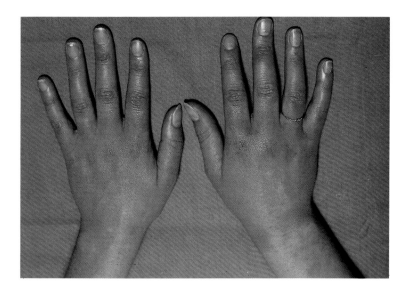

Figure 5.10b

Erythema of the backs of the hands after contacting creosote.

disease, which is considerably more common in women.

More recently minocycline has been incriminated in the cause of a lupus erythematosus-like clinical state in which arthritis or hepatitis has figured prominently.[8,9] As the condition has mostly occurred in otherwise healthy individuals with acne or rosacea, there has been a natural concern over the advisability of continuing to use the drug. Some reassurance is possible on the basis of the infrequency of this complication and its reversibility in most instances when the drug is stopped.

Fixed drug eruption

In this type of drug reaction one or several rounded, inflamed (and sometimes bullous)

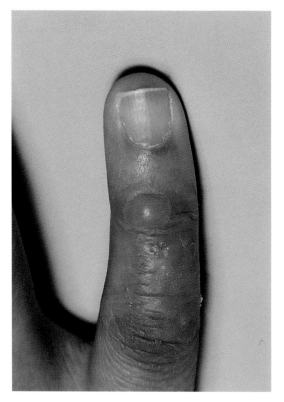

Figure 5.11

Blister on finger as part of the pseudoporphyria picture after taking frusemide.

Vasculitis

This is an unsatisfactory name for a group of disorders that are characterized by vascular damage in particular. All inflammatory reactions must have a vascular component to them—it is only when the vascular damage predominates that the term vasculitis is justified. Vasculitis can result in several quite distinct clinical pictures which depend on the types, sites and sizes of the blood vessels involved (see page 000). Systemic lesions may also occur in a variety of organs as part of a drug hypersensitivity. Three patterns have been noted to occur with drugs; all are uncommon. Rarely, polyarteritis nodosa (see page 000) can be provoked by penicillin and possibly by other drugs. A more benign variety is characterized by a dot-like, purpuric and pigmented rash appearing at first on the dorsa of the feet and the ankles, and later on the legs, which resembles the spontaneously occurring Schamberg's persistent pigmented purpuric eruption, and was at one time a not uncommon result of taking the monoureide hypnotic carbromal. It also occurred after use of the anxiolytic agent meprobamate and rarely after other agents. Probably the most frequently seen vasculitis at the time of writing is a nodular vasculitis-like eruption (see page 000) on the front of the shins as a result of thiazide sensitivity (Figure 5.13). Propylthiouracil can also cause a vasculitis.

Anticoagulant necrosis

This is fortunately rare, but deserves mention. It occurs mainly after coumarin administration,[7] but it has also been seen after heparin infusions as in the patient illustrated in Figure 5.14.[10] A large area of skin suddenly becomes painful, inflamed, congested and purpuric and this is followed by necrosis. The necrotic area sloughs off, leaving a slow-healing sloughed area. It has been suggested that it is the result of a vasculitis, but this is by no means certain.

Pigmentation

Diffuse pigmentation or pigmentation localized to particular sites is seen with several drugs.

lesions (2–10 cm in diameter) recur consistently at the same site or sites (Figure 5.12). They appear some hours to 2 days after ingestion of the drug to which the patient has become sensitive. The rash subsides after a few days, to leave faintly pigmented areas, and the degree of pigmentation of the patches increases with each attack. In many cases there are also mucosal lesions and the eruption is heralded by complaints of soreness of the mouth and anogenital mucosa. Many drugs have been incriminated in the cause of fixed drug eruption. They include phenolphthalein, dapsone, penicillin, sulphonamides, non-steroidal anti-inflammatory agents, tetracycline, the barbiturates, quinine and quinidine and the hydantoinates.

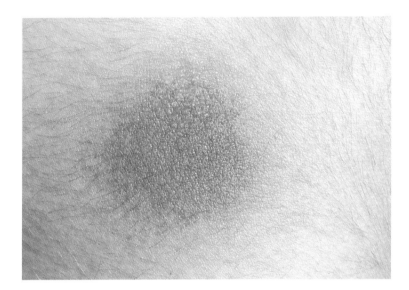

Figure 5.12a

Fixed drug eruption due to a sulphonamide.

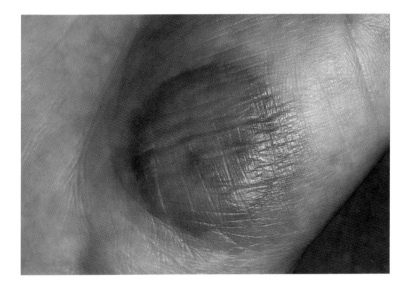

Figure 5.12b

Fixed drug eruption due to sulphonamide.

Probably the best known is the blue-grey pigmentation due to absorption of silver from nasal drops containing an antiseptic silver complex, but this is very rare now. A generalized yellow pigmentation from prolonged use of mepacrine is still occasionally seen. Mauve-purple pigmentation in the light-exposed sites owing to chronic phenothiazine administration (chlorpromazine in particular) is now uncommon. Minocycline has been found to cause a generalized, dusky pigmentation in a few individuals.[12]

Several patterns of hyperpigmentation due to minocycline have been described[13] including darkening in the skin over acne scars and disproportionate patchy pigmentation in the light

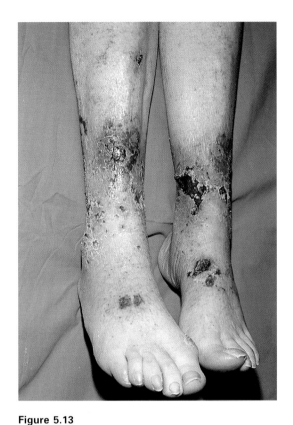

Figure 5.13

Vasculitis of lower leg after taking a thiazide.

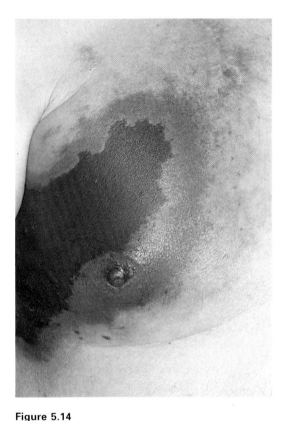

Figure 5.14

The area of necrosis on this man's chest wall developed while he was receiving a heparin infusion.

exposed areas. A patchy pigmentation in the acral sites has also been described.

Probably the most frequent drug-induced cause of pigmentation currently is amiodarone. This important anti-arrhythmic drug produces a dusky pigmentation (Figure 5.15) in the light-exposed sites in a significant proportion of the individuals taking it over a long period.[14] The pigmentation appears to be due to the deposition of a lipofuscin in the dermis and seems irreversible.

Methylsergide maleate produces a reddish discoloration of the skin, and clofazimine (an aminophenazine) used in the treatment of leprosy causes a distinctive brick-red pigmentation. ACTH (adrenocorticotrophic hormone) causes a brown-black pigmentation not dissimilar to Addison's disease.

Blistering reactions

Drug administration can produce a wide variety of blistering reactions apart from erythema multiforme and toxic epidermal necrolysis. Penicillamine, for example, has been reported to cause pemphigus and a pemphigoid type of disorder.[15] Captopril the angiotensin converting enzyme inhibitor used for hypertension is also well known to induce a pemphigus or pemphigoid like picture in a few unlucky individuals.[16] Unfortunately their skin problem doesn't always resolve when the drug is stopped. Clonidine has been found to produce a cicatricial pemphigoid-like response.[16] Nalidixic acid and frusemide have also been found to cause bullous reactions.

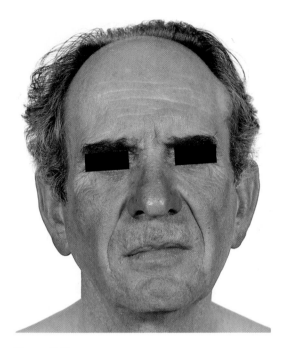

Figure 5.15

Pigmentation due to amiodarone.

Drug-induced nail defects

Photo-onycholysis implies separation of the nail plate from the nail bed caused by light exposure. The tetracyclines, and particularly demethylchlortetracycline, can cause this problem.

Several drugs can cause pigmented bands to appear in the nails—one such compound is emetine. The retinoid drugs etretinate and acitretin cause a paronychia in a few patients (Figure 5.16), shedding of the nail plates in even fewer, and nail softening in some.[17]

Acute generalized exanthematous pustulosis induced by itraconazole

This condition is a severe, generalized eruption characterized by the sudden appearance of numerous sterile pustules on a reddened oedematous background. It resembles generalized, pustular psoriasis in many ways, but is precipitated by several drugs including cephradine, norfloxacin and itraconazole.[18]

Drug-induced hair defects

Several anticancer drugs cause a predictable loss of hair in the anagen growth phase. These include cyclophosphamide, the vinca alkaloids, bleomycin and cisplatin. Heparin infusion may also cause hair loss. The retinoids etretinate and acitretin cause a dose-related reversible loss of scalp in about 30% of patients.[19] Isotretinoin also does this, but to a lesser extent.

Anabolic steroids and androgens will cause a variable degree of hirsuties in women and may also precipitate or aggravate a tendency to male pattern hair loss. Minoxidil, the peripheral vasodilator used in hypertension, also has the curious side-effect of causing distressing hirsuties in women which is not completely reversible. So striking is this that the drug has been developed as a topical agent to stimulate hair growth in those with alopecia.[20]

Miscellaneous skin effects

Dense collections of lymphocytes in the dermis causing nodules, papules and plaques as well as lymphadenopathy characterize drug-induced pseudolymphoma syndrome. Phenytoin, carbamazepine, allopurinol and amiloride are some of the drugs that have been thought responsible.[21] The range of changes due to drugs is enormous. As new drugs are introduced, new side-effects are described. For example, the retinoid drugs frequently cause a drying of the lips (cheilitis) and mucosae and occasionally peeling of the palms and soles and paronychiae (Figure 5.16).

Diagnosis

The best weapons available for the diagnosis of drug reactions remain careful history taking

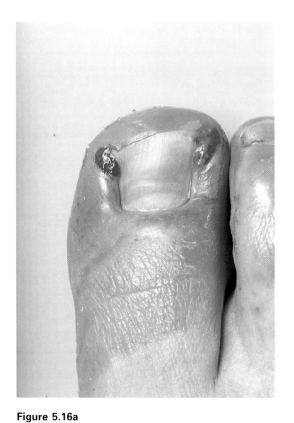

Figure 5.16a

Paronychia in a patient taking etretinate.

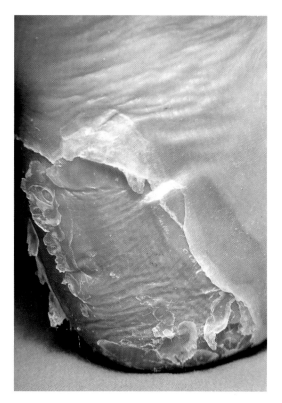

Figure 5.16b

Peeling of the heels and soles in a patient taking etretinate.

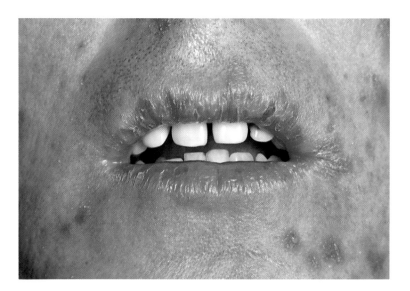

Figure 5.16c

Cheilitis from etretinate. This is the most common side-effect.

and a high index of suspicion. Most drug reactions are diagnosed through knowledge of all recent drug administration and the likelihood of each drug to cause skin disorders. Nevertheless, diagnosis in some patients is difficult and in others the confirmation of a drug hypersensitivity is of paramount clinical importance. It is for these groups in particular that the various tests described are sometimes employed. They should be used sparingly as at their present state of development they are fallible, sometimes hazardous and often expensive.

Challenge tests

The temporal relationship between drug administration (and withdrawal) and drug reaction is pivotal in the diagnosis. If the skin lesions subside after the putative drug has been withdrawn but confirmation is needed, then it is reasonable to consider administering the drug again under controlled conditions to determine whether the rash recurs. This type of challenge is justifiable and safe provided first that the initial skin disorder was not very severe or life threatening, second that the patient understands and agrees to the manoeuvre and third that the observations are properly controlled, preferably by the drug being administered while the individual is an in-patient. Clearly, if the patient had toxic epidermal necrolysis or the Stevens–Johnson syndrome it would be callous and hazardous to re-administer the suspected drug. However, it is reasonable to administer cautiously a much-reduced dose of a drug in hospital to someone who had, for example, a severe urticarial reaction, providing that there is a good clinical reason for needing to confirm the diagnosis and all possible remedial measures are on hand should an unpleasant reaction look like developing. With some drugs, such as penicillin, it is possible to avoid much of the risk of re-administering the drug using the original route by giving it intracutaneously and watching for a local response. This can be successful only if IgE antibodies are involved as these stick to mast cells locally in the skin. Minute doses are given and these are increased if no reaction occurs.[22]

Although intracutaneous tests are appropriate in some circumstances (as are scratch tests), patch tests are not. Patch tests are designed to detect delayed hypersensitivity to a complete antigen made up of a sensitizing chemical and a skin carrier protein. Clearly this type of test is only relevant to the investigation of allergic contact dermatitis.

A properly conducted challenge test, in some form, is still the most useful confirmatory test available.

Skin biopsy

The pathology of drug reactions is rarely specific but may provide supportive evidence. The presence of eosinophils is sometimes helpful, as is the absence of features known to be associated with a non-drug-induced dermatosis. In some drug-induced rashes, such as the lichenoid group, biopsy may help by demonstrating that the pathology is similar to but not quite right for the spontaneously occurring disease. If a challenge test is performed, then it is useful to biopsy any rash that is produced as a result of the challenge. This is especially important if the original rash was also biopsied, so that the two lesions can be compared.

Blood tests

Ideally, when a drug rash is suspected, a blood test should rapidly be able to confirm or refute this and also determine which of the several drugs that a patient is taking is responsible. Alas, we are a long way off this ideal. There has been much research[23] but little has emerged of real practical value. The most useful to date are the radio allergy absorbent tests (RAST) or some modification thereof for penicillin hypersensitivity, where the major and minor antigenic determinants have been characterized. Some success has been claimed for tests based on lymphocyte transformation and leukocyte migration inhibition,[24] but the problem remains that the molecular form of the drug administered that is actually responsible for the hypersensitivity is usually unknown (see later).

Other tests

In drug photosensitivity it is useful to know the patient's degree of sensitivity and the wavelengths which produce a reaction. Limited tests with artificial UVR sources are possible in most centres, but more precise investigation—for example, to determine the wavelength dependency of the reaction, requiring a Monochromator—is only possible in a relatively few centres.

Determination of the elemental composition of the skin by one of the ultrastructural analytical methods (eg, electron probe analysis in scanning electron microscopy) may be helpful in patients with diffuse pigmentation. Examples are the detection of silver in argyria and iron in pigmentation due to minocycline.

Pathogenesis

The provocative agent

In most cases of drug hypersensitivity, there is very little information concerning the identity of the actual chemical agent responsible for the problem. Apart from the native drug itself, any of the metabolic degradation or conjugation products could be responsible. The reaction could be caused not only by drug metabolites but also by minute quantities of contaminants in the formulation. To make things even more difficult, it may not be the drug at all, but a substance used in the particular drug delivery system that elicits the reaction! For example, tartrazine used as a colouring agent in capsule or tablet coverings has been found to cause urticarial reactions.

Patient susceptibility

It seems certain that there is considerable variation in an individual's susceptibility to drug reactions. As yet most of the variables that determine the ease with which a reaction develops are unknown, but in recent years some have come to light. In hydralazine-induced lupus erythematosus, patients with the human leukocyte antigens DRW3 are much more likely to be affected than others who are not of this HLA type. Women are more likely to be affected, and the acetylator status also seems to have some bearing on drug sensitivity.[25] Slow acetylators are also much more likely to develop hydralazine-induced lupus. Patients with the atopic state may be more likely to develop drug reactions, but the degree and the type of susceptibility conferred by atopy are unknown. A further interesting example of the modification of individual host susceptibility is the ampicillin-induced morbilliform rash in patients with glandular fever. This is many times more common in subjects suffering from this infection than in those given ampicillin for other infective complaints. Why this should be is unknown, but it does suggest that host factors need serious and systematic investigation before our understanding of drug reaction can substantially progress.

Mechanisms

The mechanisms responsible for drug reactions may be divided into those given in Table 5.4. It should be noted that the mechanisms quoted in the table are not necessarily mutually exclusive and that drugs often cause different reactions in different individuals. Penicillin, for example, may cause an anaphylactic reaction in one patient, a serum sickness-like illness in another and a fixed drug eruption in yet another. In all probability the commoner types of drug reaction depend on either some type of immunological mechanism, as with penicillin, or a pharmacological mechanism, as with the histamine release and urticaria caused by aspirin. Clearly the topic is both fascinating and complex.

Treatment

Once the diagnosis has been made, the only treatment usually required is to stop the drug responsible. This is hardly ever as easy as it sounds as there are often pressing reasons for the patient having that particular pharmacological agent. Another problem is that most elderly

Table 5.4 Main mechanisms of drug hypersensitivity

Mechanism	Features
Immunologically mediated	
IgE mediated	Anaphylatic shock (eg penicillins)
	Urticaria
Immune complex dependent (IgG and IgM class antibodies)	Serum sickness—with papular and urticarial rash, eg, serum products, penicillin, sulphonamides, hydantoin
Cytotoxic antibody dependent	From drug alteration of tissue components to antigenic material or drug may induce antibody that cross-reacts with tissue
	No established example
Non-immunologically mediated	
Activation of effector pathways	Direct release of mast cell mediators, eg urticaria from opiates, X-ray contrast media and polymixin B
	Direct activation of complement pathways, eg radiocontrast media may cause urticaria in this way
	Interference with arachidonic acid metabolism, eg, cyclo-oxygenase inhibition from aspirin and non steroidal anti-inflammatory agents may cause urticaria
Cumulative toxicity	Causing deposition of drug or metabolite in tissues and causing pigmentation, eg, from silver or by binding with tissue component, eg chlorpromazine
Aggravation of pre-existing disease	Withdrawal of corticosteroids precipitating attack of pustular psoriasis, or lithium aggravating psoriasis
Drug overdosage or side-effects	Exaggeration of the usual action or an expected but not desired effect, eg alopecia in cytotoxic treatments

Adapted from Wintroub and Stern[2]

patients being treated for a serious disorder are taking more than three drugs, and often as many as six or seven, which makes it extremely difficult (if not impossible) to know which agent is responsible. If the ideal of stopping all drugs is not possible, various compromises must be tried. These include stopping one drug at a time and substituting drugs that are similar pharmacologically but different chemically. If stopping the use of the drug may endanger the patient's life, it may be possible to continue the drug under a corticosteroid umbrella. This should not be regarded as a satisfactory solution, only as an emergency stop-gap measure. In fact there is no universally successful approach to the problem of drug withdrawal, and each case should be managed according to the particular circumstances.

In general, no specific local treatment is available (or needed) for the rash itself. It is kind to supply an emollient or mentholated oily calamine or even a dilute topical corticosteroid if the eruption is itchy, but mostly little else is required.

For patients with severe blistering or erosive rashes such as erythema multiforme or toxic epidermal necrolysis, a more aggressive approach may be needed. There is little evidence that systemic corticosteroids improve the prognosis of these patients, but they may have some ameliorating effect and it is certainly customary to give them. These individuals are often very sick, and need intensive supportive therapy with attention to fluid and electrolyte balance, cardiorespiratory function, renal function, heat loss and nutrition. Indeed, the more seriously affected individuals may well need nursing in an intensive care unit and need treating as though they have suffered from extensive burn injuries. The eroded areas themselves may need wet dressings and frequent bathing.

Patients with a severe anaphylactic reaction will need cardiovascular support and may also need intravenous adrenaline and corticosteroids. Systemic antihistamines are required only for the patient with an urticarial reaction. There is no other indication for antihistamines in patients with drug reactions.

References

1 Caird F E. Towards rational drug therapy in old age. *J R Coll Physiol* (Lond) (1985) **19:**235–42.

2 Wintroub B U, Stern R. Cutaneous drug reactions. Pathogenesis and clinical classification. *J Am Acad Dermatol* (1985) **13:**167–79.

3 Merk H F, Hertl M. Immunologic mechanisms of cutaneous drug reactions. *Semin Cutan Med Surg* (1996) **15:**228–35.

4 Lyell A. Toxic epidermal necrolysis (the scaled skin syndrome). A reappraisal. *Br J Dermatol* (1979) **100:**69–85.

5 Porter J, Jick H. Amoxicillin and ampicillin rashes equally likely. *Lancet* (1980) **i:**1037–8.

6 Erffmeyer J E. Adverse reactions to penicillin. Pt 1. *Ann Allergy* (1981) **47:**288–93.

7 Halevy S. Lichenoid drug eruptions. *J Am Acad Dermatol* (1993) **29:**249–55.

8 Bryne P A C, Williams B D, Pritchard M H. Minocycline related lupus. *Br J Rheum* (1994) **33:**674–6.

9 Gough A, Chapman S, Wagstaff K et al. Minocycline induced autoimmune hepatitis and systemic lupus erythematosus like syndrome. *Br Med J* (1996) **312:**169–72.

10 Nalbandian R M, Mader I J, Barrett J L et al. Petechiae, ecchymoses and necrosis of skin induced by coumarin congeners. *J Am Med Assoc* (1965) **192:**107–12.

11 Hall J C, Crockett J. Heparin necrosis. An anticoagulation syndrome. *J Am Med Assoc* (1980) **244:**1831–2.

12 Ridgway H A, Sonnex T S, Kennedy C T C et al. Hyperpigmentation associated with oral minocycline. *Br J Dermatol* (1982) **107:**95–102.

13 Basler R S W. Minocycline related hyperpigmentation. *Arch Dermatol* (1985) **121:**606–8.

14 Miller R A W, McDonald A T J. Dermal lipofuschinosis associated with amiodarone therapy. *Arch Dermatol* (1984) **120:**646–9.

15 Davies M G, Holt P J A. Pemphigus in a patient treated with penicillamine for generalized morphoea. *Arch Dermatol* (1976) **112:**1308–9.

16 Van Joost T, Faber W R, Manhel H R. Drug induced anogenital cicatricial pemphigoid. *Br J Dermatol* (1980) **103:**715–18.

17 Lindskov R. Soft nails after treatment with aromatic retinoids. *Arch Dermatol* (1982) **118:**535–6.

18 Park Y M, Kim J W, Kim C W. Acute generalised exanthematous pustulosis induced by intraconazole. *J Am Acad Dermatol* (1997) **36:**794–6.

19 Mills C M, Marks R. Adverse reaction to oral retinoids—an update. *Drug Safety* (1993) **9:**280–90.

20 Weiss W C, West D P, Fu T S et al. Alopecia areata treated with topical minoxidil. *Arch Dermatol* (1984) **120:**457–63.

21 Callot V, Roujeau J C, Bagot M, Wechsler J et al. Drug induced pseudolymphoma and hypersensitivity syndrome. Two different clinical entities. *Arch Dermatol* (1996) **132:**1315–21.

22 Parker C W. Drug therapy: drug allergy. Part 3 (no 3). *N Engl J Med* (1975) **292:**957–60.

23 Shapiro L E, Shear M. Mechanisms of drug reaction. *Semin Cutan Med Surg* (1996) **15:**217–27.

24 Rocklin R E. Clinical application of in vitro lymphocyte tests. In: Schwartz R S ed, *Progress In Clinical Immunology*, (Grune & Stratton: New York, 1974) 21–69.

25 Cameron H A, Ramsay L E. The lupus syndrome induced by hydralazine: a common complication with low dose treatment. *Br Med J* (1984) **289:**410–12.

6
The blistering diseases

Introduction

Blisters can develop in the course of a wide variety of skin disorders, but the term blistering disease is usually reserved for a disorder in which the essential underlying abnormality is one of loss of cohesion between cells or tissues resulting in blistering as a primary manifestation. However, traditionally this classification is not strictly adhered to, and a disorder such as herpes simplex, for example, which is caused by an infective agent, is not considered a primary blistering disorder. Dermatitis herpetiformis is regarded as a blistering disease because it has certain similarities to pemphigoid, despite there being a prominent vasculitic component.

Tables 6.1 and 6.2 set out the primary blistering diseases and other disorders in which blistering occurs.

The blistering disorders are among the most fascinating of skin disorders and the most recent group to be characterized. One reason for their late characterization is their propensity for a somewhat non-specific onset and their occasional mimicry of other bullous group diseases. Enormous strides in the understanding of this group have taken place in recent years, providing useful models for the elucidation of other skin disorders. Blistering disorders are particularly disabling for the elderly.

Pemphigus[1,2]

Definition

A group of spontaneously occurring disorders of skin and mucosae in which blisters and erosions form within the epidermis due to loss of intercellular contacts.

Pemphigus vulgaris

This is an uncommon serious blistering and erosive disease that affects the sexes equally and all racial groups. It occurs more frequently in Jews. In southern Arizona its incidence was 0.5 cases per 100 000 per year in 1976,[3] but there were 1.62 cases per 100 000 in Jerusalem.[4] It occurs in all age groups, but may be more common beyond middle age, most cases presenting in the sixth decade.

Clinical features

The disease usually begins insidiously, with eroded areas or flaccid blisters in the axillae, groins or around the umbilicus (Figure 6.1). Erosions in the mouth are the presenting feature in 50–60% of patients and anyway occur at some stage of the disorder in 80–90% of patients. The erosions are irregular, with ragged sloughed bases (Figure 6.2). Flaccid blisters appear anywhere on the skin surface and may be spread to involve neighbouring areas by light digital pressure (Nikolsky's sign). The disease may also affect the mucosae of the anogenital region. Occasionally the disorder starts off atypically and resembles either bullous pemphigoid or dermatitis herpetiformis. Tense blisters appear, lasting a few days to some weeks before the more typical clinical signs supervene.

When the disease affects large areas the patient becomes toxic and generally unwell. Before the advent of modern methods of treatment the disease became progressively more severe and was invariably fatal.[5] The disease is particularly unpleasant when it affects the mouth extensively. The lesions in such patients tend to spread to the nasal, laryngeal and even bronchial

Table 6.1   Primary blistering disorders

Disorder	Varieties	Site of blister formation		Major clinical features
Pemphigus	vulgaris	Basal epidermis		Flaccid blisters and mucosal erosions
	vegetans	Basal epidermis	Blisters form by breakdown of desmosomes	Blisters and vegetating erosions
	foliaceous	Superficial epidermis		Superficial scaling erosion
	erythematosus	Superficial epidermis		Lupus erythematosus-like areas and erosions
Pemphigoid	Senile bullous pemphigoid	Subepidermal		Large tense blisters
	Cicatricial pemphigoid	Subepidermal		Recurrent blisters and erosions on same sites leading to scars
	Benign mucous membrane pemphigoid	Subepidermal	Blisters form within different sites of the basal lamina	Blisters and erosions on skin and mucosae
				Pruritic tense blisters immediately before and after delivery
	Herpes gestationes	Subepidermal		Pruritus small blisters and urticarial lesions
Dermatitis herpetiformis		Subepidermal		Associated strongly with gluten enteropathy
	Linear IgA dermatosis	Subepidermal		Similar skin manifestations to above but no gluten enteropathy
Epidermolysis bullosa	Simple forms	Within basal epidermal layer		Congenital blisters on acral sites—no scarring
	Junctional and severe scarring types	Blisters form at different sites in basal lamina or below		Congenital blisters and erosions on acral sites, mucosae and at sites of trauma
	Acquired types	Blisters form at different sites in basal lamina or below		Acquired in association with systemic disease; rare; blisters on legs and at sites of trauma
Porphyria cutanea tarda		Subepidermal		Blisters and erosions with hyperpigmentation and scarring on light-exposed area owing to metabolic abnormality
	Porphyria variegata	Subepidermal		As above but with attacks of systemic disturbance

mucosa, causing hoarseness, dyspnoea, difficulty in eating and considerable discomfort.

Histopathology

The most characteristic feature is the appearance of clefts within the epidermis above the basal layer (Figure 6.3). Separated individual epidermal cells with smooth, rounded margins are found in the clefts. The rounded profiles of the cells are due to the destruction of the desmosome complexes—the same process that results in the formation of intraepidermal clefts. The intraepidermal clefting is known as acantholysis and the rounded cells are called acantholytic cells. There may be little inflammatory cell infiltrate, but in the early stage of the

Table 6.2 Other disorders in which blistering sometimes occurs

Disorder	Mechanism of blister formation
Acute eczema	Intraepidermal oedema and vesicle formation
Herpes simplex and chicken pox	Intraepidermal degeneration leading to vesicle formation
Lichen planus	Marked basal cell liquefaction and oedema at dermo-epidermal junction
Lichen sclerosus et atrophicus	Marked oedema of the papillary dermis and degenerative change in basal epidermal cells
Impetigo contagiosa	Breakdown of bonds between stratum corneum and granular layer and between cells of granular layer
Miliaria	Due to obstruction of sweat gland

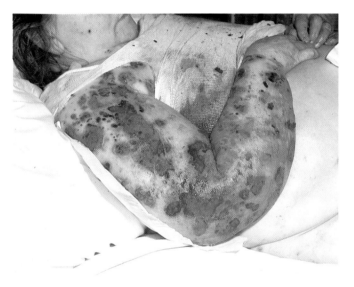

Figure 6.1a

Erosions due to pemphigus vulgaris.

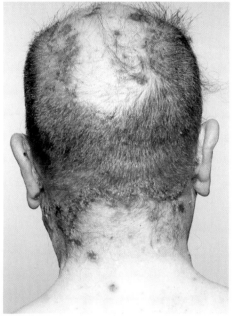

Figure 6.1b

Eroded areas on scalp and neck of an elderly man due to pemphigus vulgaris.

disease collections of eosinophils are sometimes found both within and beneath the epidermis.[6]

Immunopathology and diagnosis

The use of immunolocalization techniques has transformed the understanding of this disorder and has made accurate diagnosis much easier. It is possible to detect deposits of IgG and the complement component C3 in the intercellular areas of the epidermis around the blistered lesions[7] using either older immunofluorescence methods or newer peroxidase labelling methods (or other antibody labelling techniques) (Figure 6.4). In addition to the tissue deposits of immunoprotein, patients with active pemphigus

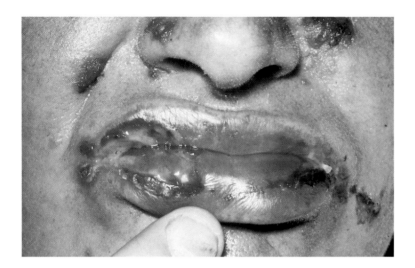

Figure 6.2

Eroded areas with ragged sloughy bases on lips of patient with pemphigus vulgaris. Lesions on the face can be seen and there were also erosions inside the mouth.

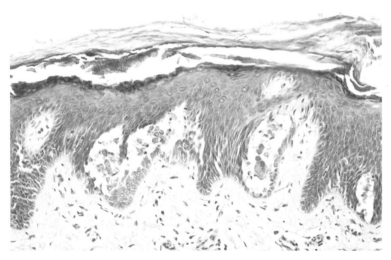

Figure 6.3

Typical histopathological changes in early lesion of pemphigus vulgaris with separation of basal layer and acantholytic cells in the intraepidermal vesicle that forms (H & E; ×90).

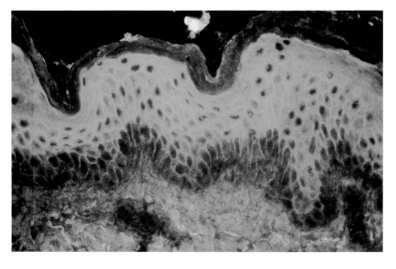

Figure 6.4

Immunofluorescence photomicrograph of biopsy from perilesional area around pemphigus erosion. Deposits of IgC are demonstrated by the pericellular fluorescence (stained with antihuman IgG reagent ×150).

have antibodies to the intercellular zone of the epidermis in the blood. These circulating antibodies have great diagnostic and prognostic importance; they are present in 90% or more of patients who have the disease and their titre is a reflection of the activity of the disease.[8] Indeed, it has been suggested that a rising titre is a reliable indicator of a relapse and may be used to plan treatment. The pemphigus antibody is also sufficiently specific to make its detection of real diagnostic value; however, it has also been found occasionally in patients with severe burns or toxic epidermal necrolysis, and in patients with lupus erythematosus and related diseases.

Aetiology and pathogenesis

The ultimate cause of pemphigus vulgaris is unknown, but the condition is thought to belong to the autoimmune group of diseases as it has associations with the so-called connective tissue disorders, particularly with myasthenia gravis and pemphigus vulgaris.

The circulating antibodies have been shown to have an important pathogenetic role. When serum containing pemphigus antibodies is put up in short-term organ culture with small explants of adult human skin, acantholysis occurs.[9] Pemphigus-type lesions have also been induced in mice by administration of IgG fractions of serum from pemphigus patients.[10] The evidence that pemphigus antibodies are themselves pathogenic is well summarized by Amagai.[11] Considerable progress has been made in characterizing the antigens to which the antibodies have been raised. Immunoprecipitation and immunoblot studies strongly suggest that the pemphigus vulgaris antigen is a 130 kDa glycoprotein and the pemphigus foliaceus antigen is a 160 kDa glycoprotein. The actual mechanism of acantholysis is not clear, although it has been suggested that plasminogen activation and plasmin production may be important.

Pemphigus is seen in all ethnic groups but appears to occur more frequently in Ashkenazi Jews than in most others. The HLA types A10,[12] AW26 and DR4[13] have been found more frequently in pemphigus patients than in normal control subjects. These considerations suggest that whatever external agency is responsible for triggering the disease, the genetic background is also important in its cause.

Treatment

Corticosteroids must be given in high dose and early in the disease for optimal effects. A dose of 200 mg prednisone daily (or even up to 400 mg daily), may be required to suppress the formation of new lesions. Low doses may actually have a deleterious effect. Surprisingly the high dose of corticosteroid seems to encourage the healing of erosions rather than impede their resolution, as may be thought on theoretical grounds. The dosage of corticosteroid must not be reduced too rapidly after initial control, and should be matched carefully with the activity of the disease, the titre of pemphigus antibody in the blood and the presence of side-effects.

Unfortunately side-effects from corticosteroid treatment for pemphigus are frequent. Vertebral collapse, peptic ulceration, diabetes and psychosis are the occasional (and sometimes fatal) result of the high dose of steroids required.

In the past 10–15 years other treatment regimens have been tried and found to be successful.[14] Addition of the immunosuppressive agent azathioprine to more moderate doses of corticosteroid drug (eg, prednisone 20 mg/day) and even azathioprine alone is used to control pemphigus with considerably fewer side-effects. Cyclophosphamide can be used for maintenance treatment, but doesn't have strong suppressive activity by itself. Cyclosporin is also used to control pemphigus. Doses of 3–5 mg/kg daily are employed. The drug does not appear to offer any special advantage in control of this disease though it is quicker acting than azathioprine and is better tolerated than other drugs by some patients.

Gold can also be used to treat patients with pemphigus. Pennys et al[15] reported that injections of gold aurothiomalate produced improvement in their patients after several weeks. Reports of treatment with the new oral gold compound auranofin have not yet appeared.

Of theoretical interest and occasional practical importance for the severely ill patient are reports of remission after plasmaphoresis.[16] Presumably the pathogenic antibodies are removed by this procedure.

How long treatment for pemphigus needs be continued has not been adequately resolved; and it used to be lifelong to forestall recurrence of the disease. This can no longer be accepted, as the author and many dermatologists know of individual patients who are no longer receiving treatment. Indeed, some reports suggest that a substantial number of patients go into prolonged remission following adequate treatment.[17] Regrettably there are no data as yet to indicate either the mean length of treatment required or the likelihood of recurrence after apparent complete remission.

Variants of pemphigus vulgaris

These are much less common than pemphigus vulgaris in Europe and North America.

Pemphigus vegetans[18]

Two types of pemphigus vegetans are recognized—the Neumann and the Hallopeau types. Pemphigus vegetans of the Neumann type occurs primarily in the flexures of affected individuals. The mouth is usually involved as in pemphigus vulgaris. Blisters are uncommon, and thickened, sloughed erosions are the hallmarks of the disorder. In the Hallopeau type the lesions start as pustules and progress into vegetating plaques. The course of the disease in the Neumann type is similar to that of pemphigus vulgaris, with remission and relapses, but the Hallopeau type seems to consist of one attack without the tendency to relapse. Histologically the characteristic suprabasal cleft is evident but the base of the cleft appears irregularly thickened with the formation of villi. In addition, intra-epidermal collections of eosinophils, polymorphs and other inflammatory cells are usually seen. Treatment is as for pemphigus vulgaris.

Superficial types of pemphigus

The acantholysis takes place at a much more superficial level within the epidermis in these disorders—within the granular cell layer. Two forms are recognized: pemphigus foliaceous and pemphigus erythematosus.

Pemphigus foliaceous

The disorder is as common or a little less so than pemphigus vulgaris in Europe and North America. However, in areas of South America a severe variety of the disease is not uncommon and seems to spread in epidemic proportions (Fogo selvagem) resembling an arthropod-borne infection. Clinically, blisters are rare and the typical lesions are moist, pink, superficial scaly patches which appear over the head, neck and trunk (Figure 6.5). Mucosal lesions are much less frequent than in pemphigus vulgaris and altogether the disorder is less disabling in most cases. Diagnosis is aided by the presence of circulating antibodies which bind preferentially to the intercellular zones of the upper epidermis. IgG and complement is found fixed in the upper epidermis in skin around lesions by immuno-localization procedures. Histological diagnosis may be difficult as the superficial cleft may be missed by the inexperienced and confused with damage to the skin surface sustained during the histological preparation.

Treatment

Systemic treatment with corticosteroids and/or immunosuppressive agents may be needed for severely affected patients, but the same high dosage of steroids is not usually needed. Some patients in whom the disorder is confined to a few sites only can be managed by the use of potent topical corticosteroids alone.

Pemphigus erythematosus (Senear-Usher syndrome)[19]

This disorder appears to be an overlap syndrome in which there are features of both cutaneous lupus erythematosus and superficial pemphigus. The lesions are more fixed and redder than in

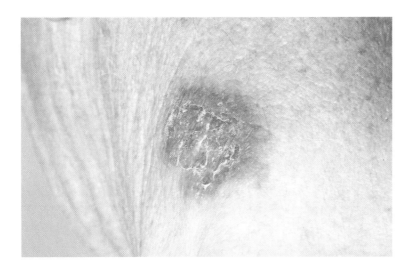

Figure 6.5a

Scaling pink patch due to pemphigus foliaceous on the neck of an elderly man.

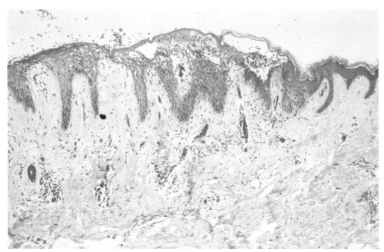

Figure 6.5b

Histopathology of pemphigus foliaceous. There is a subcorneal blister that extends into the granular layer (H & E; ×45).

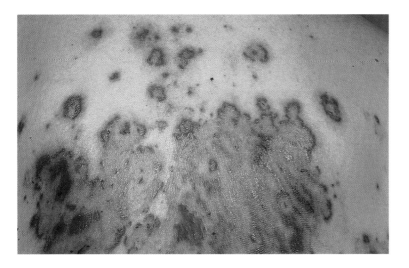

Figure 6.5c

Extensive pemphigus foliaceous in elderly woman.

pemphigus foliaceous. They are most frequently found on the face, scalp and chest. Histologically a perivascular lymphocytic infiltrate is found beneath the involved epidermis which, apart from superficial acantholysis, also demonstrates basal liquefactive degenerative change. Apart from fixed immunoglobulin and complement components intercellularly in lesions, the dermo-epidermal junction at the same site may demonstrate deposits of IgG, IgM and C3, as in lupus erythematosus. The dual nature of the disorder is also reflected in there being both circulating antibodies to the intercellular zone as in other types of pemphigus and antinuclear factors circulating in the blood.

Treatment

Treatment is as for pemphigus foliaceous.

Bullous pemphigoid (syn. senile pemphigoid)

Definition

Bullous pemphigoid is an acute severe episodic blistering disease of the skin, of unknown cause, in which the blister forms at the dermo-epidermal junction.

Clinical features

Bullous pemphigoid is primarily a disorder of later life, being uncommon below the age of 60. The disorder is not uncommon and most departments of dermatology have six or so patients with bullous pemphigoid under their care at any one time. The blisters arise on normal or reddened and urticated skin, and often develop quite abruptly (Figure 6.6). The skin is often quite itchy. A small proportion of patients present with nondescript itchy, erythematous or eczematous lesions. Mucosal lesions in bullous pemphigoid are not as frequent or as severe as in pemphigus, but localized blisters occur in approximately 25% of patients. The blisters are tense and may

reach a large size—lesions 5–10 cm in diameter are not uncommon (Figure 6.7); and the contents are often tinged with blood. The disease usually goes into remission after some months but is subject to relapse.

Differential diagnosis should exclude dermatitis herpetiformis, erythema multiforme, pemphigus and a bullous drug eruption. As mentioned at the beginning of this chapter, the diagnosis may not be immediately obvious at the onset of the disease because patients with blistering disorders quite often present with confusing and rapidly changing clinical pictures. Erythema multiforme is usually easy to diagnose having severe systemic disturbance and pronounced mucosal lesions. In dermatitis herpetiformis (see page 000) the lesions are smaller, intensely pruritic and grouped in particular sites, and as stated (page 000), the lesions in pemphigus have thin roofs or are erosions. Despite these distinguishing features, a definitive diagnosis may still be difficult, and may be reliant upon the results of histopathology and immunofluorescence studies.

Bullous pemphigoid used to be regarded as a skin marker of visceral malignancy, but several studies have thrown this supposed association into doubt. It appears that in most patients with bullous pemphigoid there are no sinister implications for visceral malignancy and there is no indication for a series of tests to hunt the cancer. There does, however, appear to be a small subgroup of patients in whom there may be a true association. In particular, patients with severe, poorly responsive disease who have severe mucosal lesions seem more likely to have an underlying malignancy.[20]

Histopathology

In bullous pemphigoid the blisters form subepidermally. Ultrastructurally it can be seen that the split occurs in the lamina lucida of the basal lamina. Polymorphs and eosinophils are found in the floor of the blister at the sides of the lesions and in the blister fluid (Figure 6.8). Eosinophils, neutrophils and lymphocytes collect subepidermally.[21] The lesion may be difficult to distinguish from an old lesion of dermatitis herpetiformis or from erythema multiforme (see page 91). After

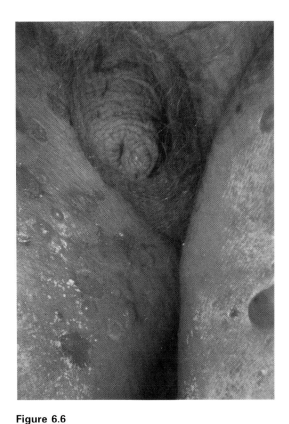

Figure 6.6

Blisters often arise from reddened skin in pemphigoid

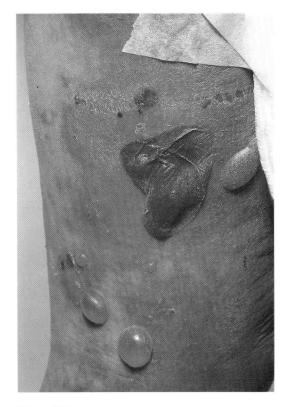

Figure 6.7

The tense blisters may be blood-stained, as in one large blister in this patient with pemphigoid.

24–48 hours, re-epithelialization may be sufficiently advanced to suggest to the inexperienced that the blister is intra-epidermal (Figure 6.9). Restricting biopsy to new lesions should prevent the possibility of this mistake. In early lesions the eosinophil is often the predominant inflammatory cell type. The absence of both papillary tip abscesses and nuclear fragments due to leukocytoclasis distinguishes the histopathological picture of pemphigoid from that of dermatitis herpetiformis.

Immunopathology

There are antibodies in the blood of some 80% of pemphigoid patients that are directed against the basement membrane of the normal epidermis.[22] They can be detected quite readily with indirect immunolocalization procedures using immunofluorescence or immunoperoxidase detection techniques. The titre of the antibodies usually reflects the severity of the skin disorder, but not predictably so and are associated with components of the hemidesmosome and have molecular weights of 180 kDa and 230 kDa.[23,24] There is little other firm information about the function of this substance or the reason for the appearance of the antibody.

The skin at the sides of the lesions contains deposits of IgG and the complement component C3, and these can be demonstrated by employing the direct immunolocalizing technique with either an immunofluorescence or immunoperoxidase method. As in pemphigus, these findings

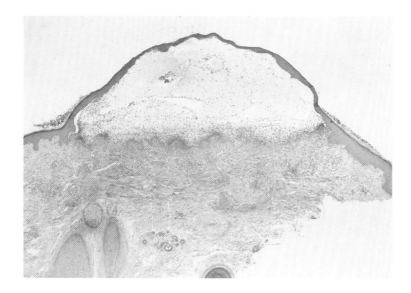

Figure 6.8

Subepidermal blister in senile pemphigoid. Note the inflammatory cells at the base of the blister, among which neutrophils and eosinophils are prominent (H & E; ×25).

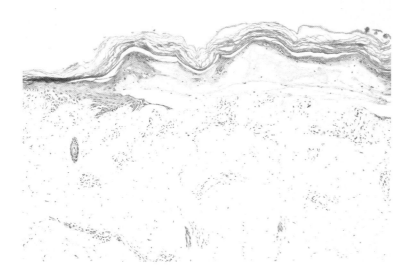

Figure 6.9

This lesion was biopsied some 36 hours after the blister formed and re-epithelialization had begun. If biopsied a little later, the process may be almost complete so that the blister appears to be intraepidermal (H & E; ×45).

are of considerable diagnostic value and should always be sought if the diagnosis is suspect.

Aetiology and pathogenesis

The circulating antibody does not quite have the status of the intercellular antibody found in pemphigus as it does not seem capable of inducing a dermo-epidermal split *in vitro*. The antibody appears to be directed against a glycoprotein component of the lamina lucida of the basal lamina (the pemphigoid antigen).

Treatment[25]

Systemic steroids are usually effective in suppressing the disease and doses less than those required for pemphigus are sufficient. A frequently prescribed regimen is 60 mg prednisone daily. Unfortunately the blistering often returns when the steroids are reduced too quickly and it is advisable to bring the dose down gently after the first 2 weeks. Patients with pemphigoid go into remission after some weeks or a few months, but relapses are frequent. To avoid the inevitable unpleasant side-effects of systemic steroids in the elderly, many clinicians favour administration of immunosuppressant agents at the start of the disease, alongside the steroids. Interestingly, it has been demonstrated that patients in whom biopsies show increased numbers of eosinophils in the sub-epidermal zones respond quickest to steroid treatment.[26] Azathioprine (100–150 mg/day) is the immuno-suppressant usually given. This will allow the dose of steroid to be greatly reduced after the first 2 or 3 weeks and possibly stopped altogether shortly afterwards. The new immunosuppressant cyclosporin has also been used, but at the time of writing experience is too limited to report on its effectiveness. Some patients who have proved resistant to the treatment outlined above have responded to treatment by plasmapheresis.

Variants of pemphigoid

There are several disorders in which the basic disease process appears similar to if not the same as that in ordinary bullous pemphigoid, but the clinical manifestations are different.

Benign mucous membrane pemphigoid

This disorder is much less common than bullous pemphigoid, but like the latter, it occurs mainly in the elderly. Blisters and erosions occur in the mouth, on the conjunctivae and less commonly in the nose. In addition, a limited number of blisters may appear on the skin of the head and neck and upper trunk in 20–30% of patients. Scars often result, especially on the mucosae, and may result in conjunctival synechiae and interference with vision. The disorder tends to be less explosive in onset but more persistent than in bullous pemphigoid.

Cicatricial pemphigoid (Perry–Brunsting type)

This variant is also very uncommon and mostly a disease of the elderly. Erosions, irritant vesicles and sometimes blisters appear on one or two sites on the head and neck and recur unpredictably, leaving scars (Figure 6.10). Involvement of the mucosae is much less frequent than in the mucous membrane type. Linear deposits of IgG at the dermo-epidermal junction were found in the six patients described by Michel et al.[27]

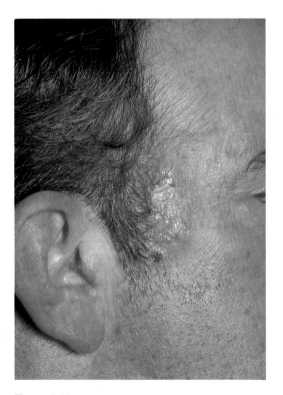

Figure 6.10

Eroded area on temple of late-middle-aged man with cicatricial pemphigoid. This site has shown intact blisters on some occasions and the disorder has been present for at least 10 years.

Desquamative gingivitis

This is yet another very uncommon variant of bullous pemphigoid in which the brunt of the disorder falls on the gingival mucosa.

Juvenile pemphigoid, bullous disease of infancy, linear IgA dermatosis

Whether these are variants of pemphigoid or of dermatitis herpetiformis is not certain. They are characterized by subepidermal blistering and deposits of IgA at the dermo-epidermal junction. As they are diseases of children or younger adults, they are mentioned only for the sake of completeness.

Immunopathology and treatment of pemphigoid variants

Deposits of immunoglobulins and complement components are found in and around the lesions as in bullous pemphigoid, although much less regularly except for cicatricial pemphigoid. Detection of circulating antibodies to the basement membrane region is uncommon. These tests are rarely of assistance in diagnosis of pemphigoid variants.

Treatment should depend on the severity of the disorder and its progress, and it is unusual to require systemic therapy of the sort needed for bullous pemphigoid. Potent topical steroids may be of assistance especially for cicatricial pemphigoid. Those with conjunctival involvement should be seen by an ophthalmologist.

Dermatitis herpetiformis

Definition

Dermatitis herpetiformis is an uncommon, persistent pruritic disorder of unknown cause characterized by vesicular and urticarial lesions and strongly associated with gluten enteropathy.

Clinical features

Dermatitis herpetiformis (DH) can present at any age from infancy to old age. However, first attacks are uncommon over the age of 30. It is seen in most racial groups and in both sexes. Its prevalence is uncertain but it is probably slightly more common than bullous pemphigoid and much more so than pemphigus vulgaris.

Characteristically DH starts insidiously though exceptions to this are not rare. The typical lesions are small vesicles, papulovesicles or reddened urticaria-like patches which occur symmetrically (Figures 6.11 and 6.12). At times there are many typical lesions scattered over the skin, but in some patients there are a few non-descript spots only and the clinical diagnosis is

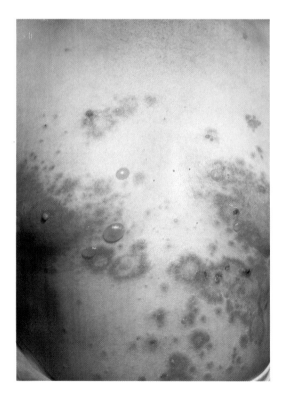

Figure 6.11

Vesiculo bullous rash of dermatitis herpetiformis.

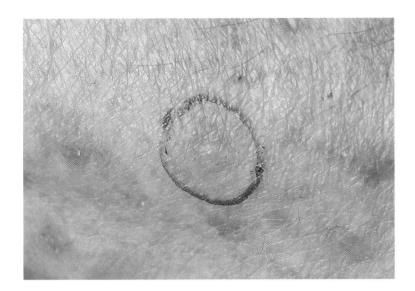

Figure 6.12

Papules and papulovesicles over knee in dermatitis herpetiformis.

quite difficult. The sites most often affected are the elbows, knees, buttocks, shoulders and scalp, though any body site may be involved. DH is an extremely itchy disease in which the quality of the pruritus is distinctive; patients complain of the intensity of the irritation and sometimes of its burning quality. Lesions may occur in the mouth but this is uncommon. DH is a persistent disease but is subject to remission and relapse.

A small proportion of DH sufferers have clinical evidence of intestinal malabsorption but a very much larger proportion of patients (perhaps two-thirds or even three-quarters) have laboratory evidence of gluten enteropathy. In most of these patients the major abnormal finding is decreased height of intestinal villi, flattening of the epithelial cells and infiltration of the submucosal tissue with lymphocytes—a picture known as partial villous atrophy.[28,29] Subtotal villous atrophy—the mucosal state in most patients with symptomatic gluten enteropathy or coeliac disease—is infrequently seen in DH. Functional consequences of this intestinal mucosal disorder in patients with DH are not often prominent. Formal tests of small intestinal absorption such as the xylose tolerance test or the faecal fat content are only occasionally abnormal. However, it is not uncommon for there to be some laboratory evidence of an absorptive defect. For example, a flattened glucose tolerance test or minor degrees of anaemia are not uncommon. The mucosal abnormality in DH patients appears to be the result of a genuine gluten enteropathy, although the reason for its low profile compared with the situation in coeliac disease remains unclear.

Patients with DH appear to have an increased risk of developing malignant disease, particularly tumours of the gastrointestinal tract—notably lymphoma, particularly reticulum cell sarcoma of the small bowel.[30] Apart from the association with gluten enteropathy the disease has also been reported to be associated with autoimmune disorders. Overlap cases between DH and lupus erythematosus have been reported, and the incidence of rheumatoid arthritis and other putative autoimmune disorders appears to be increased in DH patients.[31,32]

Histopathology[33,34]

If reddened urticaria-like lesions or very early vesicles are biopsied, microabscesses of neutrophil polymorphs are often seen at the tips of the dermal papillae (Figure 6.13). These papillary tip microabscesses are quite characteristic of

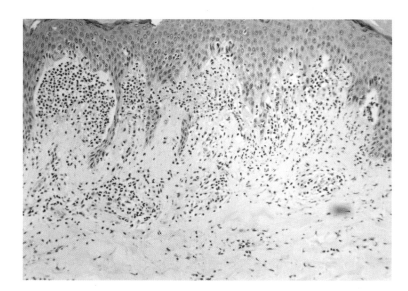

Figure 6.13

Papillary tip abscesses of neutrophils in dermatitis herpetiformis.

DH and, although they may not be completely specific, they are very important in diagnosis. They are sometimes found at the sides of the vesicles which form subepidermally in DH. Presumably the microabscesses enlarge and coalesce to form the vesicular lesions.

Other typical changes are found in the upper and mid-dermis. Around the deeper vessels there are lymphocytes closely applied to the vascular walls. The vasculature of the upper dermis just below the dermal papillae is surrounded by extravasated red blood cells, neutrophils, eosinophils and neutrophil dust (fragments of nuclei from neutrophils). Endothelial damage is not seen but in other respects the changes resemble a leukocytoclastic angitis.

Immunopathology

Unlike pemphigus or bullous pemphigoid there are no circulating antibodies in DH that can be used diagnostically. An antireticulin antibody is found in 20% of patients, an antigliadin antibody is found in 50% and an antiendomysial antibody is found in 70%—not enough to be diagnostically useful.[35] Immunolocalizing techniques, however, are of diagnostic help if uninvolved skin near lesions is examined.[35] Deposits of IgA are found at the papillary tips in about 80–85% of cases. In 15–20% of patients, IgA deposits are found in a linear band at the dermo-epidermal junction. These latter patients may have a slightly different disease (linear IgA dermatosis) as they do not appear to have an associated gluten enteropathy and they are less dramatically dapsone responsive (see later).

Aetiology and pathogenesis

The ultimate cause of the disease is unknown but any hypothesis should account for its persistent but remittent nature, the IgA deposits, the associated gluten enteropathy and the association with autoimmune diseases. The significance of the various antibodies found in DH (see earlier) is not certain, but it has been suggested that reticulin and gluten may share antigenic groups, so that there is cross-reactivity to reticulin after sensitization to gluten. In any event is seems that at least one component of the disorder is mediated by immune complexes being deposited in the endothelium of the small vessels of the dermis.

Treatment

The distressing itch of DH can be dramatically suppressed with the sulphonamide type drug dapsone (diaminodiphenyl sulphone). The relief from symptoms and lesions is so dramatic and so characteristic that some dermatologists use the response as a diagnostic test. The dose of dapsone required to suppress DH varies from 50 to 300 mg per day. It is usual to start with 100 mg per day and increase this by 50 mg per day every third day until relief occurs. The correct dose of dapsone is the dose that suppresses the rash and the itch—no more and no less. Unfortunately there are dose-related side-effects, and few patients can tolerate doses as large as 300 mg for long. Most of the side-effects are in the blood. Sulphaemoglobinaemia and methaemoglobinaemia occur in a dose-related way in all patients who receive the drug. These chemical alterations in the blood give patients headaches, make them feel generally unwell and look a curious dusky blue-grey colour. Dapsone also causes haemolysis of the older red cells in the blood, so that the haemoglobin level in patients taking 100 mg per day is usually around 12% and there is a reticulocytosis of 2–4%. Occasionally the haemolysis is more severe and treatment has to be discontinued. Rarely, dapsone causes marrow depression and agranulocytosis.

Non-haematological side-effects of dapsone include rashes—particularly fixed drug eruption and peripheral neuropathy.

Some other sulphonamides—notably sulphapyridine and sulphamethoxypyridazine—have the same effects as dapsone, and may be given if dapsone is not tolerated. The former is probably more suitable for the purpose than the latter, which can cause serious toxic side-effects.

Another approach to the treatment of DH is with a gluten-free diet as for coeliac disease. This improves not only the gastrointestinal problem but also the skin disorder.[36,37] It may take several months of strict diet for the rash to improve and it is reasonable to give dapsone (in a decreasing dose) until the diet has had time to have a beneficial effect. A gluten-free diet is difficult to prepare and restrictive socially, so some patients prefer to take dapsone rather than put up with this inconvenience. However, as with coeliac disease, a gluten-free diet may give some protection against the development of malignant disease.[35,38]

Patients with the linear IgA dermatosis variant of DH do not appear to benefit from a gluten-free diet.

Neither topical nor systemic corticosteroids are of much help to patients with DH.

Epidermolysis bullosa

Definition

This is a group of rare congenital (and, rarely, acquired) disorders in which subepidermal blistering occurs in response to trauma.

Genetic types

Although these disorders are congenital, they are occasionally encountered in old age.

Epidermolysis bullosa simplex

In this dominantly inherited disorder the defect appears to be at the base of the epidermal basal cells. Blisters form on the hands, feet, knees and elbows and are worse in the summer-time. In one variant, blisters and hyperkeratotic areas occur on the soles of the feet after trauma from footwear (Cockayne type). The blisters heal without scarring and the disorder rarely causes severe problems. Molecular genetics studies have shown that this disorder is due to mutations in keratin genes 5 or 14.[39]

Dystrophic forms and junctional forms of epidermolysis bullosa

These disorders may be recessively or dominantly inherited. Blistering occurs spontaneously and after trauma on skin and mucosae. The defects are within the junctional area or below the basal lamina. Scarring and severe deformity occur as a result of the blistering.

Junctional epidermolysis bullosa (EB) tends to be less severe, but can be as dramatically destructive and disabling as the dystrophic forms. The tissue destruction in dystrophic EB and attempts at healing cause disorganisation and webbing between the fingers and toes and eventual loss of digits is common. The terribly scarred and mutilated stumps are prone to the development of squamous cell carcinoma. Similar destruction and scarring occur in the mouth and oesophagus. Survival to old age is uncommon with the more severe types of dystrophic epidermolysis bullosa. No treatment appears to control the tendency to blistering in response to minor traumata and devoted nursing is still the best form of management. The essential defect appears to be in the anchoring fibrils just below the lamina densa of the basal lamina, and mutational defects have been described in the gene for collagen type VII.[40] In junctional EB the molecular defects appear to be in constituents of the keratinocyte basal lamina complex, ie, laminin 5, integrin $\alpha6\beta4$ and BP180.[41]

Acquired epidermolysis bullosa

This is an extremely rare disease in which blistering occurs spontaneously or in response to injury on the limbs in middle or old age. In many of the reported cases there has been an accompanying systemic disorder—often an inflammatory bowel disorder.[42] There are many similarities to senile pemphigoid, and in some cases a circulating antibody directed against a component of the lamina lucida can be detected. Colchicine by mouth was found very helpful in a series of four patients.[43]

Porphyria cutanea tarda

Definition

Porphyria cutanea tarda is a metabolic disorder of porphyrin metabolism in which blisters form subepidermally in skin exposed to sunlight or after trauma.

Clinical features

Often patients with porphyria cutanea tarda present after an episode of exposure to the sun with blistering of the backs of the hands and the forehead. The affected areas are also easily injured by minor mechanical stimuli. Eventually exposed areas become scarred and pigmented and develop milia. Hirsuties and skin thickening also occur. The latter may give rise to a pseudosclerodermatous picture (Figure 6.14).

This form of porphyria is in most cases associated with liver damage due to alcohol. Although the consumption of alcohol appears to be important in the development of the disease the amount needed varies and may not be very great. It has been suspected that there is an inherited predisposition to the development of the disease. Rarely porphyria cutanea tarda may occur in association with liver tumours and other types of liver disease. Even more uncommonly, no underlying liver disorder is found. The diagnosis is based on the typical clinical signs and the finding of abnormal levels of uroporphyrin III and coproporphyrin III in stools and urine, and isocoproporphyrin in the stools. Depressed blood levels of the enzyme uroporphyrinogen decarboxylase are also characteristic, but the test is not available in all laboratories (see later). Demonstration of abnormal sensitivity to irradiation with UVR in the 400–410 nm waveband is confirmatory.

Pathology and pathogenesis

There appears to be a defect in uroporphyrinogen decarboxylase, leading to abnormal levels of uroporphyrin and coproporphyrin III.[44] These molecules may be detected in excess in the urine and stools. The uroporphyrin appears to be the photosensitizing molecule responsible and after irradiation with light containing the 400–410 nm waveband (the 'Soret band') tissue damage occurs. The enzyme defect is probably genetically determined in most cases, but the mode of inheritance and the reasons for the irregularity in phenotypic expression are unclear. Individuals with the defect seem to be precipitated into clinical disease by liver damage and in particular by alcohol-induced liver damage. The blisters form

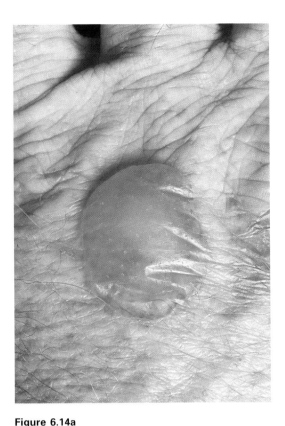

Figure 6.14a

Blister on back of hand in patient with porphyria.

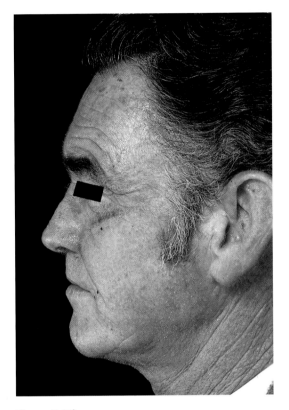

Figure 6.14b

Suffusion and thickening of skin of temple and periocular region with hirsuties in patient with porphyria cutanea tarda.

subepidermally and when mature may be difficult to distinguish from other disorders causing dermo-epidermal separation, although the absence of a marked cellular infiltrate at the base is helpful. There is a periodic acid Schiff reagent positive band around the dermal blood vessels in most cases.

Treatment

Avoidance of alcohol is an important component of treatment and may be all that is required in mildly affected individuals. Regular venesection (1 pint in alternate weeks) is the mainstay of most treatment regimens and is successful in most patients. Administration of hydroxychloroquine can also rapidly dispose of large amounts of porphyrins and is used by some clinicians although this can make patients feel quite unwell.[45]

Other miscellaneous primary bullous disorders

Blisters can occur rarely in the course of diabetes (bullosa diabeticus);[46] they are usually few and on the lower legs. They form subepidermally and arise either spontaneously or in response to minimal trauma.

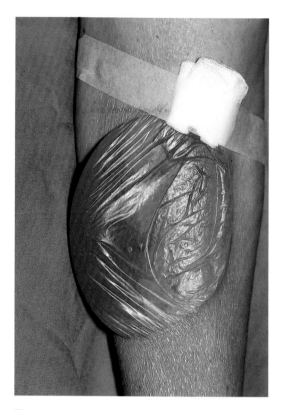

Figure 6.15

Large haemorrhagic bulla of leg in elderly patient with congestive cardiac failure.

Several drugs can cause blistering reactions. The most notorious of these are penicillamine and captopril which can result in either a pemphigus or cicatricial pemphigoid-like picture[47,48] (see page 103). Nalidixic acid and frusemide can also cause blistering (see Chapter 5).

Blisters sometimes arise on oedematous lower legs in the elderly affected by congestive cardiac failure (Figure 6.15). The mechanism is uncertain, but the blister appears to be subepidermal.

Transient acantholytic dermatosis (Grover's disease) is an unusual disorder characterized by the appearance of brown keratotic papules or papulovesicles over the trunk.[49] These show acantholysis and a pathology similar to Darier's disease or Hailey–Hailey disease. It is most common in middle-aged and elderly men, but

certainly can occur in other groups. Mostly it lasts weeks or months, but it can be recurrent.

References

1 Amagai M. Pemphigus: autoimmunity to epidermal cell adhesion molecules. In: James W D, Cockerell C J, Dzubow L M et al, eds, *Advances In Dermatology*, (Mosby, 1996) 317–42.

2 Nishikawa T, Hashimoto T, Shimizu H et al. Pemphigus: from immunofluorescence to molecular biology. *J Dermatol Sci* (1996) **12:**1–9.

3 Lynch P, Gallego R E, Saied N K. Pemphigus—a review. *Ariz Med* (1976) **33:**1030–7.

4 Pisanti S, Sharav Y, Kaufman E et al. Pemphigus vulgaris: incidence in Jews of different ethnic groups according to age, sex and initial lesion. *Oral Surg* (1974) **38:**382–7.

5 Roenigk H H Jr, Deodhar S. Pemphigus treatment with azathioprine. *Arch Dermatol* (1973) **107:**353–7.

6 Crotty C, Pittelkow M, Muller S A. Eosinophilic spongiosis: a clinicopathologic review of seventy one cases. *J Am Acad Dermatol* (1983) **8:**337–43.

7 Cormane R H, Asghar S S. *Immunology & Skin Disease*, (Edward Arnold: London, 1981).

8 Golan D, Gilhar A, Shmuel Z et al. Autoantibodies to epithelial cells (intercellular substance) and their clinical correlation with clinical activity of pemphigus vulgaris. *Dermatologica* (1984) **169:**339–41.

9 Morioka S, Naito K, Ogawa H. The pathogenic role of pemphigus antibodies and proteinase in epidermal acantholysis. *J Invest Dermatol* (1981) **76:**337–41.

10 Anhalt G J, Labib R S, Voorhees J E et al. Introduction of pemphigus in neonatal mice by passive transfer of IgG from patients with the disease. *N Engl J Med* (1982) **306:**1189–96.

11 Amagai M. Adhesion molecules I: Keratinocyte interactions, cadherins and pemphigus. *J Invest Dermatol* (1995) **104:**146–52.

12 Krain L S, Terasaki P I, Newcomer V D. Increased frequency of HL-A10 in pemphigus vulgaris. *Arch Dermatol* (1973) **108:**803–5.

13 Park M S, Terasaki P I, Ahmed A R. HLA-DRw4 in 91% of Jewish pemphigus vulgaris patients. *Lancet* (1979) **ii:**441–2.

14 Huilgol S C, Black MM. Management of the immunobullous disorders II pemphigus. *Clin Exp Dermatol* (1995) **20:**283–93.

15 Pennys N S, Eaglestein W H, Frost P. Gold sodium thiomalate treatment of pemphigus. *Arch Dermatol* (1973) **108:**56–60.

16   Swanson D L, Dahl M V. Pemphigus vulgaris and plasma exchange: clinical and serological studies. *J Am Acad Dermatol* (1981) **4:**325–8.

17   Lever W F, Schaumberg-Lever G. Treatment of pemphigus vulgaris. Results obtained in 84 patients between 1961 and 1982. *Arch Dermatol* (1984) **120:**44–7.

18   Ahmed A R, Blose D A. Pemphigus vegetans. Neumann type and Hallopeau type. *Int J Dermatol* (1984) **23:**135–41.

19   Americin M L, Ahmed A R. Pemphigus erythematosus. *J Am Acad Dermatol* (1984) **10:**215–22.

20   Venencie P Y, Rogers R S M, Schroeter A L. Bullous pemphigoid and malignancy: relationship to indirect immunofluorescent findings. *Acta Derm Venereol* (Stockh) (1984) **64:**316–19.

21   Weeden D. The vesiculobullous reaction pattern. In: Weedon D, ed, *Systemic Pathology*, Vol 9, 3rd Edn, (Churchill Livingstone: Edinburgh, 1992) 127–80.

22   Hadi S M, Barnetson R St C, Gawkrodger D J et al. Clinical, histological and immunological studies in 50 patients with bullous pemphigoid. *Dermatologica* (1988) **176:**6–17.

23   Lin M S, Mascaro J M, Espana A, Diaz L A. The desmosome and hemidesmosome in cutaneous autoimmunity. *Clin Exp Dermatol* (1997) **107** (suppl 1):9–15.

24   Pas H H, Kloosterhuis G J, Heeres K, Van der Meer J B, Jonkman M F. Bullous pemphigoid and linear IgA dermatosis sera recognise a similar 120 KD keratinocyte collagenous glycoprotein with antigenic cross reactivity to BP 180. *J Invest Dermatol* (1997) **108:**423–9.

25   Huilgol S C, Black M M. Management of the immunobullous disorders. I. Pemphigoid. *Clin Exp Dermatol* **20:**189–201.

26   Yu L, Gonzalez M, Marks R. Eosinophilia may be an indicator for glucocorticoid therapy responsiveness in bullous pemphigoid. (Submitted for publication, 1997).

27   Michel B, Bean S F, Chorzelski T et al. Cicatrical pemphigoid of Brunsting-Perry. *Arch Dermatol* (1977) **113:**1403–5.

28   Marks J, Shuster S, Watson A J. Small bowel changes in dermatitis herpetiformis. *Lancet* (1977) **ii:**1280–2.

29   Marks R, Whittle M W, Beard R J et al. Small bowel abnormalities in dermatitis herpetiformis. *Br Med J* (1968) **i:**552–5.

30   Leonard J N, Tucker W F G, Fry J S et al. Increased incidence of malignancy in dermatitis herpetiformis. *Br Med J* (1968) **286:**16–18.

31   Davies M G, Marks R, Wilson-Jones E. Dermatitis herpetiformis: a skin manifestation of a generalised disturbance of immunity. *Q J Med* (1978) **186:**221–48.

32   Reunala T, Collin P. Diseases associated with dermatitis herpetiformis. *Br J Dermatol* (1997) **136:**315–18.

33   Conner B I, Marks R, Wilson-Jones E. Dermatitis herpetiformis: histopathologic correlates. *Trans St John's Hosp Dermatol Soc* (1972) **58:**191–8.

34   MacVicar D N, Graham J H, Burgoon C F Jr. Dermatitis herpetiformis erythema multiforme and bullous pemphigoid: a comparative histopathological and histochemical study. *J Invest Dermatol* (1963) **41:**289–300.

35   Fry L. Dermatitis herpetiformis. *Baillières Clin Gastro* **9:** 371–93.

36   Marks R, Whittle M W. Results of treatment of dermatitis herpetiformis with a gluten free diet affter one year. *Br Med J* (1969) **iv:**772–5.

37   Fry L, Leonard J N, Swain F et al. Long term follow-up of dermatitis herpetiformis with and without dietary gluten withdrawal. *Br J Dermatol* (1982) **107:**631–40.

38   Holmes G K T, Prior P, Lane M R et al. Malignancy in coeliac disease—effect of a gluten free diet. *Gut* (1989) **30:**333–8.

39   Rothnagel J A. The role of keratin mutations in disorders of the skin. *Curr Opin Dermatol* (1996) **3:**127–36.

40   Lim K K, Su W P D, McEvoy M T, Pittelkow M R. Generalised gravis junctional epidermolysis bullosa: case report, laboratory evaluation and review of recent advances. *Mayo Clinic Proceedings* (1996) **71:**863–8.

41   Dunnill M G S, McGrath J A, Richards A J, Christiano A M, Uitto J, Pope F M, Eady R A J. Clinicopathological correlations of compound heterozygous COL7A1 mutations and recessive dystrophic epidermolysis bullosa. *J Invest Dermatol* (1996) **107:**171–7.

42   Gammon W R, Briggaman R A, Woodley D T et al. Epidermolysis bullosa acquisita—a pemphigoid like disease. *J Am Acad Dermatol* (1984) **11:**820–32.

43   Cunningham B B, Kirchmann T T, Woodley D. Colchicine for epidermolysis bullosa acquisita. *J Am Acad Dermatol* (1996) **34:**781–4.

44   Disler P B, Blekkenhorst G H, Eales L. The biochemical diagnosis of the porphyrias. *Int J Dermatol* (1984) **23:**2–10.

45   Petersen C S, Thomsen K. High dose hydroxychloroquinone. Treatment of porphyria cutanea tardis. *J Am Acad Dermatol* (1992) **26:**614–19.

46   Bernstein J E, Mendenica M, Soltani K et al. Bullous eruption of diabetes mellitus. *Arch Dermatol* (1979) **115:**324–5.

47   Shuttleworth D, Graham-Brown R A C, Hutchinson P E et al. Cicatricial pemphigoid in D-penicillamine treated patients with rheumatoid arthritis: a report of 3 cases. *Clin Exp Dermatol* (1985) **10:**392–7.

48 Bialy-Golan A, Brenner S. Penicillamine induced bullous dermatoses. *J Am Acad Dermatol* (1996) **35:**732–42.

49 Parson J M. Transient acantholytic dermatosis (Grover's disease): a global perspective. *J Am Acad Dermatol* (1996) **35:**653–66.

7

The autoimmune and other inflammatory disorders

The terms connective tissue disease, collagen-vascular disease and autoimmune disorder are used to describe a group of conditions which appear to owe their pathogenesis to some form of perverted immune process in which tissue components are no longer recognized as self and excite an immune and destructive response. All these terms are hopelessly inadequate and about as apt as describing the results of major trauma as bone disease. Autoimmune diseases are either multisystem disorders or organ-specific. Although the skin is a major target in several autoimmune disorders of the multisystem type, it is not affected in all. Those in which involvement of the skin plays a prominent role clinically include lupus erythematosus, scleroderma and dermatomyositis and their variants, as well as overlap states between these conditions. The organ-specific autoimmune diseases, in which the skin is the 'organ', are less well established but may include vitiligo, alopecia areata, morphoea and lichen sclerosis and discoid lupus erythematosus. The status of polyarteritis nodosa and related vasculitic disorders in relationship to the autoimmune group is uncertain.

Lupus erythematosus

Systemic lupus erythematosus affects the skin in 50–70% of patients at some point in their disorder, but a variety of visceral manifestations occur in all patients. Discoid lupus erythematosus typically affects the skin alone, although in some patients there may also be minor laboratory abnormalities not amounting to signs of serious systemic malfunction. It is not always easy to determine where one variety of the disease ends and the other begins.

Systemic lupus erythematosus (SLE)

This disorder classically affects young and early-middle-aged women, but it may occur in the elderly as well. Patients in the sixth decade or later account for some 12% of patients with SLE.[1] In general, older patients with SLE are more likely to have pericarditis and pulmonary abnormalities and less likely to have neuropsychiatric disorders and Raynaud's phenomenon than younger patients. Arthritis and skin lesions are common in the elderly but these are not as frequently seen as in younger patients.[1] SLE tends to have a more benign cause and seems to be accompanied by less renal disease in elderly patients than in their younger counterparts.[2] As it can affect all the body systems, SLE can cause diverse symptoms and signs; for an extensive description the reader should consult Rowell[3] and Hughes.[4]

Drugs such as hydralazine and procainamide may also cause a lupus erythematosus (LE)-like syndrome (see Chapter 5). SLE is more common in individuals with HLA haplotype B8. In recent years Minocycline has been reported to cause an LE like picture with autoimmune hepatitis and arthritis.[5,6]

SLE often starts abruptly or over 1 or 2 weeks, or even explosively over 24 hours, with weakness, weight loss, mild pyrexia, arthralgia and myalgia. Fleeting generalized erythematous rashes may occur at this time, as may more persistent lesions in the light-exposed areas of skin.

The butterfly rash involving both malar regions and the skin of the nose between (Figure 7.1) is a notorious sign of SLE, but is only seen in 20–30% of patients. The hands are also frequently involved symmetrically with reddened patches on the backs of the finger joints. The

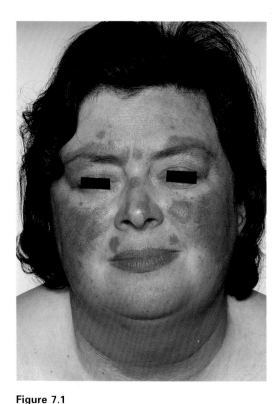

Figure 7.1

Butterfly rash of acute lupus erythematosus.

lesions are red and slightly swollen and may be urticaria-like. In fact, urticaria lesions may also occur. An arthralgia is quite common and may progress to an arthritis affecting small and medium-sized joints symmetrically with some general resemblance to rheumatoid arthritis. Raynaud's phenomenon (see Chapter 11) is seen in some patients with SLE but is a less prominent syndrome than in systemic sclerosis.

The physical signs, progress and prognosis of SLE depend on which systems are involved. The kidneys are commonly affected, the disease causing a membranous glomerulonephritis, which may progress to the nephrotic syndrome and ultimately to chronic nephritis and renal failure. Generalized lymphadenopathy is also frequently seen. The most unpleasant complication is involvement of the central nervous system causing a meningoencephalitis. This accounts for most of the fatalities from SLE, although renal failure and infection may also be responsible for

a fatal outcome. Overall the 10–year survival rate is approximately 90%.[7]

Other manifestations of SLE include a polyserositis, cardiomyopathy and endocarditis, a myopathy and a pneumonitis. The diagnosis of the disease is much aided by adherence to the criteria laid down by the American Rheumatism Association.[8]

Laboratory findings and pathology

There are several haematological signs of SLE; all of the cellular components of blood may be affected. There is often an anaemia which is usually normochromic and normocytic, but may be due to haemolysis as well. There is often a leukopaenia with reduction in both granulocytic and lymphocytic components. Thrombocytopaenia is also seen and may be sufficiently severe to result in purpura. The ESR (erythrocyte sedimentation rate) is usually raised—often to relatively high values. In many patients there is a polyclonal increase in the serum IgG, causing a hypergammaglobulinaemia. Hypocomplementaemia,[9] detectable circulating immune complexes and a positive Coombs' test are also important laboratory markers of the disease. The LE cell test is now not often performed as other tests are of more value diagnostically. The antinuclear factor test is positive in 85–95% of patients, depending on the particular substrate tissue technique used. More specific are tests for double-stranded DNA antibodies which are positive in some 80% of patients with SLE.[10] Antibodies directed to the basement zone have been detected in 16 of 21 patients examined in SLE even though there were no bullous lesions.[11]

Biopsy of acute skin lesions will reveal oedema of the upper and mid-dermis and 'cuffing' of the small upper dermal blood vessels by lymphocytes. The epidermis often shows areas of basal liquefactive degenerative change but not as markedly as in discoid lupus erythematosus. Direct immunofluorescence examination of uninvolved and normally unexposed skin is useful from the diagnostic point of view as deposits of IgG (and sometimes IgA) and the complement component C3 are found in some 60% of patients with SLE.

As our understanding of this disorder has expanded, various subsets of SLE patients have

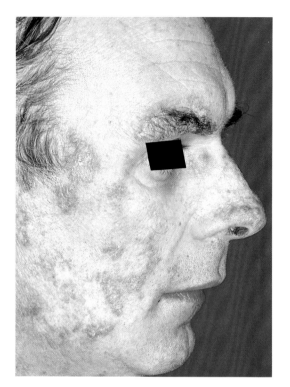

Figure 7.2a

Typical discoid lupus erythematosus affecting the face. There are scarred areas as well as active red plaques.

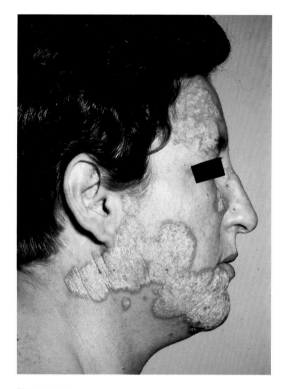

Figure 7.2b

Discoid lupus erythematosus. The patches are almost psoriasiform in their appearance.

been recognized with particular constellations of physical signs and laboratory findings. Elderly patients with SLE seem more likely to be positive to antibody Ro(SSA)—a cytoplasmic antigen—accompanied by positivity to La(SSB), and less likely to have anti-DNA antibodies.[2] Of particular interest are the SLE syndromes that occur in association with congenital complement deficiences,[12] although they are of less relevance to the elderly than to other age groups.

Treatment and prognosis

The treatment should be adjusted to the type and severity of involvement by the disease. Many elderly patients require little in the way of systemic therapy. Renal changes and involvement of the central nervous system or heart demand vigorous treatment to prevent irreversible changes. Systemic corticosteroids, with or without azathioprine, in

sufficient dosage to suppress signs of the disease, are generally administered. Patients should be discouraged from direct sun exposure as this aggravates the disease. Patients who are desperately ill may benefit from plasmapheresis.

Discoid lupus erythematosus (DLE)

This disorder is also more common in women in the reproductive years, but is also seen in men and in the elderly of both sexes.

Clinical features

The lesions of DLE typically occur on the face (Figure 7.2), but in addition are seen on the scalp, ears and neck. In severely affected individuals DLE lesions occur on the backs of the hands,

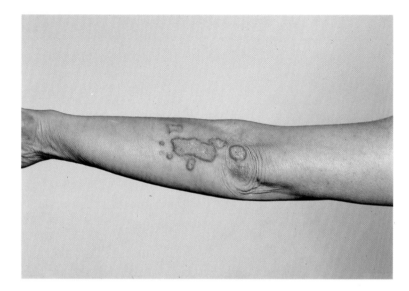

Figure 7.3a

Discoid lupus erythematosus. Plaques affecting the arm.

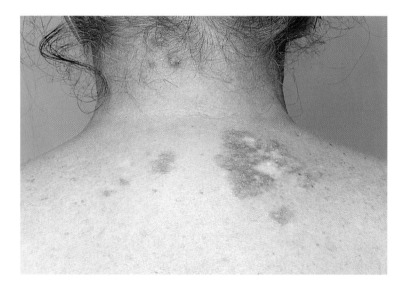

Figure 7.3b

Patches of discoid lupus erythematosus on upper back and back of neck.

arms and upper trunk (Figure 7.3). The distribution of the lesions suggests that sun exposure may play a role in their localization, and indeed exposure to the sun often precipitates and aggravates the disease. It has also been suggested that sunlight can transform the disorder to SLE, but the evidence is inconclusive on this point.

Well defined, raised, red scaling or warty plaques of irregular shape characterize the lesions of DLE (Figure 7.4). The hyperkeratosis often seems particularly to affect the follicles, so that these can be seen to be plugged with horny spines. The lesions persist for long periods and later scarring, atrophy and areas of irregular pigmentation occur (Figure 7.5) causing considerable disfigurement (Figure 7.6).

An uncommon variant is rosacea-like LE which is marked by the presence of pink papules occurring on the cheeks and looking very like rosacea (Figure 7.7). Even more uncommon is the condition known

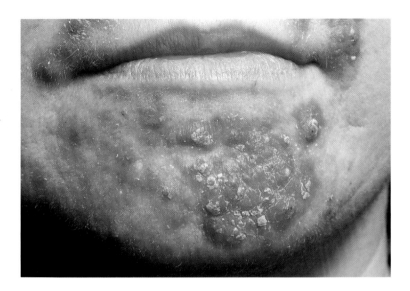

Figure 7.4

Close-up of very inflamed lupus erythematosus affecting the chin.

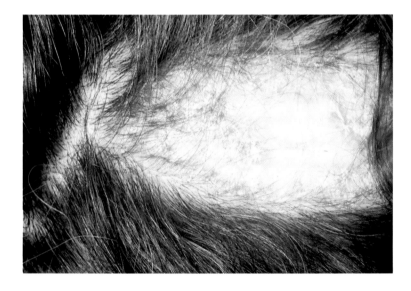

Figure 7.5

Scar on the scalp from discoid lupus erythematosus.

as lupus profundus or lupus panniculitis, where the inflammatory process is in the deep dermis and fat. In this type there are large red, deep swellings, particularly over the upper arms.

The disease is very persistent, but is quite variable and unpredictable in its course and is subject to periods of activity and spontaneous defervescence for no apparent reason.

Some 5% of patients with DLE develop SLE. Those with extensive and rapidly developing lesions seem more likely to change their character in this way.[13]

Laboratory findings and pathology

It is not unusual to find focal 'haematological' abnormalities in patients with DLE, including anaemia, leukopaenia and thrombocytopaenia

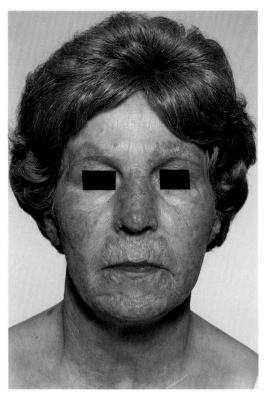

Figure 7.6

This woman has had severe discoid lupus erythematosus for many years, resulting in considerable scarring. She has a wig covering severe scarring of the scalp as well.

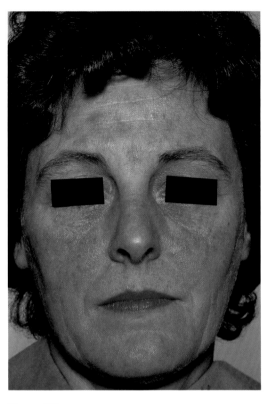

Figure 7.7

Rosaceous lupus erythematosus. The lesions in this woman were papular at first, leading to a mistaken diagnosis of rosacea.

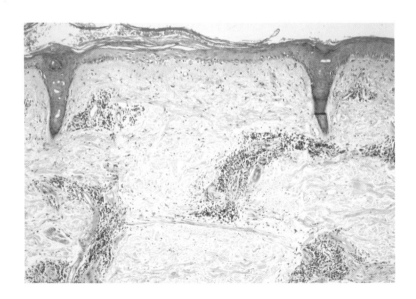

Figure 7.8

Histopathology of discoid lupus erythematosus. There is an infiltrate closely applied to the dermal blood vessels. In places there is degenerative change of the epidermis and some slight hyperkeratosis (H & E; ×45).

and a raised esr, though if these occur together the possibility of systemization should be remembered. The antinuclear factor test is positive in 30–50% of patients with discoid LE, depending on the sensitivities of the particular tests used. Anti-DNA antibodies are found in approximately 20% of patients with DLE.[14]

Histologically the changes are similar to those described above for SLE, but with less oedema and with the other features more pronounced. The epidermis shows basal liquefactive degenerative change. Often the basal cell changes are subtle and amount to no more than areas in which there is vacuolation and 'fuzziness' of the dermal margin of the cells involved. In other patients, the degenerative changes are very much more pronounced with total destruction of the basal layer focally and the formation of cytoid bodies. When this occurs there is sometimes an accumulation of mononuclear cells subepidermally so that there is a strong resemblance to lichen planus. There is also hyperkeratosis with follicular plugging and areas of hypergranulosis. The lymphocytic infiltrate around the small blood vessels is often prominent around the vasculature of the hair follicles and sweat coils (Figure 7.8). In older lesions there is epidermal atrophy, scarring and melanin pigment resulting in dermal macrophages from epidermal damage. Direct immunofluorescence examination of the lesions will demonstrate deposits of IgG, C3 and sometimes IgA and IgM in a band at the dermo-epidermal junction. There is often an irregular homogenous (pink) eosinophilic band at the dermo-epidermal junction some 3–7 µm thick which stains with the periodic acid Schiff reagent. This band presumably reflects the deposition of immunoprotein.

Treatment

In some patients the lesions can be controlled by the application of potent topical corticosteroids such as betamethasone-17–valerate or clobetasol-17–propionate, but if these are employed care should be taken to ensure that severe local atrophy does not occur. Many patients are helped by the administration of the antimalarial drugs chloroquine, hydroxychloroquine or mepacrine by mouth. Hydroxychloroquine appears to be of the

most use as it is generally well tolerated and may be less prone to cause severe ocular side-effects than chloroquine.[15] It is prudent to obtain the opinion of an ophthalmologist before starting treatment with hydroxychloroquine, but if the dose is restricted to less than 400 mg/day and treatment is for less than 1 year, retinal degenerative changes are extremely unlikely to develop. Some patients not helped by these measures have benefited from administration of an antirheumatic oral gold compound auranofin.[16] For patients whose lesions do not respond to the above measures, treatment with Thalidomide should be contemplated. This latter agent, once feared as a potent teratogen, has been resurrected because of its anti-inflammatory actions. At a dose of 50–100 mg/day it has also been employed in Behçet's disease, erythema nodosum leprosum and chronic photodermatoses. Apart from its teratogenicity it should be remembered that the drug may also cause paraesthesia and eventually a peripheral neuropathy. Patients must be instructed to avoid direct sunlight and to use a sunscreen when outdoors (see Chapter 5).

Disseminated discoid, subacute cutaneous and chilblain lupus erythematosus

These conditions are unstable varieties of LE, many transforming to SLE at some stage. In disseminated discoid LE there are numerous angry-looking lesions of DLE over face, arms and upper trunk, as well as a minor degree of systemic upset. In some patients lesions with a resemblance to erythema multiforme are seen as well as typical DLE lesions. These patients have recurrent episodes of annular erythema multiforme-like lesions and a complex of laboratory findings including an antinuclear antibody giving a speckled pattern, a positive rheumatoid factor test and anti-La antibodies. In chilblain LE the lesions occur predominantly on the backs and tips of the fingers and toes, though there may be lesions on the knees, elbows, ears, nose and elsewhere on the face as well. These latter patients may have cold agglutinins or cryofibrinogenaemia. Subacute cutaneous LE is marked by polycyclic scaling patches in the upper half of the body. More than half of these patients have photosensitivity and 75% possess anti-Ro and anti-La antibodies; about half of these patients show features of SLE.[17]

Scleroderma

Under this heading three disorders will be discussed. The first, systemic sclerosis, is a serious systemic disorder in which the skin is involved in most patients and which is mainly a disorder of maturity and middle age, but which is also the autoimmune disorder seen most frequently in the elderly. It has been pointed out that systemic sclerosis is not at all uncommon in elderly women[18] and one series of 15 patients (average age 80 years) represented 0.1% of all patients admitted under the reporting physician's care.[19] Morphoea is confined to localized areas of skin and is not associated with systemic disorder. It is seen in all age groups. Generalized morphoea is a similar but rare disorder in which large areas of the skin surface are affected by the same sclerotic process. Lichen sclerosus et atrophicus is often believed to represent a very superficial form of morphoea. A form of the disorder is found in children but it is predominantly a disorder of late-middle-aged and elderly women.

Systemic sclerosis

This multisystem inflammatory disorder is characterized by deposition of new collagen and/or an obliterative vasculitis in all sites affected. The most frequent presenting complaint is Raynaud's phenomenon, which is present in some 90% of patients with systemic sclerosis.[20] The attacks of coldness and whiteness of the fingers do not differ qualitatively from the same condition due to other causes or occurring spontaneously. However, it does tend to be more severe in patients with systemic sclerosis resulting in severe atrophic changes in the finger tips and marked tapering of the fingers and eventually absorption of the terminal phalanges, ulceration and even gangrene (Figure 7.9).

The skin is also frequently involved. The skin of the hands, fingers and forearms thickens and becomes stiff, shiny and immobile, resulting in the condition known as acrosclerosis. Calcium deposits in the skin may accompany this change when they are of long standing. The face is also often affected. The tissues stiffen and appear to contract, so that it becomes difficult to open the mouth and the facial features become pinched and bird-like (Figure 7.10). Alongside these changes telangiectatic macules often develop on the affected skin (Figure 7.11) and pigmentation occurs in about 30% of patients. The skin changes and the Raynaud's phenomenon often occur together and the combination is then known as the CRST syndrome (calcinosis, Raynaud's, sclerosis and telangiectasia). It has been suggested that there is an underlying fault in the cutaneous microvasculature in Raynaud's phenomenon in which there is a basic fault in the production and release of calcitonin gene-related peptide.[21] Some prefer the term CREST syndrome, adding oesophageal dysfunction to the symptom complex. The CREST syndrome supposedly has a slower rate of progress and a better prognosis than other types of systemic sclerosis.

As well as the skin, systemic sclerosis can affect the gastrointestinal tract, the lungs, the kidneys and the joints.[22] In the gastrointestinal tract the disease disturbs motility resulting in dysphagia and constipation. Occasionally the function of the small intestine is also affected causing a malabsorption syndrome because of stagnation and bacterial overgrowth. So far as the respiratory system is concerned, there is a progressive alveolar capillary block and ultimately hypoxaemia. Cardiac abnormalities occur, as witnessed by ECG (electrocardiogram) abnormalities. Renal decompensation and hypertension may also develop as a result of involvement of the renal vasculature. In some patients a symmetrical small joint arthropathy develops which is similar to rheumatoid arthritis. These serious systemic effects of the disease are not present in all patients and also vary in severity and speed of progress in individual patients.

Antinuclear factor (ANF) occurs in about three-quarters of patients with systemic sclerosis. A speckled pattern of ANF is found more frequently in patients with systemic sclerosis than in other disorders. Centromere staining antibody also

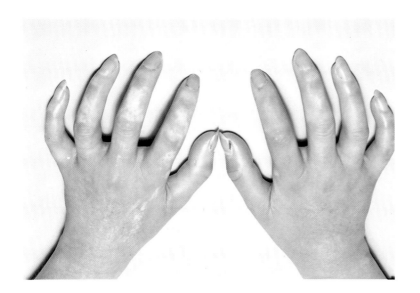

Figure 7.9a

Acrosclerosis in systemic sclerosis. The fingers appear tapered.

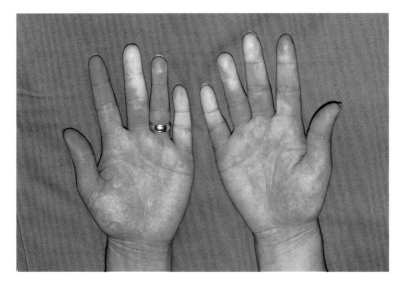

Figure 7.9b

Raynaud's phenomenon in patient with systemic sclerosis.

occurs in systemic sclerosis. At least 95% of systemic sclerosis patients have an identifiable autoantibody (see Perez and Kohn[20]: table III). While immunological tests may help classify patients into subsets and assist in the prognosis clinical criteria developed by the American College of Rheumatology are of greater use diagnostically. The diagnosis is 97% certain with one major or two minor criteria present.[23]

The available 5-year survival figures vary between 34 and 73%, and there is no doubt that

the disease substantially shortens life. The prognosis is worse in men. No currently available treatment appears to influence the progress of the disorder though penicillamine has been used extensively and some success claimed.[24] Unfortunately the side-effects of this drug are too frequent and too severe for use in any but the most severely affected patients.

Immunosuppressive treatment with azathioprine and steroids or cyclosporin has also been tried for patients with rapidly progressive

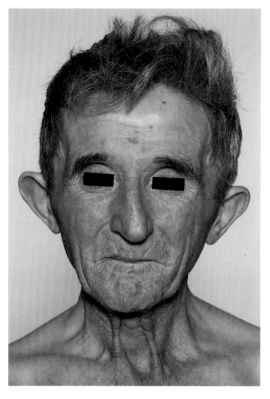

Figure 7.10

Facial appearance of elderly man with systemic sclerosis. There is some puckering around the mouth and a 'beaked' appearance.

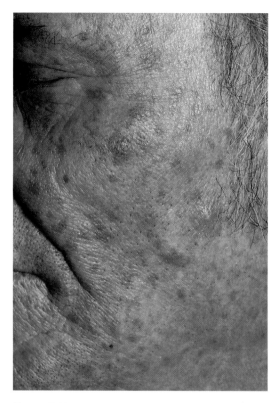

Figure 7.11

Telangiectatic macules on the face of a man with systemic sclerosis.

disease, but rarely gives much respite. Treatment with gamma interferon holds some promise. A study using three times weekly subcutaneous interferon for 1 year demonstrated that the patients' disease did not progress during this period.[25] Success has recently been reported for the technique known as 'extracorporeal phototherapy.[26] Separated white cells are subjected to UVA after the patient has ingested a psoralen as in PUVA treatment (see page 270). The results of controlled trials are as yet unavailable, but the anecdotal results available appear promising. Evaluation of response to treatment is particularly difficult in scleroderma. Attempts have been made to follow the effects of treatment using non-invasive instrumental methods—for example by measuring skin thickness with pulsed A-scan ultrasound[27] and with a suction device known as the Cutometer.[28]

Morphoea (localized scleroderma)

Large plaques of sclerotic skin characterize this disease, which remains localized to the skin. The plaques appear on the trunk and limbs mainly in the elderly (Figure 7.12), but in younger individuals they are sometimes also found in a vertical linear distribution over the face. The facial deformity produced is fancifully referred to as 'en

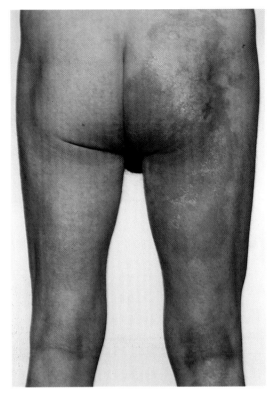

Figure 7.12

Extensive plaque of morphoea affecting the buttock and thigh of an elderly man. Notice the characteristic mauve colour in places, and whitish colour in others where the lesion is beginning to resolve.

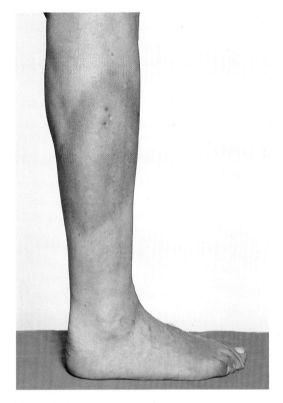

Figure 7.13

Patch of resolving morphoea of the leg, showing slight hyperpigmentation.

coup de sabre' as it has been likened to the effects of a sabre blow. They often start off by being mauve or violaceous, but later become pale and develop hyperpigmentation around them (Figure 7.13). When they resolve (as they usually do within 2 or 3 years or even less) the patches become smooth and hyperpigmented. The plaques vary greatly from 2 or 3 cm in diameter to the size of a dinner plate or even larger. The affected skin is thicker than normal and appears bound down to the surrounding skin. Histologically, in early lesions, a lymphocytic infiltrate around the blood vessels is seen, together with new thick collagen bundles which appear more homogeneous than normal and replace the fat in the deeper dermis. Generally,

morphoea causes little in the way of symptoms, though mechanical interference with movement can prove to be a problem, especially when the lesion occurs over a joint.

Rarely, large areas of the skin surface are affected by confluent plaques of morphoea. Naturally enough this is known as generalized morphoea. Unlike the localized form, the generalized variant can cause severe disability and can even be life threatening. Most of the disability results from involvement of the chest wall so that the mechanisms of ventilation are disturbed and involvement of the skin over the joints prevents full movement. There is also some evidence that patients with generalized morphoea are more likely to develop systemic sclerosis than other

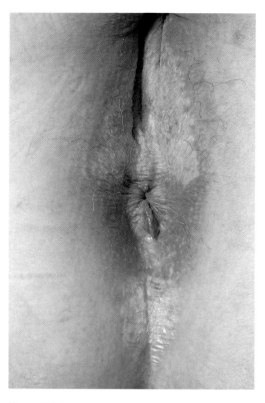

Figure 7.14

Lichen sclerosus et atrophicus of the genital area. Notice the marked white appearance of the affected area.

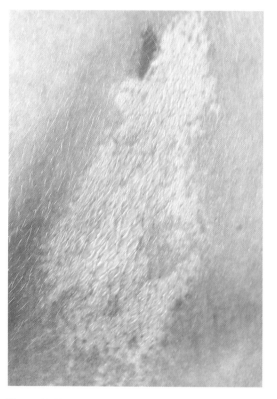

Figure 7.15

Lichen sclerosus et atrophicus of the trunk in an elderly woman. The silvery white appearance is typical, and appears to be composed of a number of separate white papules.

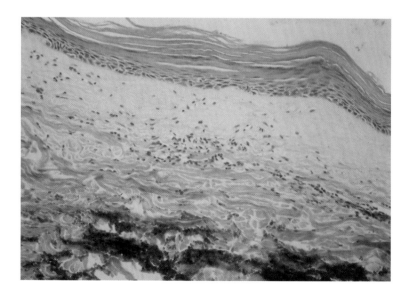

Figure 7.16

Histopathology of lichen sclerosus et atrophicus. Note the intense oedema subepidermally and the hyperkeratosis (H & E; ×45).

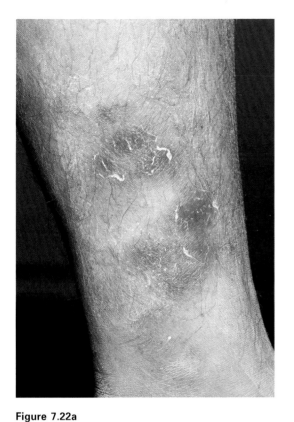

Figure 7.22a

Lesions of nodular vasculitis on the lower leg in an elderly woman.

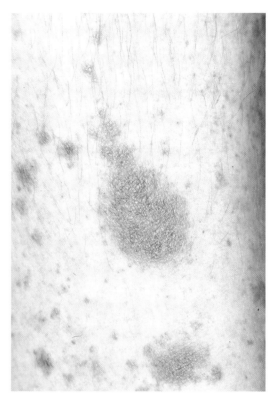

Figure 7.22b

Purpuric nodules and papules in nodular vasculitis.

as the mainstay of treatment, and more than 80% of patients survive for longer than 5 years although relapses are common.[41]

Temporal arteritis (giant cell arteritis)

Temporal arteritis mainly occurs in elderly men. It is characterized by pain and tenderness and swelling in the temporal region due to inflammation of the temporal artery. Histologically the affected vessel is infiltrated with a granulomatous infiltrate containing giant cells. Involvement of retinal and cerebral vessels may occur with unpleasant results for function. Temporal arteritis can produce a variety of ophthalmic complications including ischaemic optic neuropathy, retinal artery occlusion, retinal haemorrhages and cotton wool spots and muscle palsies. Rarely it can also cause anterior segment ischaemia and homonymous hemianopia. Rarely, ulceration of the skin occurs in the affected area. Treatment is with oral steroids.

Persistent purpuric pigmented eruptions

This is a group of disorders characterized by the development of a rash consisting of purpuric spots and subsequent pigmentation on the basis of what appears to be inflammation of the papillary capillaries, ie, a capillaritis. They probably do not represent a true vasculitis but are

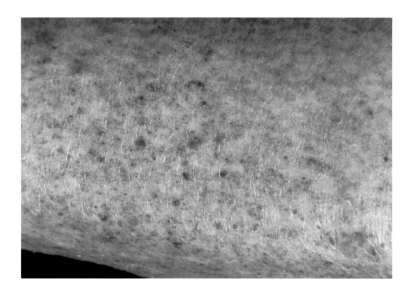

Figure 7.23

Schamberg's disease, showing many purpuric spots in a 'caynenne pepper' appearance, and some pigmentation of the lower leg in an elderly man.

Figure 7.24

Lichen aureus. There is an odd-shaped patch of golden brown pigmentation on the leg.

described here for convenience. Several clinical forms are recognized. The most often seen is a diffuse involvement of the lower legs and dorsa of the feet, known as Schamberg's disease (Figure 7.23). This is most common in men, of all ages including the elderly. Other less frequently seen types include one in which the purpura occurs in rings (purpura annularis telangiectodes of Majocchi), one associated with a lichenoid dermatitis and one in which the pigmentation is golden rather than brown (lichen aureus) (Figure 7.24). They are all benign in that there are no systemic changes and they are not associated with any functional deficit. The histological appearance is similar in all these variants and marked by a mild subepidermal lymphocytic and histiocytic cellular infiltrate, haemorrhage deposition of pigment in macrophages and swelling of the capillary endothelium. All are persistent but do eventually remit usually after some months.

Pityriasis lichenoides and lymphomatoid papulosis

These two diseases are often described together despite some doubt as to whether they actually represent the same disease process.[43]

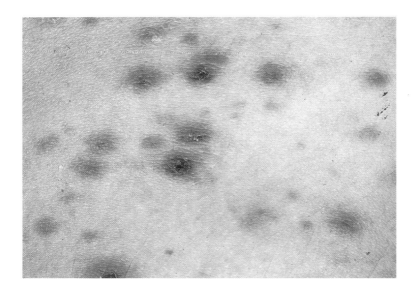

Figure 7.25

Acute pityriasis lichenoides. Many papules with central necrosis and crusting can be seen.

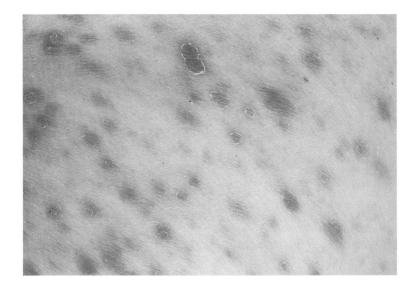

Figure 7.26

Pityriasis lichenoides chronica. There are many typical scaling papules present in this area.

Pityriasis lichenoides

This is a chronic relapsing inflammatory disease of the skin of unknown cause. The lesions are papular and two types are recognized, acute (pityriasis lichenoides et varioliformis acuta) and chronic (pityriasis lichenoides chronica), which may co-exist.[44] Acute lesions have a haemorrhagic,

crusted appearance while chronic lesions have a characteristic peripherally detached (mica-like) scale (Figures 7.25 and 7.26). The papules come in profuse crops over many years. The disorder is often found in young adults although older individuals are sometimes affected. It is not uncommon for 'acute' and 'chronic' lesions to be seen in the same patient. The trunk is mainly affected—the skin of the limbs and face being comparatively spared. The disorder has few symptoms and is surprisingly itch free. This disorder was originally classed as one of a larger group of conditions known as the parapsoriasis group,[44] which had few characteristics in common other than that they were inflammatory scaling disorders with a greater or lesser propensity to transform to malignant lymphomas. The grouping is an artificial one and there seems to be little value in retaining the term. The pathology of pityriasis lichenoides chronica is characterized by subepidermal inflammation and oedema and epidermal disturbance. The epidermis is thickened, oedematous and parakeratotic and shows individual cell necrosis. In the acute form the epidermis is eroded and crusted and there is a marked inflammatory cell infiltrate of mononuclear cells. Some of these are large and show nuclear abnormalities. These latter changes are very much more prominent in the condition known as lymphomatoid papulosis.

In the rare lymphomatoid papulosis[46] the papules may resemble those of acute pityriasis lichenoides but are larger and more irregular. They occur in crops but larger lesions may persist for months. The condition tends to occur in an older group of patients—mainly in those past middle age. Histologically the abnormal appearing cells referred to above are much more prominent so that the picture resembles that of a lymphoma. The term pseudolymphoma would be justifiable; however, a few cases are on record as having developed a frank lymphoma and it would seem prudent not to use a term that prejudges the issue.

The only form of treatment for either condition that appears to be of any benefit is some form of ultraviolet irradiation. PUVA (see page 270) has been used successfully for these disorders.

Rosacea

Rosacea is a common chronic inflammatory disorder of the facial skin of unknown cause. It is uncommon in the young and is most frequent after the age of 35. Rosacea is quite often seen in the elderly. It occurs in both sexes but may be somewhat more common in women. It is mainly a disorder of fair-skinned Caucasians from Northern Europe and is uncommon in

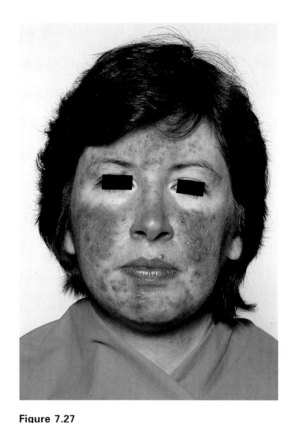

Figure 7.27

Rosacea in a youngish woman showing symmetrical erythema and papules on the cheeks, forehead and chin.

Mediterranean types, very uncommon in darker-skinned Asiatic subjects and very rare in black-skinned peoples.

Clinical features

The disorder is characterized by persistent erythema and telangiectasia of the convexities of the facial skin although other areas of the head and neck can be affected (Figure 7.27). In very severely affected patients the entire face may be involved (Figure 7.28). Rarely, particular sites are picked out, such as one cheek or just the forehead or just the bald part of the scalp (Figure 7.29). Occasionally one site is spared when there

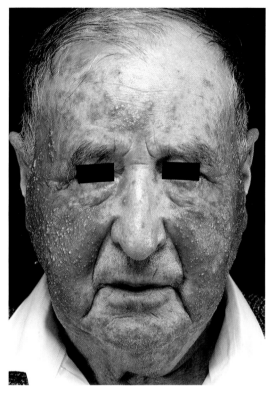

Figure 7.28

Severely inflammed rosacea in an elderly man with many papules and pustules as well as swelling of the cheeks.

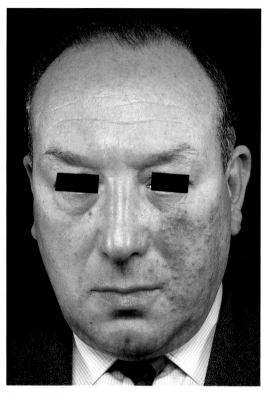

Figure 7.29

Rosacea affecting the left cheek alone.

is otherwise symmetrical involvement. The ears, front of the neck and even the front of the chest can be affected. A few cases have been reported in which peripheral sites such as the wrists and legs have been involved[47] in the course of ordinary severe rosacea.

Apart from the background of erythema and telangiectasia, the disease is punctuated by episodes of inflammation in which red or pink papules appear at the affected sites. Less commonly, pustules occur as well. These acute episodes are often accompanied by some swelling of the involved facial skin. Unlike the papules of acne, these are not tender and regularly hemispherical.

Generally the disorder runs a chronic course in which the condition subsides to a greater or lesser degree between attacks of inflammation. It is doubtful whether once established the tendency to develop the condition ever goes entirely. Rosacea causes embarrassment and depression after being present for some time. This is to be expected from a disorder which produces considerable cosmetic disability.

Differential diagnosis (see Table 7.1).

An acute red face may also be caused by allergic contact dermatitis, other forms of eczema (see Chapter 3), systemic lupus erythematosus and dermatomyositis. Superior vena caval obstruction and polycythaemia rubra vera may also cause generalized reddening of the face. Perioral dermatitis is a condition seen in younger women for the

Table 7.1   Differential diagnosis of rosacea

Disorder	Comment
Allergic contact dermatitis	Itchy, scaling, sometimes exudative disorder; does not spare flexures; appears on sites outside face and neck
Photodermatitis	Appears on light exposed sites as well as face; strict relationship to light exposure; may be scaly and exudative. Papules and pustules uncommon
Seborrhoeic dermatitis	Scaling disorder, particularly marked in flexures; scalp often affected; sites other than face frequently involved
Systemic lupus erythematosus	Systemic illness; other sites involved apart from face; papules and pustules uncommon
Dermatomyositis	Systemic illness; weakness and muscle tenderness; mauve hue to rash, particularly marked around eyes
Acne	Seborrhoea marked; inflammatory papules are tender; cysts, blackheads and scars occur; involvement of back and cheek very common
Polycythaemia rubra vera	Uniformly suffused red face; no papules or pustules.
Superior vena caval obstruction	Uniformly red face; no papules or pustules; signs and symptoms of a chest disorder

most part in which minute papulopustules occur around the mouth.[48] It should not be confused with rosacea because there is no background of erythema and telangiectasia on the affected areas and the condition has a characteristic perioral distribution, although the nasolabial grooves and the paranasal areas are sometimes affected.

Complications

Rhinophyma is an irregular hypertrophy of the soft tissues of the nose which predominantly affects men past middle age. The nose is bulbous and enlarged with a pitted and craggy surface (Figure 7.30). The pilosebaceous orifices are dilated and from them may be expressed a viscid and foul smelling substance consisting of sebum and horny debris. The colour of the affected skin is dull red or purplish. Rhinophyma is known by a collection of colourful folk-lore synonyms implying intemperate use of alcohol. These include elephantiasis des buveurs, whisky nose and grogblossom. Despite popular opinion hallowed by the drawing of attention to this supposed association by literary giants such as Chaucer and Shakespeare, there is no evidence that those affected by this disfiguring condition drink any more than anyone else.[49] Rarely the type of soft tissue enlargement noted in rhinophyma is seen on the ears, in the paranasal areas or over the chin.[50]

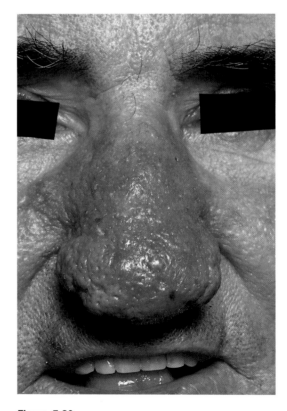

Figure 7.30

Rhinophyma, showing marked irregular hypertrophy of the soft tissue of the nose in an elderly man.

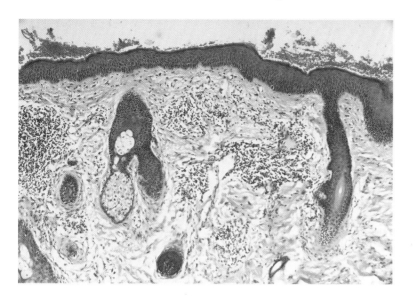

Figure 7.31

Histopathology of rosacea. There is oedema and disorganization of the upper dermal connective tissue, telangiectasia and a mixed perivascular inflammatory infiltrate (H & E; ×45).

Inflammatory disorders of the eyes are common in rosacea. Blepharoconjunctivitis may occur in as many as one-third of patients with acute rosacea. Styes, hordeolum and meibomian cysts are quite common as well. A painful keratitis is a rarer but much more dangerous complication of the disorder, more common in elderly men, which may threaten sight due to the effects on the transparency of the cornea.

Pathology

Between episodes of inflammation when there is only erythema and telangiectasia, the most noticeable change is in the quality of the dermal connective tissue. There is marked elastotic degenerative change and a loose, irregular arrangement of the upper dermis. The elastosis seems to be more prominent than may be expected after taking into consideration the site biopsied as well as the age, occupation and skin colour of the individual concerned.[51] Amidst the degenerate dermal connective tissue there are large telangiectatic blood vessels.

During episodes of inflammation a variety of cell types accumulate around the dermal vasculature (Figure 7.31). Because of the rich perifollicular plexuses of blood vessels, the follicles appear to be surrounded by the inflammatory cells. A variety of cell types are found, but lymphocytes and histiocytes predominate. Giant cells are present in about 10% of the biopsies from patients with inflamed rosacea. In some cases they may be prominent and simulate tuberculoid granulomas.

Aetiology and pathogenesis

We know much more about what does not cause rosacea than what does. The author's own studies somewhat demoted dietetic, gastrointestinal, microbial and psychological factors as contestants in the aetiological stakes.[53] However, there are some clues. Climatic injury does seem to play an important role, as witnessed by the sites affected by the disease, the occurrence of the disorder in light-skinned subjects mainly, and the dermal changes. Depressed immune responsiveness may also play a role[53,54] but it is difficult to construct a reasonable unifying hypothesis to explain how this feature is involved. Rosacea seems a complex disease and it is likely that an inherent predisposition and climatic and immunological aspects may all play a part in the cause.

Treatment

Topical treatments have very limited value in rosacea, although a topical preparation of metronidazole has been found to give some relief.[55] Studies comparing topical metronidazole (0.75 or 1.0% preparations) with systemic tetracycline suggest that these two treatments have equal efficacy. An emollient is occasionally helpful to relieve any discomfort and to satisfy the patient's urge to apply something to the skin. Topical tretinoin used over many months assisted a group of patients described by Kligman[56]—presumably via its stimulatory activity on dermal connective tissue (see page 25). Topical corticosteroids are harmful in rosacea. The urge to prescribe them for the inflammation in rosacea must be checked as their use aggravates the disease. The skin thinning potential of these agents compounds the tendency to dermal dystrophy already present in rosacea and the skin becomes redder and more telangiectatic.[52] Sunscreens should be recommended as they prevent further damage to connective tissue as well as stopping acute exacerbations.

The attacks of inflammation are best curtailed by the use of oral tetracycline.[57] As mentioned above, there is no evidence that the disorder has a microbial basis and the reasons for the efficacy of tetracycline are unclear. Usually the drug is started at a dose of 250 mg three or four times daily and continued until there are signs of improvement, when the dose is gradually reduced until it is stopped. In most patients improvement starts after 3–4 weeks and the treatment can be stopped after 3 or 4 months. However, some patients find that they need to continue with a small dose (eg, 250 mg daily or on alternate days) for long periods. Some 10 to 20% of patients fail to respond to tetracycline and erythromycin and metronidazole have been described as useful alternatives. The oral retinoid 13–cis-retinoic acid (isotretinoin) has also been used and found helpful in some individuals.[58] Isotretinoin seems to have a particularly good effect in patients with rhinophyma causing a reduction in the size and irregularity of this structure although this condition can be treated satisfactorily by surgical paring or dermabrasion or laser therapy.

Patients with rosacea also require considerable support and sympathy in an attempt to relieve their gloom at their facial appearance. It is also helpful to advise patients to avoid those things that they know make them blush. In addition they should avoid the more severe vagaries of north-west European weather and sun exposure, as these tend to aggravate the disease.

Acne vulgaris

Acne is uncommon in the elderly, and when it does occur in this age group, it is often misdiagnosed. A study by Cunliffe and colleagues described 152 women and 48 men with 'post adolescent acne' of mean age 35.5 years, 12.5% of whom were over 45.[59] The disorder is similar to that occurring in youth, but large truncal lesions predominate (Figure 7.32). Treatment of acne in the elderly is very similar to the treatment of the disease in other age groups although it tends to be more resistant to treatment and there is more dependence on systemic therapies rather than topical preparations.

Chondrodermatitis nodularis chronica helicis

This disorder is seen only in the elderly and is very much more common in elderly men with thin ears. The cause is unknown but it has been suggested that it is the result of ischaemia from the minor trauma of pressure during sleep. Interestingly it has also been described in nuns from the pressure of their whimples.

Clinical features

A painful and tender nodule up to 0.5 cm in diameter appears on the superior or posterior margin of the pinna (Figure 7.33). Less commonly lesions occur on the antihelix—especially if this structure is prominent. The skin over it is sometimes broken and occasionally pink and scaling. Despite its insignificant appearance it may cause considerable discomfort especially at

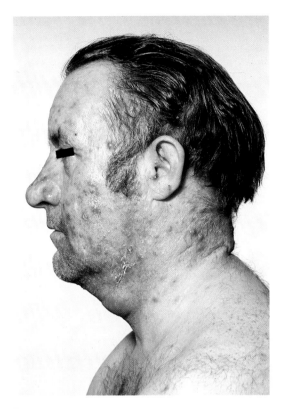

Figure 7.32

Moderately severe papular and nodulocystic acne in a man of late middle age. His acne was of late onset.

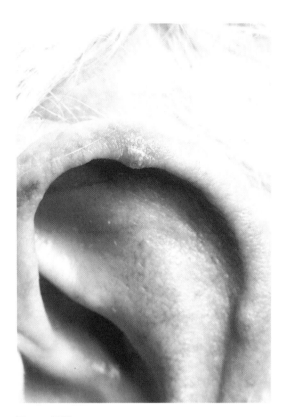

Figure 7.33

Nodules of chondrodermatitis nodularis chronica helicis on the helix of the ear of an elderly man.

night. It has to be differentiated from solar keratosis (see page 193) and gouty tophus.

Pathology

The histological picture is quite typical in that there is considerable oedema, fibrin deposition and telangiectasia in the dermis overlying an area of degenerate ear cartilage and under a thickened epidermis.

Treatment

The only suitable treatment is excision and curiously this usually provides symptomatic relief without recurrence.

References

1 Baker S B, Rovira J R, Campion E W et al. Late onset systemic lupus erythematosus. *J Am J Med* (1979) **66:**727–32.
2 Cattoggio L J, Skinner R P, Smith G et al. Systemic lupus erythematosus in the elderly: clinical and serological characteristics. *J Rheumatol* (1984) **11:**175–81.
3 Rowell N R. The natural history of lupus erythematosus. *Clin Exp Dermatol* (1984) **9:**217–31.
4 Hughes G R V. Systemic lupus erythematosus: treatment and prognosis. *Br Med J* (1979) **2:**1019–22.
5 Gough A, Chapman S, Wagstaff K et al. Minocycline included autoimmune hepatitis and systemic lupus erythematosus like syndrome. *Br Med J* (1996) **312:**169–72.
6 Crosson J, Stillman T. Minocycline related lupus erythematosus with associated liver disease. *J Am Acad Dermatol* (1997) **36:**867–8.

7   Mills J A. Systemic lupus erythematosus. *New Engl J Med* (1994) **330:**1871–7.

8   Tan E M, Cohen A S, Fries J F et al. The 1982 revised criteria for the classification of systemic lupus erythematosus. *Arthritis Rheum* (1982) **25:**1271–7.

9   Tsutsui K, Imai T, Hatta N, Sakai H, Takata M, Takehara K. Widespread pruritic plaques in a patient with subacute cutaneous lupus erythematosus and hypocomplementemia: response to Dapsone therapy. *J Am Acad Dermatol* (1996) **35:**313–15.

10 Hochberg M C. Systemic lupus erythematosus. *Rheum Dis Clin North Am* (1990) **16:**617–39.

11 Ishikawa O, Zaw K K, Miyachi Y, Hashimoto T, Tanaka T. The presence of anti basement membrane antibodies in the sera of patients with non bullous lupus erythematosus. *Br J Dermatol* (1997) **136:**222–6.

12 Osterland C K, Espirioza L, Parker L P et al. Inherited C2 deficiency and systemic lupus erythematosus: studies on a family. *Ann Int Med* (1975) **82:**323–8.

13 Beck J S, Rowell N R. Discoid lupus erythematosus. A study of the clinical features and biochemical and serological abnormalities in 120 patients with observations on the relationships of this disease to lupus erythematosus. *Q J Med* (1966) **35:**119–36.

14 Tuffanelli D L. Discoid lupus erythematosus. In: *Clinics in Rheumatic Diseases* **8:**(2) 327–42 (WB Saunders: London, 1982).

15 Dubois E L. Antimalarials in the management of discoid and systemic lupus erythematosus. In: Moschella S L ed, *Dermatology Update, Review for Physicians*, (Elsevier: New York, 1982) 153–84.

16 Dalziel K, Going S, Cartwright P H et al. Treatment of chronic discoid lupus erythematosus with an oral gold compound. *Br J Dermatol* (1986) **115:**211–16.

17 Sontheimer R D, Thomas J R, Gillian J N. Subacute cutaneous lupus erythematosus. A cutaneous marker for a distinct lupus erythematosus subset. *Arch Dermatol* (1979) **115:**1409–15.

18 Rodnan G P. A review of recent observations and current theories on the aetiology and pathogenesis of progressive systemic sclerosis (diffuse scleroderma). *J Chronic Dis* (1963) **16:**929–49.

19 Hodgkinson H M. Scleroderma in the elderly with special reference to the CRST syndrome. *J Am Geriatric Soc* (1971) **19:**224–8.

20 Perez M I, Kohn S R. Systemic sclerosis. *J Am Acad Dermatol* (1993) **28:**525–47.

21 Bunker C B, Goldsmith P C, Leslie T A et al. Calcitonin gene-related peptide, endothelin-I, the cutaneous microvasculature and Raynaud's phenomenon. *Br J Dermatol* (1996) **134:**399–406.

22 Rowell N R. Systemic sclerosis. *J R Coll Physicians (Lond)* (1985) **19:**23–9.

23 Drake L A, Dinehart S M, Farmer E R et al. Guidelines for care of scleroderma and scleroder-moid disorders. *J Am Acad Dermatol* (1996) **35:**609–12.

24 Hunzelman N, Anders S, Fierlbeck G et al. Systemic scleroderma. Multicenter trial of 1 year of treatment with recombinant interferon therapy. *Arch Dermatol* (1997) **133:**609–13.

25 Rodnan G P. Progressive systemic sclerosis and penicillamine. *J Rheumatol* (1981) **7**(Suppl): 116–20.

26 Rook A H, Freundlich B, Jegasothy B V et al. Treatment of systemic sclerosis with extracorporeal phototherapy. *Arch Dermatol* (1992) **128:**337–46.

27 Serup J. Quantification of acrosclerosis, measurement of skin thickness and skin phalanx distance in females with 15 Mhz pulsed ultrasound. *Acta Derm Venereol* (Stockh) (1987) **64:**35–40.

28 Enomoto D N H, Mekkes J H, Bossayt P M M et al. Quantification of cutaneous sclerosis with a skin elasticity meter in patients with generalised scleroderma. *J Am Acad Dermatol* (1996) **35:**381–7.

29 Hunzelman N, Anders S, Fierlbeck G et al. Double-blind placebo controlled study of intralesional interferon gamma for the treatment of localised scleroderma. *J Am Acad Dermatol* (1997) **36:**433–5.

30 Stege H, Berneburg M, Humke S et al. High dose UVA, radiation therapy for localised scleroderma. *J Am Acad Dermatol* (1997) **36:**938–44.

31 Bohan A, Peter J B. Polymyositis and dermatomyositis (part I), *New Engl J Med* (1975) **292:**344–7.

32 Bohan A, Peter J B. Polymyositis and dermatomyositis (part II), *New Engl J Med* (1975) **292:**405–7.

33 Walton J. The inflammatory myopathies. *J R Soc Med* (1983) **76:**998–1010.

34 Kitchiner D, Edmonds J, Bruneau C et al. Mixed connective tissue disease with digital gangrene. *Br Med J* (1975) (Feb 1): 249–50.

35 Diaz-Perez J L, Winkelmann R K. Cutaneous periarteritis nodosa. *Arch Dermatol* (1974) **110:**407–14.

36 Sack M, Cassidy J T, Bole G G. Prognostic factors in polyarteritis. *J Rheumatol* (1975) **2:**411–20.

37 Tancrede-Bohin E, Ochinsky S, Vignon-Pennamen M D et al. Schönlein-Henoch purpura in adult patients. *Arch Dermatol* (1997) **133:**438–42.

38 McCluskey R T, Fienberg R. Vasculitis in primary vasculitides granulomatoses and connective tissue diseases. *Human Pathol* (1983) **14:**305–15.

39 Baselga E, Margall N, Barnadas M A et al. Detection of mycobacterium tuberculosis DNA in lobular granulomatous panniculitis (erythema induration–nodular vasculitis). *Arch Dermatol* (1997) **133:**457–62.

40 Po C T, Holt M E, Denny P et al. Deposition of eosinophil cationic protein in granulomas in allergic granulomatosis and vasculitis: the Churg Strauss syndrome. *Br Med J* (1984) **289**:400–2.

41 Savage C O S, Harper L, Adu D. Primary systemic vasculitis. *Lancet* (1997) **349**:553–8.

42 Burden A D, Tillman D M, Foley P, Holme E. IgA class anticardiolipin antibodies in cutaneous leukocytoclastic vasculitis. *J Am Acad Dermatol* (1996) **35**:411–15.

43 Willemze R, Scheffer E. Clinical and histological differentiation between lymphomatoid papulosis and pityriasis lichenoides. *J Am Acad Dermatol* (1985) **13**:418–28.

44 Marks R, Black M M, Wilson-Jones E. Pityriasis lichenoides: a reappraisal. *Br J Dermatol* (1972) **86**:215–25.

45 Lambert W C, Everett M A. The nosology of parapsoriasis. *J Am Acad Dermatol* (1981) **5**:374–95.

46 Karp D L, Horn T D. Lymphomatoid papulosis. *J Am Acad Dermatol* (1994) **30**:379–95.

47 Marks R, Wilson-Jones E. Disseminated rosacea. *Br J Dermatol* (1969) **81**:16–28.

48 Marks R. Rosacea, flushing and perioral dermatitis. In: Champion R H, Burton J L, Ebling F J G, eds, *Textbook of Dermatology*, 5th Edn, (Blackwell Scientific Publications: Oxford, 1992) 1851–63.

49 Marks R, Beard R J, Clark M L et al. Gastrointestinal observations in rosacea. *Lancet* (1967) **i**:739–43.

50 Jansen T, Plewig G. Rosacea: classification and treatment. *J R Soc Med* (1997) **90**:144–50.

51 Marks R, Harcourt Webster J N. The histopathology of rosacea. *Arch Dermatol* (1969) **100**:683–92.

52 Marks R. Rosacea: hopeless hypothesis, marvellous myths and dermal disorganisation. In: Marks R, Plewig G, eds, *Acne & Related Disorders*, (Martin Dunitz: London, 1989) 293–9.

53 Manna V, Marks R, Holt P J A. Involvement of immune mechanism in the pathogenesis of rosacea. *Br J Dermatol* (1982) **107**:203–8.

54 Nunzi E, Rebora A, Hamerlinck F et al. Immunopathological studies on rosacea. *Br J Dermatol* (1980) **103**:543–51.

55 Schmadel L K, McEvoy G K. Topical metronidazole: a new therapy for rosacea. *Clin Pharmacol* (1990) **9**:94–101.

56 Kligman A M. Topical tretinoin for rosacea: a preliminary report. *J Derm Treat* (1993) **4**:71–3.

57 Marks R, Ellis J. Comparative effectiveness of tetracycline and ampicillin in rosacea. *Lancet* (1971) **ii**:1049–52.

58 Hoting E, Plewig G. Treatment of rosacea with isotretinoin. *Int J Dermatol* (1986) **25**:660–3.

59 Goulden V, Clark S M, Cunliffe W J. Post adolescent acne: a review of clinical features. *Br J Dermatol* (1997) **136**:66–70.

8
Infections and infestations of the skin

Immune defences in the elderly

If any reader believes that this topic is straight-forward and has a 'one line, take home message', he or she should consult recent reviews by Nagel[1] and Finkelstein.[2] It seems any conclusion is difficult other than that the immune defence mechanisms are less efficient in old age. The major problems in drawing firm conclusions over the effects of ageing on immunity in humans include the obvious difficulties in performing longitudinal studies on the same population group (compared with the less infor-mative cross-sectional types of investigation), and the doubtful relevance of studies performed in mice. These difficulties are compounded by an incomplete understanding of the immune function and its control in young and mature subjects and by incompletely validated testing techniques. It is clear that there are age-related alterations in immune function, that they are subtle and that little is known as to the reasons for these changes or their clinical significance. In general, T-lymphocyte function seems more affected by the ageing process than B-cell function, but changes occur in both. Total lymphoid tissue seems to decrease with advanc-ing age but total blood lymphocyte counts remain constant. The *in vitro* mitogen respon-siveness of T cells decreases with age and the cell-mediated killing of allogenic tumour cells is decreased in aged mice.[3]

The number of positive reactions to intracuta-neously injected anamnestic antigens is decreased in apparently fit elderly individuals compared with a cohort of young subjects.[4] Furthermore, the ability to mount a delayed hypersensitivity response is depressed when this is tested by exposure to a powerful sensitizing agent such as dinitrochlorobenzene or rhus oleoresin.[5] However, the effector response is also depressed in the aged,[6] so that apparent decreased immunological reactivity has to be interpreted cautiously. There is also a drop in the density of antigen presenting Langerhans cells within the epidermis in the elderly and this will decrease the ease of sensitization.[7]

The levels of circulating immunoglobulins are little changed in the elderly. There is some drop in the level of circulating IgM, possibly a small drop in IgG, but no decrease in the IgA or IgE levels. There is certainly an adequate response to polyvalent pneumococcal antigen and although the levels of antibody may not reach the high points attained in younger folk the protection against influenza by vaccination in the elderly is good.[8]

The complement system appears intact in the elderly and there does not seem to be any decrease of phagocytic capacity either by the reticuloendothelial system[9] or by circulating monocytes.[10] Neutrophil killing of *Staphylococcus aureus* appears similar in young and old.[11]

In general, the aged certainly are able to respond with an immune response to an infection, but it is slightly less speedy and efficient than in younger individuals and their ability to develop protective skin inflammation is diminished.

Virus infections of the skin

Varicella zoster

Infection with the varicella zoster virus is the most important virus infection of the skin in the elderly. Primary infection causes chickenpox (varicella) and is essentially a disorder of child-hood, although young adults who have not previously encountered the virus may develop the disease. After this primary infection the virus takes refuge in the dorsal root ganglia. This latent infection becomes manifest only after many years as herpes zoster in a small proportion of individuals when host defences are for some reason weakened. It is for this reason that you cannot catch herpes zoster, although it is quite possible to catch chickenpox from someone with herpes zoster if there has been no previous infection with the virus. This has to be remembered when a patient with herpes zoster is taken into hospital, as nursing and medical staff who have not had chickenpox previously do not take too kindly to developing the disease.

Herpes zoster (shingles) is mostly a disorder of the elderly and usually no precipitating cause can be found. In a small proportion of patients the disorder is a complication of an acknowledged cause of depressed immunity, involving occult neoplasia HIV disease or immunosuppressive drugs. In these latter patients the disease can be very severe and even life threatening.

Clinical features

The first signs of the disorder are paraesthesia and discomfort in the area to be involved. After 2–4 days there is fever and general malaise followed by a rash in the affected zone. Characteristically the rash is confined to the innervation of the affected dorsal root ganglion, although more than one dorsal root is sometimes involved. Certain zones are more often affected than others. The fifth nerve ganglion seems particularly frequently affected, causing the condition of herpes ophthalmicus if the ophthalmic branch of the fifth nerve is involved (Figure 8.1). The maxillary branch is sometimes affected but rarely the mandibular branch in the distribution of herpes. Cervical and thoracic dorsal nerve roots are quite frequently involved sites. When the thoracic roots are involved the distribution of the rash follows the rib line, giving rise to the term zoster, derived from the Greek word for a girdle.

The rash itself is identical to chickenpox. Red, oedematous papules become papulovesicles and then crusted pustules, the whole sequence taking some 14–21 days (Figure 8.2). The entire area may be red and swollen. Generally all the lesions are at the same stage of development although

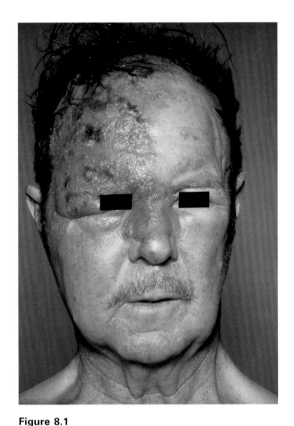

Figure 8.1

Herpes ophthalmicus. Herpes zoster affects the right side of the forehead, scalp and temporal region in this man.

in the early stages of the disease fresh crops of lesions may occur.

Although the disorder is mainly confined to the distribution of one or sometimes two dorsal nerve roots, a few typical lesions may occur outside these areas—rarely these outlying lesions may be so prolific as to simulate chickenpox itself.

Herpes zoster always causes considerable discomfort and may be extremely painful. It is especially uncomfortable when the ophthalmic region is affected as the cornea and the eyelids become involved. Often the whole region is very swollen and the eye is shut. The discomfort and pain does not automatically abate when the rash subsides and post herpetic neuralgic pain and unpleasant paraesthesia are found in perhaps

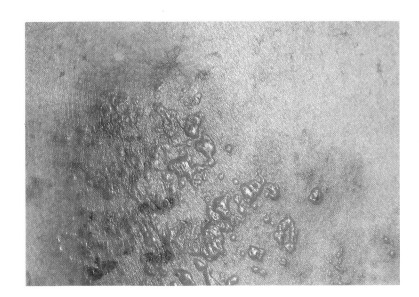

Figure 8.2

Close-up of the early vesicular lesions of herpes zoster.

one-third of patients. The reasons for the persistence of the symptoms is not entirely understood but it has been suggested that fibrotic changes occur in the nerve terminals. It may be so severe as to make life utterly miserable for some older patients. The area of skin affected may also be left with whitish scars, although the typical pock marks of chickenpox are rarely observed.

More than one attack of herpes zoster is not uncommon, and seems to have no special significance.

Treatment

Provided that affected individuals are not very ill and that there is someone at home to care for them, hospitalization is not necessary. The affected area needs frequent bathing with either saline or an antiseptic solution such as dilute potassium permanganate (1 in 8000), or povidone-iodine aqueous solution, until it is no longer exudative.

Analgesics are required to relieve the discomfort and aspirin, dihydrocodeine or paracetamol is usually sufficient. If the pain is not relieved by simple measures, then more potent analgesics should be prescribed.

Some physicians have suggested that early treatment with systemic corticosteroids reduces the risk of post-herpetic neuralgia by decreasing the amount of neural damage and subsequent fibrosis.[12] Prednisone is given at 60 mg per day for 2–4 weeks and then gradually reduced to zero over the next 4–6 weeks. The treatment does not appear to increase the morbidity or mortality of the disease but, although attractive in concept, it has not been adequately validated.

The antiviral drug acyclovir, given intravenously in the early stages of the disorder, appears to reduce the duration and severity of the disease and should be seriously considered for the very old and sick patient.[13] It is given in a dose of 5 mg/kg body weight over 1 hour, 8–hourly. Oral acyclovir 800 mg, five times daily is an alternative for less severely sick patients. Famciclovir is an alternative analogue for patients with herpes zoster who present early on in the disease.

Herpes simplex

Two antigenic types are recognized: herpes simplex I, the type causing common cold sores around the mouth and nose, and herpes simplex

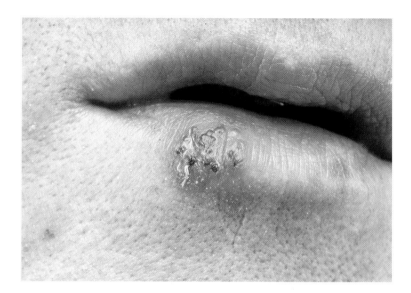

Figure 8.3a

Typical herpes simplex of the lower lip. This not often seen in elderly subjects.

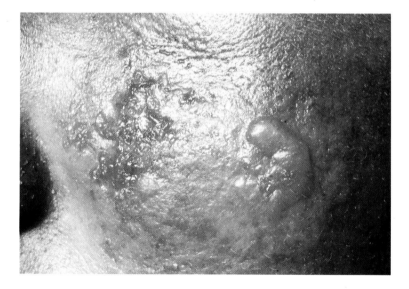

Figure 8.3b

Unusual and quite severe herpes simplex affecting the cheek.

II, causing herpes genitalis.[14] For reasons that are unclear, neither type is at all frequent in old age. Occasionally during a severe febrile illness cold sores break out around the mouth in the elderly (herpes febrilis) (Figure 8.3). If this should happen, very little is required other than to keep the affected area clean and dry. If the attack of herpes is severe and the condition presents early, topical acyclovir may reduce the duration and severity of the complaint. Famciclovir (a pro-drug of the agent penciclovir) is similar in action and effect to acyclovir. Foscarnet is yet another agent that has anti-herpes simplex effects, but does not appear as active as acyclovir.[14]

Warts

The human papilloma virus exists in more than 70 antigenic types,[15] particular clinical types of

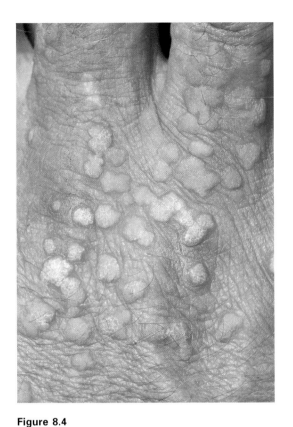

Figure 8.4

Multiple warts of the hand affecting an elderly patient on immunosuppressive therapy.

wart being associated with particular antigenic varieties. Warts are mainly a clinical problem in the young, although genital warts are quite common in the sexually active middle aged. All varieties of wart are transmitted by direct contact. None the less, ordinary viral warts are occasionally found in the elderly. When such lesions do occur they are either solitary or few, and are often suspected of being squamous cell carcinoma, keratoacanthoma or seborrhoeic warts. The commonest variety clinically in the elderly is the sessile warty nodule occurring on the hands. Plane warts, plantar warts and ordinary genital warts are very unusual in the elderly. If an elderly subject presents with large numbers of warts some form of immunosuppression should be suspected (Figure 8.4). Rarely it is the manifestation of a lymphoreticular neoplasm. Treatment when needed for these lesions should be the least destructive possible. Salicylic acid or podophyllin preparations are often sufficient. When something more vigorous is required, freezing with liquid nitrogen or solid carbon dioxide or curettage and cautery may be used.

One papilloma virus-induced lesion that is almost specific to the elderly is the giant condyloma of Buschke. This is an exuberant warty nodule which develops on the external genitalia or the perianal region (Figure 8.5). It behaves like a slow growing invasive squamous cell carcinoma and is best regarded as such. Certainly

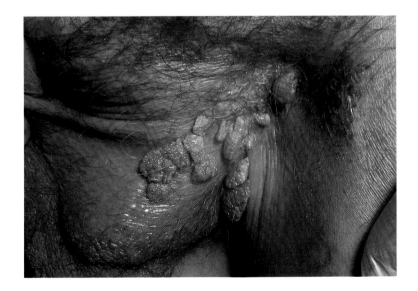

Figure 8.5

Large exuberant warts affecting the scrotal region. Lesions such as these can transform into invasive epitheliomatous growths.

from the histological viewpoint the distinction between benign warty hyperplasia and a slow growing, well differentiated squamous cell carcinoma can be very difficult. For this reason it is of great interest that antigenic type 6 of the papilloma virus has been identified in such lesions.[16] There is growing interest in the involvement of HPV in human neoplastic disease and it is quite evident from experience with wart like lesions in renal transplant patients and the condition known as bowenoid papulosis that certain of the antigenic types of HPV virus may be more deeply involved than we have believed previously.[17]

Treatment of the giant condyloma of Buschke is either by a straightforward surgical excision or by cryotherapy.

Mollusca contagiosa

This belongs to the pox virus group of infections and like other members of this group is a large DNA virus. It causes small umbilicated pearly nodules, the centre of which contains a whitish, cheesy or waxy material that can be expressed out by pressure on the sides of the lesion. Multiple small lesions occur over the face, in the flexures or on the trunk in the young, and, as with warts, are transmitted by direct skin contact. Odd giant solitary lesions, or a myriad of tiny lesions, may rarely arise in the elderly. Individual lesions may be treated by expression of the softish central contents or by light cautery.

Orf

This infection is also caused by a member of the pox virus group. It is essentially a disease of sheep and calves, causing a condition in them known as contagious pustular dermatitis. It is transmitted by contact with the infected animal and is seen in farm hands of all ages (Figure 8.6). The lesions generally occur on the fingers as painful, swollen, exudative pustular areas with a variable amount of systemic upset. It generally remits spontaneously after 14–28 days but is followed in a surprisingly large number of patients (perhaps 30–50%) by an attack of erythema multiforme.

Acquired immunodeficiency syndrome (AIDS)

The prevalence and incidence of HIV infection and AIDS have increased steadily in the past 10 years, but now seem to have reached a plateau and a short note on the disorder as it affects the skin is appropriate here. The disorder is caused by a virus known as the human immunodeficiency virus (HIV). HIV is transmitted in a similar way to hepatitis B virus—via direct inoculation of blood and body fluids. The disease has caused fear and gained notoriety because of its lethal nature. It is not yet known what proportion of HIV patients will develop ARC (AIDS related complex). At present it appears that 15–20% of HIV-infected patients develop AIDS per year. Some 70% of haemophiliacs who received pooled factor VIII concentrates have developed HIV antibodies.[18]

Few elderly patients have been seen with AIDS as yet, but it is to be expected that more will present in the future.

The major effect of the infection is to cause a profound immunosuppression, allowing opportunistic infections to gain a foothold and causing an increase in certain neoplastic disorders. So far as skin manifestations are concerned, the best known is the rapidly spreading type of Kaposi's idiopathic haemorrhagic sarcoma, which has been the cause of death in many AIDS patients. A form of seborrhoeic dermatitis is also quite frequent in AIDS patients (Figure 8.7). In addition, odd follicular and acneiform eruptions seem to be quite common and patients have been described who have developed a particularly virulent form of psoriasis. Other skin disorders resulting from the immunosuppression will almost certainly be described and those interested should consult monographs and reviews on the topic.[19,20]

Dermatophyte infections

Ringworm infections

In general, only certain sorts of ringworm infection are particularly common in the elderly.

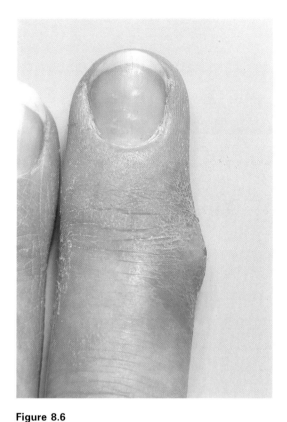

Figure 8.6

Lesion of orf on the finger.

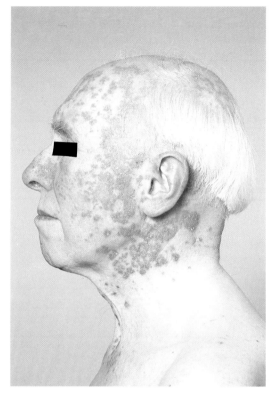

Figure 8.7

Extensive seborrhoeic dermatitis in a haemophiliac with HTLV-III virus infection and depressed immunity. This cleared after treatment with topical miconazole.

Tinea corporis (body ringworm)

The micro-organisms responsible for this form of ringworm include *Trichophyton rubrum, Trichophyton mentagrophytes* and *Epidermophyton floccosum*. Typically, well-defined, round, red scaling patches occur, which have the tendency to central clearing (Figure 8.8). Diagnosis is confirmed by identification microscopically of the fungal mycelium in scales or skin surface biopsies[21] and by culture. Mistreatment of small unrecognized patches of ringworm with potent topical corticosteroids can lead to the development of the condition of 'tinea incognito'.[22] The suppression by the corticosteroid of the usual eczematous response to the infecting ringworm fungus allows the micro-organism to proliferate and gives rise to unusually large involved areas of skin, often with a bizarre appearance (Figure 8.9). This clinical presentation is by no means uncommon in the elderly and often causes first considerable diagnostic confusion, followed by professional embarrassment.

Tinea cruris

Most of the rashes in the groins of elderly men referred to as tinea cruris are in fact due to seborrhoeic dermatitis. This common condition can be

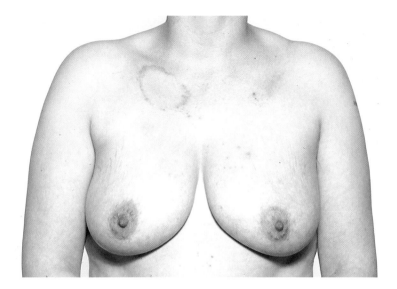

Figure 8.8a

Ringworm infection of the upper trunk

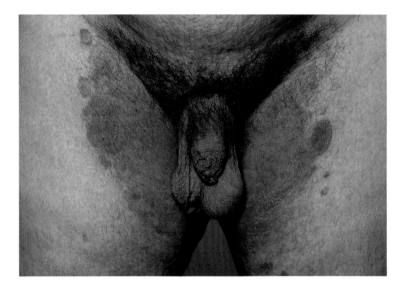

Figure 8.8b

Extensive tinea cruris in an elderly man.

distinguished from ringworm by the symmetrical nature of the former disorder and by its diffuse irregular margin compared with the latter (Figure 8.8). It is none the less a wise precaution to take scrapings from any eruption in the groin, just to confirm the absence of fungal elements. Both seborrhoeic dermatitis of the groins and tinea cruris have to be distinguished from erythrasma (page 173), which tends to be less angrily inflamed and to cover larger areas of skin.

As with tinea corporis, misdiagnosis and treatment with potent topical corticosteroids results in 'tinea incognito'.

Tinea capitis

Scalp ringworm due to infections of the scalp with small spore ectothrix fungi—*Microsporon audouinii* and *Microsporon canis*—is essentially a

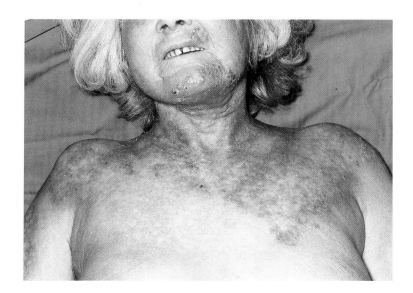

Figure 8.9

Tinea incognito. This elderly woman, who had systemic sclerosis, developed a rash on her shoulders, which was treated with topical corticosteroids. The rash spread and was found to be due to a ringworm infection.

disorder of prepubertal children. However, other types of fungus may infect the scalp of adults causing inflammation of the scalp skin and focal hair loss. Although not common in the elderly, cases in which scalp infection with *Trichophyton tonsurans* has mimicked seborrhoeic dermatitis have been described.[23] *Trichophyton schoenleinii* can also infect the elderly, causing the condition known as favus, giving rise to a more exudative eruption with crust formation. In recent years this has been rare in the UK, though it has been seen in socially deprived immigrant groups. Uncommonly animal ringworm can cause ringworm of the scalp in adults.

Kerion

This is an acute inflammatory disorder of the scalp or other hair-bearing areas due to an animal ringworm or other virulent dermatophyte species. Clinically a boggy swelling is the result, which may exude pus. It is usually self limiting, lasting at most 4 weeks.

Tinea pedis

The interdigital variety of tinea pedis (Figure 8.10) and the acute vesicular forms of tinea pedis are much more common in young adults. A persistent scaling variety of ringworm of the feet affecting the soles of the feet (and sometimes the palms too) is occasionally seen in older patients. The ringworm fungus responsible for this type of infection is *Epidermophyton floccosum, Trichophyton rubrum* or *Trichophyton mentagrophytes*. The affected areas are usually only mildly pink but have a characteristic dry, silvery scale. Occasionally only one foot (or palm) is involved. The condition usually continues for many years with few symptoms and is usually misdiagnosed initially as eczema. It has been suggested that the non-inflammatory nature and the persistence of these infections in middle-aged and elderly men is due to a specific immunological anergy to the infecting micro-organism.[24]

Tinea unguium

Persistent infection of the toe-nail plates by ringworm infection is quite common in the elderly male population and is sometimes seen in elderly women too. The involved nail plate is thickened, opaque and discoloured, brown or yellow, and is irregular (Figure 8.11). Usually a few nails are affected: occasionally finger nails may be involved as well. The clinical diagnosis

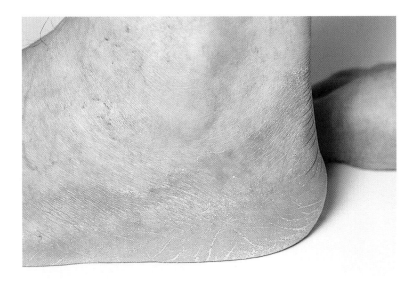

Figure 8.10

Ringworm on sole and side of foot.

is not necessarily straightforward. Toe nails affected by psoriasis sometimes appear similarly altered. The toe nails of the elderly may anyway become yellowed, thickened and irregular (dystrophic) for no apparent reason and this again closely simulates tinea unguium. Other types of nail infection, for example, candida infection, including *Candida parapsilosis* and *Scopulariopsis brevicaulis* can also give rise to a similar appearance. Dermatophytes account for 90%, candida accounts for 6% and non-dermatophyte moulds account for 3% of the pathogens responsible for onychomycosis.[25] It is essential to confirm the diagnosis by microscopic examination of toe-nail clippings after they have been softened in 20% potassium hydroxide for 30 minutes and by culturing of the nail fragments.

Treatment of ringworm infections

For localized areas of skin infection, topical treatments are adequate. The various imidazole preparations (miconazole, isoconazole, clotrimazole and econazole) all seem effective and have very few side-effects. Old-fashioned Whitfield's ointment consisting of 6% each of salicylic and benzoic acids is also effective but is irritant and

messy to use. Topical treatments should be used daily or twice daily for at least 3 weeks.

When the infection is extensive and the nails are also involved, systemic treatment may be required. Griseofulvin (250 mg 6–hourly for 4–6 weeks) is often adequate for skin infection. Unfortunately it is not very effective for toe-nail infections—perhaps only one-third of patients being cleared after 1 year of continuous treatment. Griseofulvin is a moderately safe drug, though it has caused rashes in a few patients. A new imidazole compound, tioconazole, used topically on the nails of patients with tinea unguium, it claimed to be effective in conjunction with griseofulvin given by mouth. Ketoconazole, an imidazole drug, is designed for systemic administration and has a much broader spectrum of antifungal activity than griseofulvin (which is active only against ringworm fungi). However, it has caused serious hepatotoxicity, particularly in the elderly, and many clinicians now reserve it for serious systemic fungal infections. Terbinafine is an allylamine type of drug which is suitable for both oral and topical tretinoin administration. It is effective against ringworm, but less so against yeast like microorganisms such as *Malassezia furfur*. At a dose of 500 mg daily most cases of nail ringworm are cleared after 3 months treatment; some patients may need a further month of treatment. It is

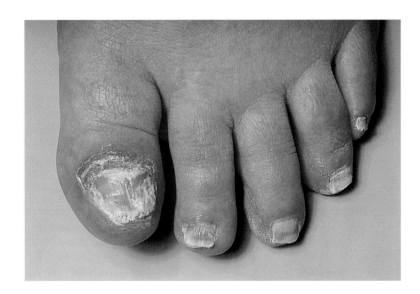

Figure 8.11a

Tinea unguium affecting all the toenails.

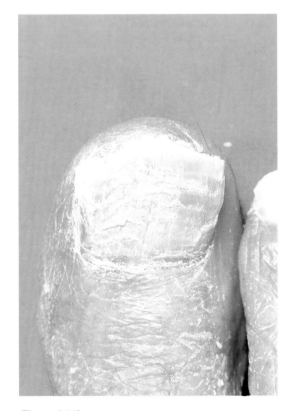

Figure 8.11b

Close-up of big toe nail affected by ringworm infection. It is thickened, yellow and crumbling, as well as deformed.

relatively non-toxic, although drug-induced hepatitis has been recorded.[26]

Terbinafine (250 mg daily) is now the oral antifungal agent of choice. It is effective in tinea unguium in some 70–80% of patients after 3 months treatment and in tinea capitis and corporis in shorter periods. An alternative is itraconazole (a 'triene') but this is mainly employed for candidiasis and pityriasis versicolor.

Itraconazole is an orally administered triazole active against both yeast-type pathogens and ringworm fungi. Short courses (7–14 days) of 100 mg/day are effective against pityriasis versicolor. Longer periods of treatment are needed for ringworm.

Pityriasis versicolor

This disorder is caused by an overgrowth of a normal microaerophilic lipophilic yeast-type denizen of the hair follicles known as *Pityrosporum ovale* or *Malassezia furfur*. The organism at times becomes pathogenic and causes a widespread pink-brown macular scaling disorder of the upper trunk (Figure 8.12). In some patients the rash also affects the arms and even the face. The light fawn colour of the eruption is

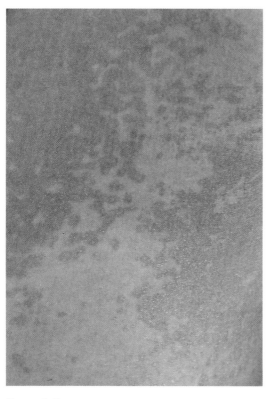

Figure 8.12

Pityriasis versicolor, showing typical pinky-fawn, slightly scaly, well defined patches on the trunk.

quite typical but in some patients the affected areas appear lighter than the surrounding skin. The diagnosis is easily confirmed by examination of skin scrapings or skin surface biopsies and finding a mass of pseudohyphae and collections of round spores, giving the well-recognized 'spaghetti and meatball' appearance in the stratum corneum (Figure 8.13). Observation of the skin in long-wave ultraviolet light (using a Wood's light) often reveals the affected areas as having a delicate lemon-green fluorescence. The condition is most common in young adults but is certainly not unusual in the elderly.

Treatment is usually with a topical preparation of one of the imidazole derivatives. Topical treatment should continue for at least 4 weeks and even then recurrences are frequent. It should be noted that after resolution, depigmented areas persist at the sites of infection for several weeks or even months.

Candidiasis (moniliasis)

This disorder is caused by the widespread yeast *Candida albicans*. It is often present in the bowel and on the mucosae as a commensal but becomes pathogenic when the local defences or the systemic immune defences are compromised. In

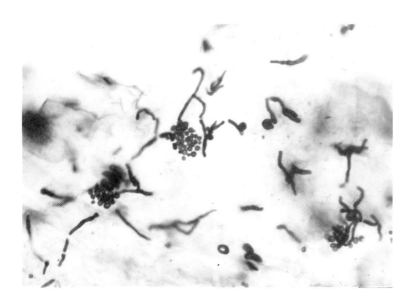

Figure 8.13

Pityriasis versicolor, showing pseudo mycelium and clusters of spores in a skin surface biopsy. (Periodic acid Schiff stain; ×40).

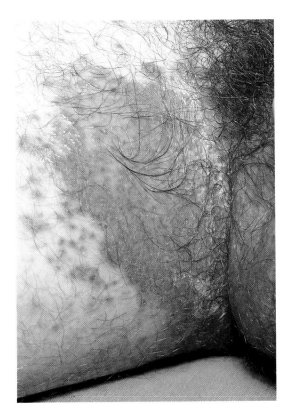

Figure 8.14

Candidiasis in the inguinal region. There are many outlying papules and pustules.

the older members of the population the commonest type of skin involvement by candida is in flexural intertrigo (Figure 8.14). The obese are particularly at risk, especially in the retromammary region in obese elderly women with pendulous breasts. The affected area usually has a glazed, red appearance and is studded with white pustules. Whether the candida micro-organism is a primary pathogen in this clinical situation or merely an aggravating secondary invader is unknown.

The candida micro-organism may also cause infection of the nail plate and has a role in the perpetuation and possibly precipitation of chronic paronychia, although mechanical factors are also believed to be of importance in the latter. In chronic paronychia the paronychial tissues are swollen and red and the cuticle is lost (Figure 8.15). Pus occasionally oozes from beneath the

folds. Continual maceration of the tissues by the trapping of water under the nail fold is believed to be of importance aetiologically.

Thrush is the clinical term often used for mucosal candidiasis. In the elderly it occurs in the mouth in the course of severe illness, especially when oral feeding is curtailed or salivary function diminished. The affected area is usually bright red and sore looking, but has white plaques superimposed. There is a not dissimilar appearance of the vaginal mucosa in vulvovaginal thrush—occasionally a problem in elderly women especially if they have diabetes. Candidal balanoposthitis is rare in elderly men. Mucocutaneous candidiasis with monilial granulomata due to some type of immunoparesis is a very rare problem in the elderly.

Systemic candidiasis always has to be considered as a possible complication of widespread candidiasis of skin or mucosae, but is not within the scope of this book.

Most of the agents used topically for ringworm infections are also effective for candidiasis, but others are also available, including nystatin, 5–fluorocytosine, amphotericin B and fluconazole. Many of the latter have no effect in other types of skin infection, but fluconazole has found a particular place in the treatment of immunocompromised patients with systemic candidiasis such as those with AIDS. Nystatin solutions are particularly helpful for mucosal candidiasis.

Trichomycosis axillaris

This mild infection of the axillary hairs is now somewhat uncommon as a result of improved hygiene. The hair shafts are granular and discoloured according to the pigment-producing capacity of the various fungi responsible. Shaving the affected sites and instruction on adequate washing is usually sufficient.

Bacterial infections

Erythrasma

The exact taxonomic status of the micro-organism causing this disorder is uncertain. It seems to

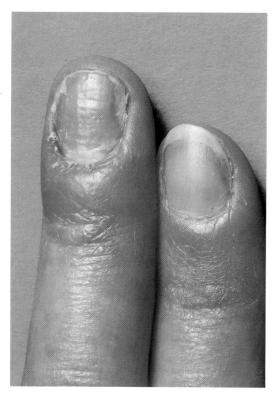

Figure 8.15a

Chronic paronychia. Notice the heaped up paronychial tissues.

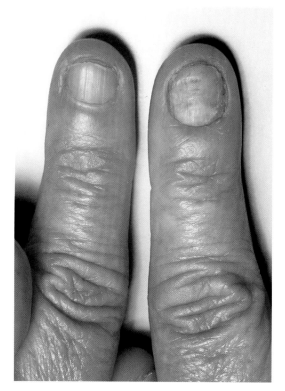

Figure 8.15b

Chronic paronychia of one finger. Notice the absence of eponychium and the deformed nail plate.

fit in more with the Propionibacterium group than any other and has been called *Corynebacterium minutissimum*. The disorder affects the flexures predominantly, causing slightly pink and scaly patches (Figure 8.16). It occurs in those individuals who do not wash frequently and is not uncommon in socially deprived elderly men. It has to be differentiated clinically from ringworm and seborrhoeic dermatitis but as the condition causes less inflammation and involves larger areas than either of these there is generally little difficulty in its identification. A Wood's ultraviolet lamp shone on the affected zone will often reveal a characteristic coral pink fluorescence (Figure 8.17). If skin surface biopsies are taken from the affected region and stained with periodic acid Schiff reagent, microcolonies of small rod-like structures will be evident (Figure 8.18). Often these have an angulated arrangement like Chinese lettering. The micro-organism can sometimes be cultured from skin scrapings using special culture media.

The condition is responsive to the same topical agents as ringworm as well as the use of detergent antibacterial products when washing such as povidone iodine and hexachlorophane-containing materials. There was a vogue for the use of systemic antibiotics as the disorder also responds to these, but in reality systemic treatments are unnecessary.

Erysipelas

Before antibiotics were available, this was a much feared disorder that sometimes killed old

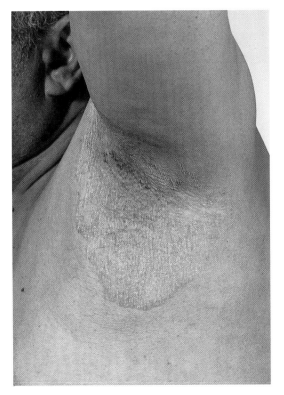

Figure 8.16

Erythrasma infection of the axillary region in an elderly man.

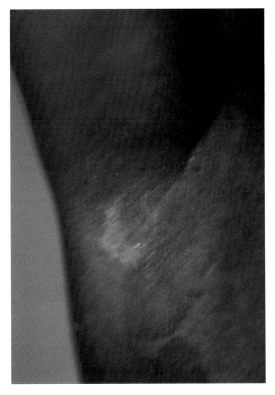

Figure 8.17

Coral pink fluorescence due to erythrasma.

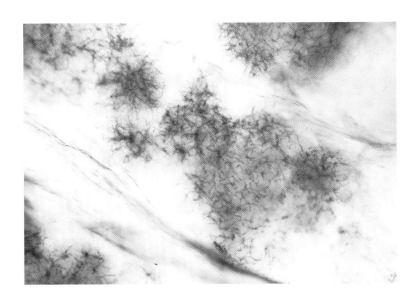

Figure 8.18

Microcolonies of the micro-organism causing erythrasma, seen in a skin surface biopsy. (Periodic acid Schiff stain; ×90).

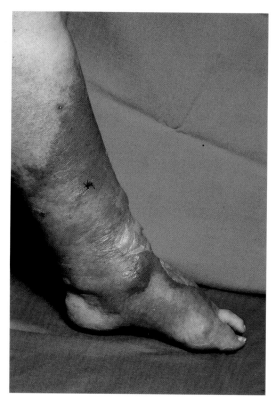

Figure 8.19

Erysipelas affecting the lower leg. This patient was quite severely ill with the disorder. Note the large blister above the ankle.

marked by extreme tissue oedema and haemorrhage. In recent years erysipelas has been increasing in frequency especially in the elderly and the immunocompromised.[27]

Treatment is at first with large doses of penicillin. Local treatment directed to the exudative or necrotic area will also be required.

Erysipeloid

This infective condition, caused by an organism known as *Erysipelothrix rhusiopathiae*, must now be considered rare. Classically it causes areas of intense erythema and swelling after minor injury and was seen particularly in butchers. It responds rapidly to penicillin or other antibiotics.

Cellulitis

Cellulitis is a non-specific term indicating subcutaneous soft tissue infection. It often occurs around leg ulcers and if untreated can spread to cause septicaemia. The affected area is diffusely swollen, pink and tender. There is more or less systemic upset dependent on the virulence of the micro-organisms involved and the size of the area affected. On the legs, care should be taken to distinguish cellulitis from the effect of a deep vein thrombosis or superficial thrombophlebitis. It may be necessary to inject ^{131}I-tagged fibrinogen and 'scan' the limb to determine whether there is a deep vein thrombosis.

It is rarely possible to ascertain which micro-organism is involved and it is wise to start treatment with broad spectrum antibiotics. A frequent initial regimen is a combination of cephradine and cloxacillin. Subsequent treatment depends on the patient's response.

Boils and carbuncles

These are essentially forms of folliculitis of varying degrees of severity. They are usually caused by a pyogenic *Staphylococcus aureus*. Crops of lesions may be due to colonization of the nose or

people. The disease is now much less common but is still sometimes seen and can cause serious illness. It appears to be caused by a virulent beta haemolytic streptococcus. It is very difficult to recover the micro-organism from the lesion and the intense inflammation may represent a hypersensitivity reaction to small numbers of cocci.

The condition seems to be most common on the face and legs, although anywhere may be affected. At first the infected site is swollen, well-defined, red, tender and painful, and there is fever and malaise. Within a day or two the area spreads, becomes haemorrhagic and sometimes bullous and exudative. When severe, tissue necrosis occurs that can be extensive and destructive enough to require subsequent grafting (Figure 8.19). Histologically the condition is perineum with a particularly unpleasant staphylococcus that has decided to take up residence. A carbuncle is a massive colliquative area of inflammation that usually starts off as an angry boil. At one time the disorder had an appreciable mortality in the elderly. It is now less frequently seen and is usually responsive to antibiotics. However, antibiotic resistance of the staphylococcus is quite common and the organism should be cultured for its antibiotic sensitivities.

Impetigo contagiosa

This is a superficial infection of the skin by either a staphylococcus or a combination of a staphylococcus and a streptococcus. It occurs in minor epidemics amongst schoolchildren but the adult population appears immune.

Syphilis

This venereal disease, caused by the spirochaete known as *Treponema pallidum*, is now uncommon in the UK. It is, however, still occasionally seen in ports and among the homosexual population. The primary chancre and the secondary forms are rare for obvious reasons in the elderly population, but the tertiary form is worth a brief mention as elderly persons may present with this stage of the disease, having been infected many years before. In the skin the tertiary form (syphilitic gumma) is a slowly progressive ulcer, indurated plaque or nodule containing destructive areas of chronic inflammation, which causes the eventual ulceration. The diagnosis is confirmed by serological tests and by biopsy. Treatment is with a prolonged course of penicillin, but for details the reader is referred to King et al.[28]

Cutaneous tuberculosis

Although tuberculosis was considered under control, there is now an alarming world-wide increase in the disease and fresh cases continue to occur. The older population seems particularly at risk from reactivation of long-standing quiescent foci when their immunological defences are in some way compromised. This reactivation generally concerns the lungs, or occasionally the kidneys. The skin is not usually involved. Very rarely such reactivated lesions become progressive and cause miliary tuberculosis and then small inflammatory lesions of tuberculosis may appear in the skin. Immunocompromised patients, such as those with AIDS or those receiving immunosuppressive treatment for organ transplants or autoimmune disease are especially at risk of contracting the disease.

Patients with long-standing lupus vulgaris still occasionally present in the clinic, their lesions having been continuously present for the previous 30 or 40 years or longer. This condition is a slowly progressive area of destructive granulomatous inflammation of the skin caused by *Mycobacterium tuberculosis* and hypersensitivity to it. Any area of skin may be affected but the face seems to be particularly at risk. Although ulceration of the skin is not usual in lupus vulgaris, the tissue necrosis that occurs causes unpleasant scarring. When the disease was rife the scarring was a major cause of facial disfigurement. The lesions are large, red, irregular plaques which may contain areas of thin atrophic scar tissue (Figure 8.20). Pressure with a glass slide makes the area blanch, leaving brownish-yellow nodules ('apple jelly nodules') within the lesion. Biopsy reveals a characteristic pathological appearance with tuberculoid granulomata but little caseation necrosis. Special staining techniques to identify the mycobacterium are sometimes successful but there are often remarkably few bacteria in the lesions of lupus vulgaris and they are difficult to find.

It used to be said that it was perfectly in order to treat lupus vulgaris with isoniazid alone, that there was no danger of bacterial resistance developing and the therapeutic response was gratifying. It now appears prudent to ignore this older approach and institute formal anti-tuberculosis combination therapy.[29]

Other forms of cutaneous tuberculosis

Warty tuberculosis (tuberculosis verrucosa cutis) is rare and not often seen in the elderly, although

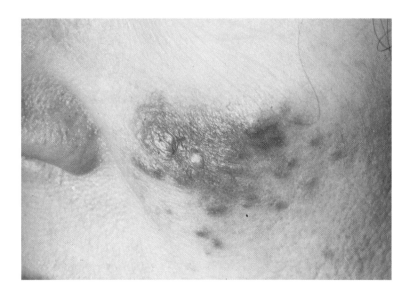

Figure 8.20a

Lupus vulgaris affecting the cheek.

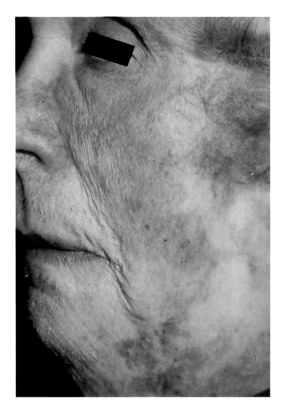

Figure 8.20b

Severe scarring and irregular pigmentation of the face in a woman who had had lupus vulgaris.

elderly post-mortem attendants used to contract this type of tuberculous infection from handling infected cadavers (prosectors' warts). Tuberculous ulcers and sinuses are now also rare and hardly ever seen in the elderly.

Other mycobacterial disorders

Occasionally infection of the skin occurs with micro-organisms similar in many respects to those causing tuberculosis. Those of particular relevance to Europe and possible importance for the elderly include *Mycobacterium balnei*, causing swimming bath granuloma, and various types of avian mycobacteria. Swimming bath granulomata are areas of granulomatous infection that develop on the knees and elbows, in particular at the site of minor abrasions sustained during swimming— a sport often encouraged in the elderly. Avian tuberculosis can infect the skin of those looking after cage birds and as the elderly are often keen on this pastime this possibility should be borne in mind in the case of an odd persistent inflamed swelling on the fingers (or lips: one famous patient fed her canary from her own lips).

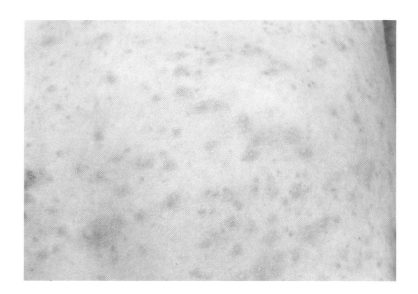

Figure 8.21a

Irregular papules and vesicles on the trunk due to scabies.

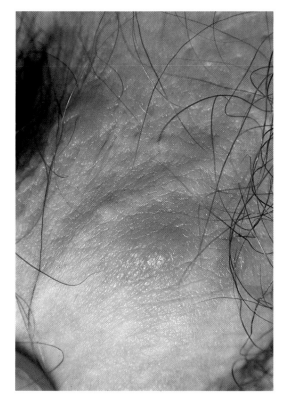

Figure 8.21b

Large persistent papules on the genitalia due to scabies.

Scabies

Scabies is due to infestation with the mite *Sarcoptes scabiei*. The responsible mite is specific to humans and usually contracted by intimate skin-to-skin contact. As this implies venereal contact, it may be thought that the disease is uncommon in the elderly, but this is not the case. Scabies is often a family disease and affectionate friendly familial contact appears sufficient to contract the disorder. In addition, the disease occasionally runs riot in an old persons' home or a geriatric ward—presumably nursing contact is sufficient to spread the mite.[30]

In the late 1960s and early 1970s there was a pandemic of scabies and the disease was extremely common. In recent years it has settled down to modest endemic proportions, being uncomfortably common at times but rare at others. Colloquially the disease is known with considerable justification as 'the itch'. The itch that it produces is severe and constant but worse at night. The scratching caused by the itching is responsible for most (but not all) of the rash that appears, particularly over the wrists, elbows, shoulders, buttocks, genitalia, knees and ankles, although anywhere below the neck can be affected. The rash consists mainly of crusted excoriations, but there is also a primary eczematous component that may be due to hypersensitivity to the products of the mite (Figure 8.21). In addition,

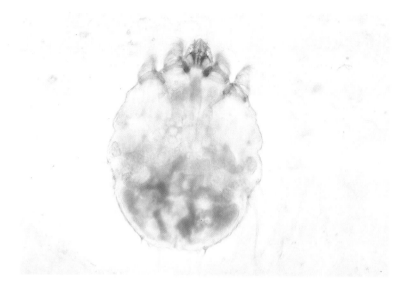

Figure 8.22

Scabies mite.

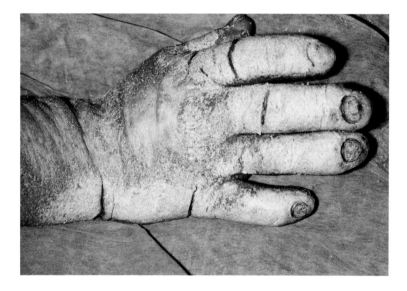

Figure 8.23

Thickened, crusted lesions due to severe infestation with scabies ('Norwegian scabies').

the burrows (runs) of the female scabies mite can also be seen at the sites detailed above and often over the palms and soles and at the sides of the fingers. Diagnosis is confirmed by identification of the female mite or its eggs from one of the burrows. These are extracted with a needle (an impressive skill of older dermatologists) or scraped off the skin with a scalpel blade and the debris examined, or the skin surface sampled using the skin surface biopsy technique using a quick bonding cyanoacrylate adhesive (Figure 8.22).

A variant of ordinary scabies that may be relevant to the older population is known as Norwegian scabies. It occurs particularly in immunosuppressed individuals and those who for some reason are too inert to scratch efficiently. Vast numbers of the mites inhabit crusted accretions on the skin, giving a bizarre clinical appearance. The condition is extremely contagious and nursing and medical staff of old persons' homes afflicted by this problem are often also affected (Figure 8.23).

The treatment of scabies has been based on one of the miticidal agents benzyl benzoate, gammexane or malathion. They are equally effective and safe if used properly, although the former may be slightly more irritating to the skin than the others. Permethrin, a recently introduced synthetic analogue of pyrethrum, is a probably more effective and safer option.[31] All are used as lotions that are painted on to the skin all over the body (literally all over, regardless of where the lesions appear to be) apart from the head and neck. It is usual to ask those to be treated to take a bath first then to paint on the chosen application. After the application has dried, a second application is made. Nothing more is done then until 24 hours later, when a further application is used. All members of the household (or ward) in which there is an affected member should be treated simultaneously to prevent those who are incubating the infestation from developing it and spreading the problem further. Although the regimen described should eliminate the mite it does not eliminate the itch for 3–4 weeks, so that it is a kindness to give patients some type of antipruritic topical application for use after the miticidal applications have been employed. Oily calamine lotion with 0.25% menthol is usually appreciated.

Pediculosis

Head lice are mostly found in children and are rare in old age. Pediculosis pubis (caused by crab lice) is essentially a venereal disorder and again, extremely uncommon in old age. Pediculosis corporis is in general uncommon, but is occasionally seen in the elderly vagrant. The louse and its eggs can be identified on body hair and on the clothes. Treatment is by disinfestation of the clothes and applications of permethrin to the patient, who often requires social assistance.

References

1 Nagel J E. Immunology. In: *Review of Biological Research In Ageing*, (Alan R Liss: New York, 1983) 103–60.

2 Finkelstein M S. Defences against infection in the elderly: the compromises of ageing. *Triangle* (1984) **23:**57–64.

3 Shigemoto S, Kishimoto S, Yamamura Y. Change of cell mediated cytotoxicity with ageing. *J Immunol* (1975) **115:**307–9.

4 Grossman J, Baum J, Gluckman J et al. The effect of ageing and acute illness on delayed hypersensitivity. *J Allergy Clin Immunol* (1975) **55:**268–75.

5 Lejman E, Stoudemayer T, Grove G et al. Age differences in poison ivy dermatitis. *Contact Dermatitis* (1984) **11:**163–7.

6 Grove G L, Lavker R M, Hölzle E et al. Use of non intrusive tests to monitor age associated changes in human skin. *J Soc Cosmetic Chem* (1980) **32:**15–26.

7 Thiers B H, Maize J C, Spicer S S et al. The effect of ageing and chronic sun exposure on human Langerhans cell populations. *J Invest Dermatol* (1984) **82:**223–6.

8 Howells C H, Vesselinova-Jenkins C K, Evans A D. Influenza vaccination and mortality from bronchopneumonia in the elderly. *Lancet* (1975) **ii:**381.

9 Palmer D L, Rifkind D, Brun D W. [131]–Labelled colloidal human serum albumin in the study of reticuloendothelial system function II. Phagocytosis and catabolism of a test colloid in normal subjects. *J Infect Dis* (1971) **123:**457–64.

10 Teller M N. Age changes and immune resistance to cancer. *Adv Gerontol Res* (1972) **4:**25–9.

11 Phair J P, Kauffman C A, Bjornson A et al. Host defences in the aged: evaluation of components of the inflammatory and immune responses. *J Infect Dis* (1978) **138:**67–73.

12 Eaglestein W H, Katz R, Brown J A. The effects of early corticosteroid therapy on the skin eruption and pain of herpes zoster. *J Am Med Assoc* (1970) **211:**681–3.

13 Bean B, Braun C, Balfour H H Jr. Acyclovir therapy for acute herpes zoster. *Lancet* (1982); 118–21.

14 Pereira F A. Herpes simplex: evolving concepts. *J Am Acad Dermatol* (1996) **35:**503–20.

15 Jablonska S, Orth G. Human papoviruses. In: Rook A, Maibach H I, eds, *Recent Advances in Dermatology*, Vol 6, (Blackwell: Oxford, 1983) 1–36.

16 Woodruff J D, Braun L, Cavalieri R et al. Immunological identification of papillomavirus antigen in paraffin processed condyloma tissues from the female genital tract. *Obstet Gynaecol* (1980) **56:**727–32.

17 Majeivski S, Jablonska S. Human papillomavirus-associated tumours of the skin and mucosa. *J Am Acad Dermatol* (1997) **36:**658–85.

18 Kitchen L W, Barin F, Sullivan J L et al. Aetiology of AIDS antibodies to human T cell leukaemia

virus (type III) in haemophiliacs. *Nature* (1984) **312:**367–9.

19   Farthing C F, Staughton R C D, Rowland Payne C M E. Skin disease in homosexual patients with acquired immunodeficiency syndrome (AIDS) and lesser forms of human T cell leukaemia virus (HTLV.III) disease. *Clin Exp Dermatol* (1985) **10:**3–12.

20   James W D, Redfield R R, Lupton G P et al. A papular eruption associated with human T cell lymphotropic virus type III disease. *J Am Acad Dermatol* (1985) **13:**563–6.

21   Marks R, Dawber R P R. In situ microbiology of the stratum corneum. *Arch Dermatol* (1972) **105:**216–21.

22   Ive A F, Marks R. Tinea incognito. *Br Med J* (1968) **3:**149–52.

23   Moberg S. Tinea capitis in the elderly. A report on two cases caused by Trichophyton tonsurans. *Dermatologica* (1984) **169:**36–40.

24   Svejgaard E. Immunologic investigations of dermatophytes and dermatophytosis. *Semin Dermatol* (1985) **4:**201–21.

25   Eleweski B E. Diagnostic techniques for confirming onychomycosis. *J Am Acad Dermatol* (1996) **35:**S6–S9.

26   Odom R. New therapies for onychomycosis. *J Am Acad Dermatol* (1996) **35:**S26–S30.

27   Bratton R L, Nesse R E. St Anthony's Fire: diagnosis and management of erysipelas. *Am Fam Phys* (1995) **5:**401–4.

28   King A, Nicol C, Rodin P. *Venereal Diseases*, 4th Edn (Balliere Tindall: London, 1981).

29   Grosset J H. Present status of chemotherapy for tuberculosis. *Rev Infect Dis* (1989) **11**(suppl 2): 347–52.

30   Jimenez-Lucho V E, Fallon F, Caputo C, Ramsay K. Role of prolonged surveillance in the eradication of nosocomial scabies in an extended care veterans affairs medical centre. *Am J Infect Control* (1995) **23:**44–9.

31   Schulz M W, Gomez M, Hansen R C et al. Comparative study of 5% permethrin cream and 1% lindane lotion for the treatment of scabies. *Arch Dermatol* (1990) **126:**167–70.

9
Neoplastic disorders of skin

The skin contains many different cell types and virtually all are subject to neoplastic transformation.

Neoplastic disease of the epidermis

Skin tumours composed primarily of epidermal tissue are the most common neoplastic lesions of humans. Viral warts and mollusca contagiosa, which can rightfully claim a place in this section, are dealt with in the chapter on skin infections.

Benign epidermal tumours

Seborrhoeic warts (basal cell papillomas)

Most elderly people have a few of these benign excrescences. They increase in numbers with the passing of the years like barnacles on a rusting hulk. Some unfortunate patients have vast numbers of these lesions and their sudden appearance has been thought of as a form of acanthosis nigricans and associated with visceral malignant disease.[1] They may occur anywhere on hair-bearing skin but are especially common in light-exposed sites. So called 'senile lentigines' are a well recognized mark of chronic photodamage and should be known as solar lentigines. These flat brown macules often have features of seborrhoeic warts and it is interesting to speculate on the relationship of thicker more obvious basal cell papillomata with persistent sun exposure.

Seborrhoeic warts vary in colour from a dull fawn or even skin colour to jet black, but mostly are a uniform light brown. As their name implies, they have a warty or at least a roughened surface (Figure 9.1). They vary in size from 2 or 3 mm in diameter to large plaques 2 or 3 cm across (Figure 9.2).

Typically they appear to be stuck on to the skin surface although some lesions become extruded and papillomatous. Others remain flat, especially those on the back of the hand (Figure 9.3). These are sometimes known as senile lentigines or by the more fanciful French term, *les medallions de cimitière*. Similar lesions are seen in the temporal region. They gradually increase in size over the years. They may suddenly enlarge and become inflamed if irritated. Generally they do not give rise to symptoms but are a nuisance cosmetically. Occasionally they may irritate or become sore if irritated but more frequent reasons for complaint are fear that they are some form of cancer or that they catch in the patient's clothes.

Pigmented lesions often give rise to problems in clinical diagnosis. Even the most experienced of dermatologists can claim at best an accuracy of only about 70%.[2] Malignant melanoma, lentigo maligna, benign melanocytic naevus, pigmented basal cell carcinoma, histiocytoma and solar keratosis have all to be differentiated from seborrhoeic warts. Generally the history, the uniformity of pigmentation and the crumbling horn on the surface allow a positive diagnosis, but bear in mind that with this type of lesion confidence in diagnosis is a sign of inexperience. Flat, brown, pigmented lesions over the sides of the face also cause difficulties in clinical diagnosis. Even the experienced dermatologist may not be able to distinguish a flat seborrhoeic wart, a lentigo, a lentigo maligna and a pigmented solar keratosis. Even histologically the diagnostic category may

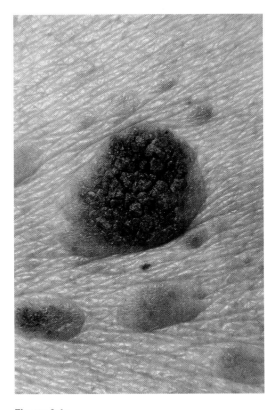

Figure 9.1a

Typical seborrhoeic wart.

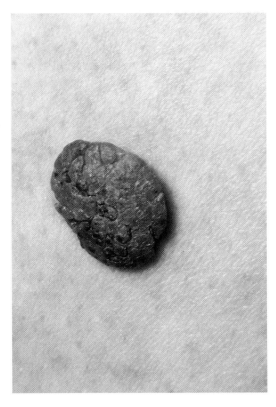

Figure 9.1b

Typical seborrhoeic wart with more pedunculated appearance.

not be clear cut.[3,4] The main differential diagnoses of a warty lesion and of a pigmented lesion are set out in Tables 9.1 and 9.2 respectively.

Pathology

There is a well-defined area of epidermal thickening surmounted by warty hyperkeratosis. The cells are small or medium-sized and basophilic. The tumour contains rounded cyst-like structures of lamellated horn and sometimes areas of degenerative change (Figure 9.4). When irritated there may be areas with many mitotic figures in which the cells are irregularly arranged. These may be mistaken for squamous cell carcinoma. The epidermal surface of seborrhoeic warts is irregular and often thrown up into a series of peaks. The base of the lesion is also irregular and often infiltrated with inflammatory cells.

Very little is known of the origin of these common benign epithelial tumours. Their appearance at photodamaged sites may suggest that they arise in skin in which growth controls have been damaged.

Treatment

If there is no doubt as to the diagnosis but the patient would still like to have the lesion removed, the simplest and least damaging ablative procedures should be used. Curettage and light cautery are the most suitable, but cryotherapy may also be used.

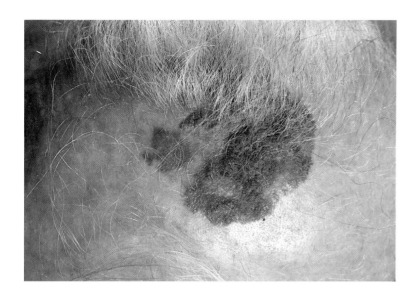

Figure 9.2a

Flat plaque-like seborrhoeic wart. These lesions can reach large sizes.

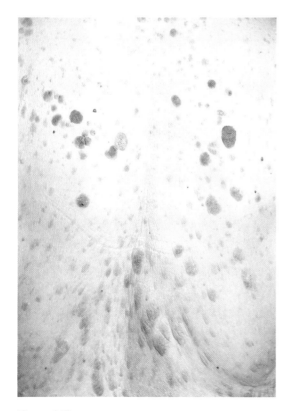

Figure 9.2b

Multiple seborrhoeic warts on the back of a man aged 82.

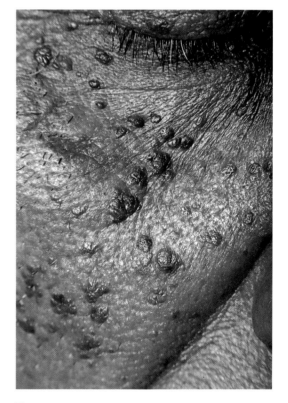

Figure 9.2c

Dermatosis papulosa nigra. Black, slightly warty papules on the cheek of an elderly black patient. These lesions are thought to be similar to seborrhoeic warts.

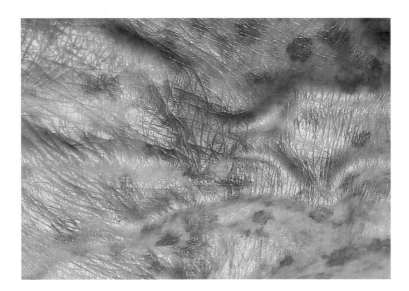

Figure 9.3

Flat, lentigo-like seborrhoeic warts affecting the back of the hand.

Table 9.1   Commoner warty tumours

Lesion	Distinguishing features
Seborrhoeic wart	Flat, stuck on appearance is typical with uniform pigmentation in older population
Viral warts	Usually multiple and non-pigmented, mostly in younger age groups
Keratoacanthoma	Rapidly enlarging nodule with central horn-filled crater
Squamous cell carcinoma	Rapidly growing warty plaque or nodule in older individuals
Solar keratoses	Slightly raised scaling or warty lesions with diffuse margins; may have slight pigmentation
Bowen's disease	Warty or scaling reddened plaque (often psoriasiform) on limbs or trunk
Epidermal naevus	Linear or zosteriform or plaque like lesion slowly enlarging in infancy only

Table 9.2   Differential diagnosis of malignant melanoma

Lesion	Distinguishing features
Seborrhoeic wart	Lesion is warty and usually uniformly pigmented
Pigmented basal cell carcinoma	Slow-growing smooth nodule usually flecked by pigment although sometimes uniformly pigmented
Histiocytoma	Firm intracutaneous brown nodule; may have scaly or hard surface
Inflamed mole	Often is hairy brown nodule; no change in pigmentation
Pyogenic granuloma	Vary rapidly enlarging sessile nodule without pigmentation

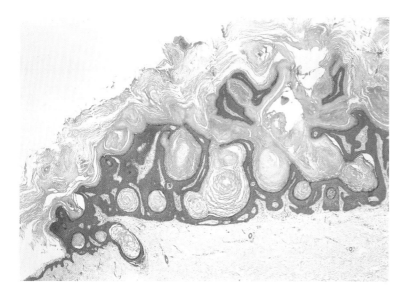

Figure 9.4

Pathology of seborrhoeic wart, showing typical 'stuck-on' appearance, warty surface and horny cysts (H & E; ×15).

Skin tags

The true nature of these extremely common excrescences is uncertain. Many seem to be extruded seborrhoeic warts but others have no sign of any warty thickening and may bear no relation to these lesions. Skin tags occur in the elderly obese subject in the flexural areas and around the front of the neck. They are unsightly and may cause irritation. If required, they can be removed by cautery.

Inverted follicular keratoses

Although many consider that these lesions are a type of hair follicle tumour, they have several histological features suggestive of seborrhoeic warts. There is a similar histological appearance to that of an irritated seborrhoeic wart but the bulk of the tumour is below the general epidermal surface unlike the ordinary seborrhoeic wart, which appears to be stuck on. They generally occur on the face around the nose as small dome-shaped nodules in older individuals. They were thought to arise from follicular structures—hence their name. They are often mistaken for squamous cell carcinomas because of their irritated appearance (see earlier) and because they are generally subsurface.

Degos acanthoma (clear cell acanthoma)

Degos acanthoma is an uncommon, benign epidermal tumour occurring predominantly on the limbs of middle aged and elderly individuals. The surface often appears pink and moist and they are frequently mistaken for amelanotic melanoma or pyogenic granuloma. They have the curious property of persisting unchanged for several years. Several patients have been described in whom multiple lesions have developed.[5]

Histologically Degos acanthoma may bear an uncomfortable resemblance to psoriasis. The thickened epidermis is very psoriasiform and is infiltrated by neutrophils. Staining with periodic acid Schiff reagent reveals that the cells of the lesions are loaded with glycogen. Treatment is by surgical removal or cryotherapy.

Warty epidermal naevus

These are not uncommon, benign, congenital epidermal tumours which occur in a number of clinical forms. Consultation for these lesions occurs generally in childhood or adolescence, although they usually persist throughout life.

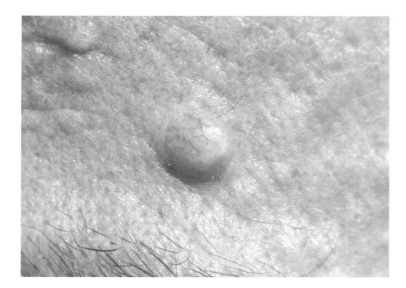

Figure 9.5

Trichoepithelioma. This lesion looked a little like a basal cell carcinoma, but was found to be a trichoepithelioma.

They are often linear or zosteriform. Apart from the cosmetic problems that they may cause, squamous cell carcinoma or basal cell carcinoma can develop within their substance. Some epidermal naevi are psoriasiform and strangely inflammatory.

Treatment is by surgical excision. Cryotherapy and curettage and cautery may also be employed.

Naevus sebaceous of Jadassohn

This lesion is a variety of epidermal naevus in which all epidermal elements may be involved, but in particular there is gross and irregular enlargement of the sebaceous glands. The great majority of these lesions occur on the scalp as small orange, occasionally warty nodules. Although these are more often a management problem in the paediatric clinic, they are subject to neoplastic change in later life and are worthy of description here for this reason if for no other. Basal cell carcinoma and adnexal tumours such as syringocystadenoma papilliferum arise in perhaps 10–25% of the lesions of naevus sebaceous.[6] Treatment is by surgical excision.

Benign adnexal tumours

Tumours arising from the hair follicles and the eccrine or apocrine glands are referred to as adnexal tumours. Although clinical diagnosis is possible in some instances the true nature of many lesions is revealed only by histological examination. A brief outline is included here and for a full description the reader is advised to consult standard histological texts such as Lever and Schaumberg–Lever[7] and Pinkus and Mehregan.[8]

Tumours with hair follicle differentiation

Trichoepithelioma

These may be single or multiple. When multiple they may occur in large numbers over the scalp and sometimes the face (Figure 9.5). They are mostly slow growing, skin-coloured intracutaneous nodules 3 mm to 1 cm in size, but may be mistaken for nodular basal cell carcinoma as sometimes they have a more translucent appearance. Histologically they may also be difficult to distinguish from basal cell carcinoma. Typically they consist of rounded masses of basaloid cells that show antler-like branching and contain tiny horny cysts.

Trichofolliculoma

These rare, solitary lesions emulate hair follicle structures more closely than other hair follicle derived tumours. They consist of branching, epithelial-lined, sinus-like structures which open in a pore at the skin surface.

Pilomatrixoma (calcifying epithelioma of Malherbe)

Clinically, pilomatrixoma is a solitary, skin-coloured or slightly bluish nodule consisting of basaloid cells that undergo a characteristic type of mummification. In the lesion there are lobules with a rim of basaloid cells that become abruptly transformed into a faintly basophilic homogeneous substance containing ghost-like outlines of the epithelial cells towards the centre. The condition is often said to be strongly associated with solar damage, but the evidence for this is scanty.

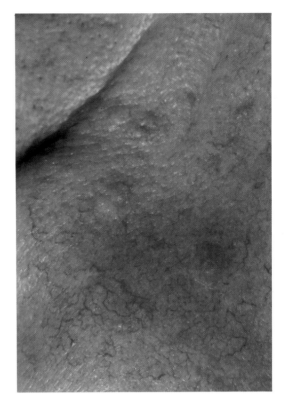

Figure 9.6

Small nodules of sebaceous gland hyperplasia.

Sebaceous adenoma

These are very unusual, slowly growing nodules of abnormal sebaceous gland tissue in the elderly. They mostly develop over the face as orange or yellowish smooth nodules.

Sebaceous gland hyperplasia

This condition is not strictly neoplastic but is described here for convenience. It is a common disorder of elderly skin that mainly affects the face. It occurs after the age of 60 but is occasionally seen in the fifth and sixth decades. Skin-coloured or slightly yellowish nodules which may have a central pore appear (Figure 9.6). They grow very slowly to 2–5 mm in diameter and cause no symptoms. Their main importance apart from their appearance is the fact that they are frequently mistaken for nodular basal cell carcinoma. In general they are less translucent in appearance and are not traversed by telangiectatic blood vessels so that, with care, distinction from basal cell carcinoma is usually possible. They consist of sebaceous gland lobules which are often quite high in the dermis and which are abnormally large but of normal appearance. No adequate explanation has been advanced for their development. They do not appear to be associated with sun damage.[9]

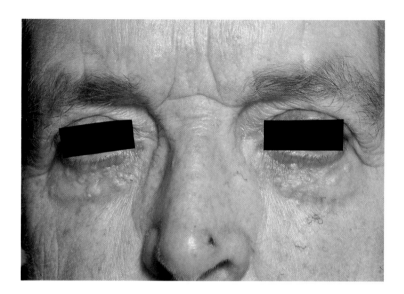

Figure 9.7

Syringoma. There are small white papules beneath the eyes in this elderly patient.

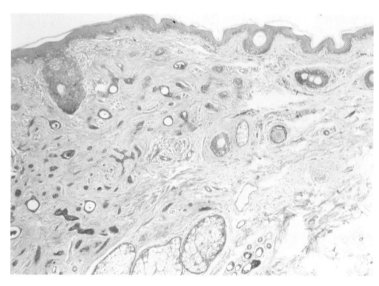

Figure 9.8

Pathology of syringoma. There are many small comma-shaped and angulated epithelial structures as well as several small cystic structures in the upper dermis (H & E; ×15).

Tumours with differentiation towards sweat glands

Syringoma

Syringomata are more often multiple than solitary and mostly present between the ages of 20 and 40 but tend to persist unchanged. They have the propensity of developing in large numbers quite rapidly over the face, particularly beneath the eyes, and over the front of the lower trunk, when they are known as hidradenome eruptif. The lesions are small (1–3 mm) and milky white (Figure 9.7). Around the eyes they are often mistaken for milia. Their histological appearance is typical, consisting of short, comma-shaped epithelial structures, branching tubular structures and tiny horn filled cysts (Figure 9.8). The connective tissue surrounding the epithelial structures

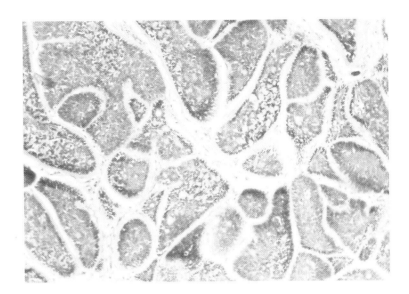

Figure 9.9

Pathology of cylindroma. There are many lobules of basaloid epithelial cells which seem to fit together in a jigsaw type of pattern. Some of the lobules are surrounded by a pinky 'colloid' type of material; many others contain small areas of cystic degenerative change (H & E; ×45).

has a distinctive quality in places, as it does in most of the sweat gland tumours, with material of eosinophilic homogeneous appearance. Occasionally morphoeic basal cell carcinoma may have a similar histological appearance.

Nodular hidradenoma

These are skin-coloured, solitary nodules that consist of relatively undifferentiated lobules of basaloid cells interspersed with some larger clear cells and with a few slit-like ductular spaces. If they consist of clear cells predominantly they are known as clear cell hidradenomas.

Eccrine poroma

This and a deeper variant known as the dermal duct tumour consist of a mass or masses of small basaloid cells. Although solitary lesions are the rule, patients have been described with large numbers of lesions. They are often but not always found on the sole of the foot and palm of the hand.

Eccrine spiradenoma

This rare nodular lesion consists of lobules of eccrine derived epithelium among which are numerous vascular channels. It has the doubtful distinction of being one of the few benign tumours of skin that may give rise to pain spontaneously.

Syringocystadenoma papilliferum

This unusual lesion often arises from a pre-existing epithelial naevus of the scalp but may arise de novo elsewhere over the trunk, particularly in women, on the mons pubis. It consists of a central cavity whose walls have two cell layers and develop pouching opening on to the skin surface. The stroma usually has many plasma cells.

Cylindroma

Although not common, these are among the least infrequent of adnexal tumours. The tumours usually arise over the scalp in moderately large numbers as skin-coloured nodules 3–10 mm in diameter (turban tumours). Histologically they are unmistakable, consisting of lobules that are irregular but faceted together like a jigsaw puzzle (Figure 9.9). There are two cell types in the lobules—small dark cells and larger clear cells. Around each lobule there is a band of pale pink homogeneous clear colloid-like material. The tendency to develop these is in some cases inherited as a dominant characteristic.

Hidrocystomas

These are rare, cyst-like epithelial structures containing ductular elements which occur over the face. They may have a bluish appearance clinically.

Common cysts derived from epidermis

Epidermoid cysts

These are common at all ages. Clinically they are plainly cystic, variable in size (up to 2 or 3 cm in diameter) and are subject to episodes of inflammation with pain and tenderness. They occur virtually anywhere over the skin surface. They contain lamellated horn, the arrangement resembling that of an onion. The lining epidermis is very similar to normal interfollicular epidermis with a prominent granular cell layer.

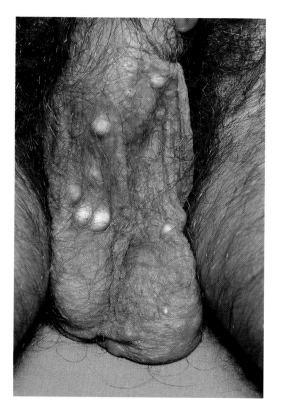

Figure 9.10

Typical pilar scrotal cysts.

Milia

Milia are tiny intracutaneous epidermoid cysts that arise from damaged adnexal structures. They frequently occur in skin affected by blistering and are commonly found after the blisters of porphyria cutanea tarda, epidermolysis bullosa or pemphigoid have subsided. They are particularly common around the eyes.

Pilar cysts (trichilemmal cysts)

Pilar cysts are formed by epithelium derived from the hair follicle external root sheath. They are often multiple. Individual lesions clinically resemble epidermoid cysts. They are sometimes inherited as a dominant trait. They are mostly found on the scalp and often occur in the elderly. They are also found on the scrotum (Figure 9.10). They are also subject to episodes of inflammation with pain and tenderness. Differences from epidermoid cysts are that in pilar cysts the horn is less clearly lamellated and the lining epithelium of the cyst wall has no granular cell layer and transformation into horn is more gradual.

Proliferating pilar cysts

These are an uncommon complication of ordinary pilar cysts which are mostly found in elderly women. The cyst wall becomes hyperplastic and lobulated, sometimes producing a large tumour of the scalp. Occasionally they become truly invasive and neoplastic.

Steatocystoma multiplex (sebocystoma multiplex)

It should be noted that the solitary lesions commonly referred to as sebaceous cysts are misnomers. The term is used incorrectly to describe epidermoid cysts whose centre decomposes, producing a foul smelling, viscid, greyish necrotic material incorrectly assumed to be derived from sebum. True sebum-containing cysts are uncommon. They are usually multiple—sometimes occurring in large numbers. The lesions are small (2–4 mm in diameter), dome-shaped, skin-coloured or bluish nodules. Histologically the cystic spaces are lined either by epidermal cells producing horn or by sebaceous gland cells. Often nodules of sebaceous glands are present in the wall of the cysts. The condition of steatocystoma multiplex is in some cases heritable.

Treatment

Treatment of all the benign adnexal lesions is similar. Surgical excision is indicated if there is any doubt as to the nature of the lesion, if the lesion impairs function or it is a cosmetic nuisance. Other forms of removal are less satisfactory although there are advocates of cautery, diathermy, laser ablation or cryosurgery.

Premalignant and malignant disease of the epidermis

Solar (senile) keratoses

Solar keratoses are extremely common premalignant lesions that occur in the light-exposed areas of the skin of elderly individuals with increasing frequency after the age of 60. In one Australian survey they were found to occur in 56.9% of the population over 40 in one town.[10]

They are much more common in fair-skinned individuals and those of Celtic ancestry. In one survey in South Wales solar keratoses were found in approximately 25% of those over 60 and were also more common in the fair-skinned types.[11] There is no doubt as to their relationship with cumulated damage from solar UV radiation (see also Chapter 2) as the prevalence of these lesions is directly related to the total dose of solar energy received.[12,13] They are much more common in sunny climates and in those who are occupationally or recreationally continually exposed to the sun. None the less they may also occur at sites of chronic heat injury and are a well known complication of erythema ab igne[14] (the reticulate patterning seen on the legs of the elderly from sitting in front of the fire). They were also quite often seen as a side-effect of the chronic medicinal use of arsenic when this was in vogue.[15]

Although premalignant, only a very small proportion of keratoses transform to frank squamous cell carcinoma. This was estimated at 20% by one author, but experienced clinicians will know that it is much less than this. A quite recent study has estimated a transformation rate of solar keratoses to squamous cell carcinomata of less than 0.1%. Much more work must be completed before any one estimate can be accepted—indeed some lesions seem to spontaneously regress.[16]

Clinically solar keratoses are small, pink or grey, scaling or warty nodules or plaques (Figures 9.11 and 9.12). In some instances they give rise to horn-like protuberances producing bizarre looking lesions (cutaneous horns) (Figure 9.13). Uncommonly there is only a little scaling but pronounced redness, so that on the face it is difficult to tell the lesions apart from the lesions of discoid lupus erythematosus (Figure 9.14). Solar keratoses are most common on the face, especially the nose, ears and forehead, the bald area of the scalp and on the backs of the hands; in badly sun-damaged individuals they may be profuse.

Histologically there is considerable variation in the degree of abnormality found. Some lesions require the eye of an expert to tell them apart from normal elderly skin. Others are so frankly abnormal that they are a hair's breadth from squamous cell carcinoma. The major diagnostic discriminant is the presence of abnormal

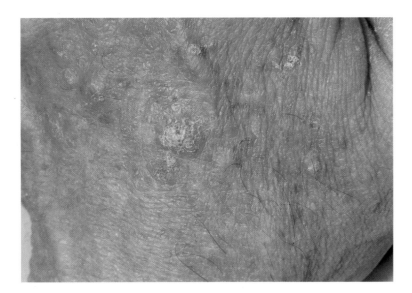

Figure 9.11

Several small keratoses on the back of the hand of an elderly man.

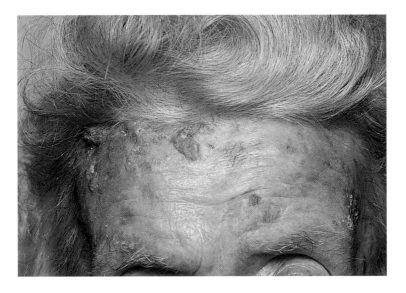

Figure 9.12

Severe flat scaly and hyperkeratotic solar keratoses are present on this women's forehead.

(dysplastic) epidermal cells in the basal regions of the epidermis (Figure 9.15). These dysplastic cells are larger than usual and have enlarged, irregular, hyperchromatic nuclei. They occupy the basal epidermal zone and in places form downward projections into the dermis. The overlying stratum corneum is mostly parakeratotic and there is usually a mixed inflammatory cell infiltrate of variable density (Figure 9.16). In some cases there is focal destruction of the basal epidermal cells with a dense band-like inflammatory infiltrate and the pathological picture may bear an uncanny resemblance to lichen planus. Cytoid bodies are also observed underlining the resemblance. Not unnaturally these have come to be known as lichenoid keratoses.[17] The upper dermis always demonstrates marked solar elastotic degenerative change.

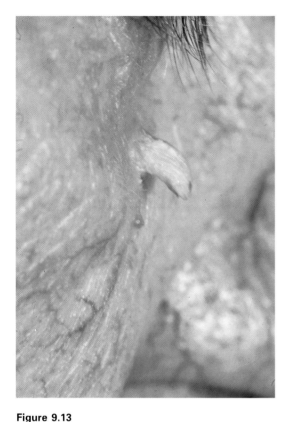

Figure 9.13

Cutaneous horn due to solar keratosis.

Keratoses caused by chronic heat injury are found at the traumatized site—usually the front of the shins. Keratoses due to arsenic are now very uncommon but were found in a variety of sites, including palms and soles.

Patients who are immunosuppressed seem especially prone to develop solar keratoses (and even squamous cell carcinoma). Patients who have received a renal transplant, are taking immunosuppressive drugs and who have had considerable solar damage may be particularly at risk.[18] The subject of solar keratoses and related premalignant lesions has been extensively reviewed by Schwartz.[19]

Treatment

Solitary lesions on the face or back of the hand can be dealt with by curettage and cautery, cryosurgery or straight excision. When there are multiple lesions in sun battered elderly subjects the problem may be quite difficult. Clearly the larger lesions should be excised, and several of the smaller can be treated at one sitting with cryotherapy. Topical 5-fluorouracil (5% ointment) is effective in many patients. The material is applied twice daily for 10–14 days or even longer.

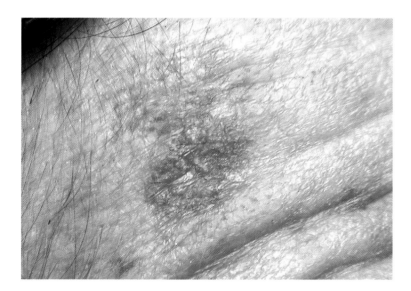

Figure 9.14

Lupus erythematosus-like keratoses on the jaw line of an elderly lady.

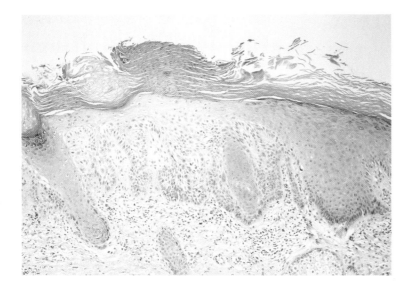

Figure 9.15

Histopathology of solar keratosis. There are many large cells with abnormal nuclei within the epidermis, and parakeratosis (H & E; ×90).

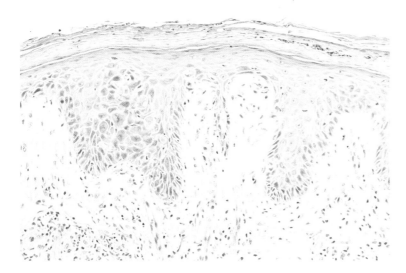

Figure 9.16

Pathology of solar keratosis. There is marked parakeratotic scale and inflammatory cell infiltrate, and an abnormal population of epidermal cells in this section (H & E; ×45).

If successful, the treated areas may become inflamed, especially if the treated area has been exposed to the sun and many clinicians prescribe a corticosteroid to be used after the application of 5-fluoruracil to damp down this inflammatory episode. However, when the lesions are numerous this approach is inadequate. Furthermore, even the clinically normal-looking skin may be abnormal in these people.[20] For this group of patients further solar damage should be prevented by advice and the use of sunscreens, and regular follow-up arranged for removal of any lesions that enlarge. In addition there is a body of opinion that these patients may benefit from the use of oral retinoids. Certainly there have been several reports describing their effectiveness for epidermal premalignancies and malignancy (eg, see Peck[21] and Kingston and Marks[22]).

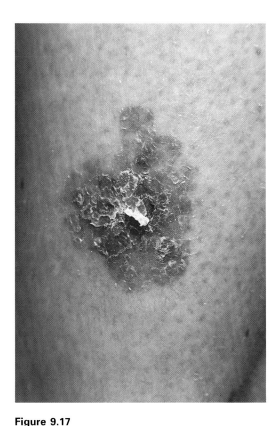

Figure 9.17

Bowen's disease on the skin of a lady of 67.

Unfortunately their use is associated with inconvenient side-effects and not all elderly patients can tolerate them. Topical retinoids also appear to reduce the number and size of solar keratoses.[23] They may also discourage the emergence of new lesions. Other experimental techniques for the treatment of these lesions include photodynamic therapy[24] and dermabrasion.[25]

Bowen's disease (intraepidermal epithelioma)

These lesions are examples of carcinoma *in situ* and can be regarded as having taken one step further along the pathway to malignancy compared with solar keratoses. They are less strictly related to solar exposure than solar keratoses and are frequently found on usually non-sun exposed sites such as the legs or trunk. Clinically they are thickened red scaling patches of up to several centimetres in diameter and may appear similar clinically to a patch of psoriasis (Figure 9.17). Less commonly they present as cutaneous horns. On the glans penis the reddened area has a glazed appearance and is less scaly than at the other sites. In this situation the disorder is known as erythroplasia of Queyrat and must be distinguished from benign inflammatory penile conditions (balanoposthitis) (Figure 9.18).

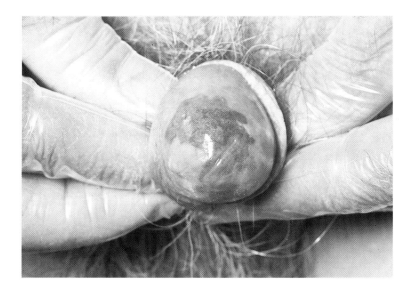

Figure 9.18

Erythroplasia of Queyrat, This velvety red patch had been present for the previous six months.

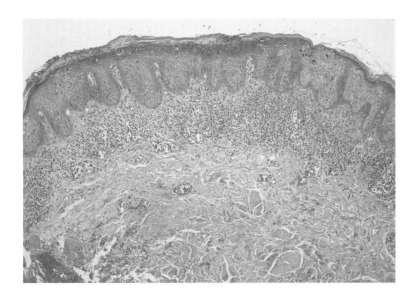

Figure 9.19

Pathology of Bowen's disease showing a psoriasiform picture overall. The epidermis contains many large abnormal epidermal cells and there is parakeratotic scaling and a heavy inflammatory cell infiltrate (H & E; ×25).

The one condition most likely to cause diagnostic difficulty is plasma cell balanitis of Zoon. This tends to be less raised and slightly browner in colour.

Histological appearance

Histologically dysplastic cells are present throughout the width of the thickened (often psoriasiform) epidermis. They are often bizarre, justifying the apt (figurative) French term *cellules monstreuses* (Figure 9.19). As with solar keratoses there is a variably dense mixed inflammatory cell infiltrate and a parakeratotic stratum corneum.

Treatment

Usually there is only one or a limited number of lesions of Bowen's disease so that in most cases surgical excision is perfectly adequate. Some may be treated by cryotherapy or by topical 5-fluorouracil if removal cannot be arranged for some reason. Radiotherapy may also be used if the other modalities are for some reason inappropriate.

Keratoacanthomas[26]

These are also sometimes known as self-healing epitheliomas, although this term is also given to a rare familial disorder in which similar but larger lesions occur (Ferguson Smith disease). Keratoacanthomas can occur anywhere but are more common on light-exposed skin. Their biological status is uncertain but they have histological similarities to squamous cell carcinomas and are presumed to be an odd type of non-progressive neoplasia. Clinically they occur singly for the most part although multiple lesions are also seen. The typical keratoacanthoma is a nodule with steep walls and a central horn-filled invagination (Figure 9.20). Most lesions expand rapidly over 4–12 weeks and then regress eventually to leave a scar. The histological appearance suggests a large and deformed hair follicle with hyperplastic epithelium for the most part, but with some dysplastic changes at the periphery. There is a variable mixed inflammatory cell infiltrate. The most important differential diagnosis is squamous cell carcinoma. A slow-growing carcinoma can be very similar clinically and can be difficult to distinguish histologically. It therefore takes the eye of experience to distinguish these entities when the lesion has the general architecture of

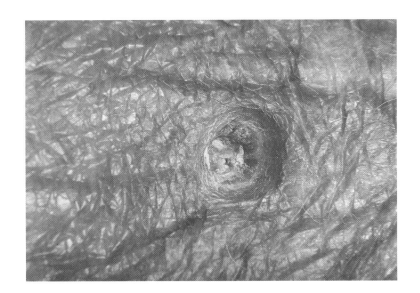

Figure 9.20a

Typical keratoacanthoma on the back of the hand.

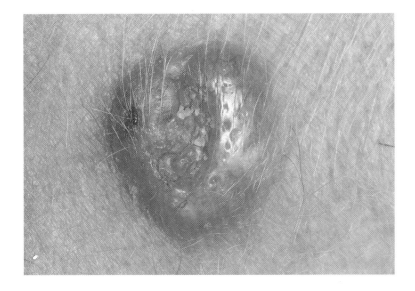

Figure 9.20b

Keratoacanthoma. Note central horn filled crypt.

a horn-filled hyperplastic epithelial cup. The treatment of choice is excision.

Squamous cell carcinoma

This malignant disorder of the epidermis arises either *de novo* or from premalignant solar keratoses or Bowen's disease. It is a common neoplasm in the elderly on sun-damaged skin. It is particularly common on the face and backs of the hands and the lower legs of fair-skinned people living in sunny climates. As with keratoses, heat injury and arsenic can also be provoking stimuli. In addition, squamous cell carcinoma can arise from areas treated by X-rays and from pre-existing benign skin lesions, including chronic discoid lupus erythematosus, lupus vulgaris, chronic gravitational ulcers, warty naevi and genital warts. In the latter, some antigenic strains of the wart virus have been incriminated in the aetiology.[27] Squamous cell carcinoma is well reviewed by Robin Marks.[28]

Clinical appearance

They may present either as warty plaques or nodules or raised ulcerated lesions, often with proud margins which characteristically have a rolled and everted appearance (Figures 9.21 and 9.22). Their rate of growth is variable but a size of 3 cm diameter reached in as many months would not be unusual. Metastasis from squamous cell carcinoma is uncommon, although lesions on the penis and lip have a bad reputation. An overall rate of metastasis from all sites in all patients with squamous cell carcinoma in the UK is probably of the order of 1–3%, although accurate figures are not available. Metastasis is primarily via lymphatic pathways.

Histological appearance

There are many abnormal dysplastic epidermal cells, some of which show individual cell keratinization (malignant dyskeratosis). Although the epidermal abnormalities are also seen in Bowen's disease and to a lesser extent in solar keratoses and keratoacanthoma, the distinctive feature of a squamous carcinoma is that clumps of cells have invaded the dermis and become separated from their point of origin in the epidermis (Figure 9.23). The degree of inflammatory reaction around the lesion depends to some extent on whether there is ulceration at the surface.

Treatment

Most small lesions are satisfactorily handled by excision with an adequate margin. Cryotherapy, cautery and superficial X-ray treatment are other modalities that have been used successfully. When metastatic spread has occurred chemotherapeutic agents may be indicated. Oral

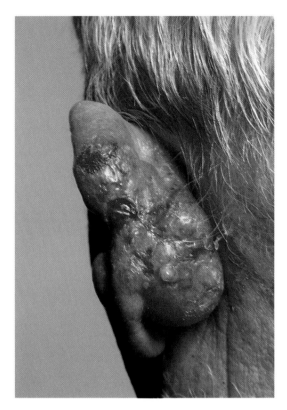

Figure 9.21

Large nodular plaque of squamous cell carcinoma.

retinoids have been used and are of help on some occasions.[29] They have also been employed in combination with interferons and IL-2 (interleukin-2). The latter have also been used by themselves, cytotoxic agents including cisplatin and bleomycin have also been employed.

Paget's disease[28,29]

Paget's disease represents an unusual variety of intraepidermal carcinoma in which the abnormal intraepidermal cells are from a ductular structure that opens at the surface. Two varieties are recognized—the mammary and extramammary forms. The mammary form (Paget's disease of the nipple), which is the least uncommon,

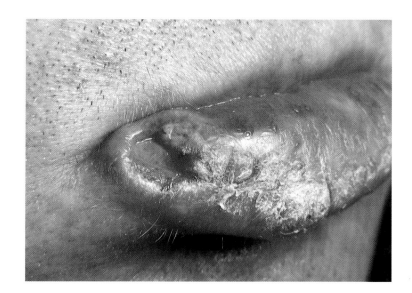

Figure 9.22a

Ulcerated lesions of squamous cell carcinoma affecting the lip.

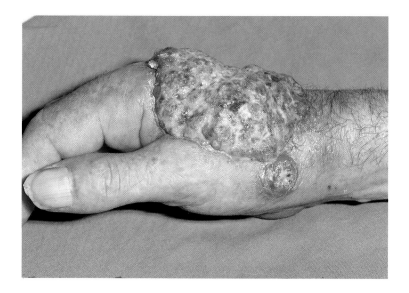

Figure 9.22b

Eroded fungating plaque on back of the hand of a 66-year-old ex-welder and keen gardener, present for the previous 9 months.

presents on the nipple areola as an eczematous-looking eruption and is due to the spread into the epidermis of an intraductal carcinoma of the breast (Figure 9.24). Extramammary Paget's disease occurs perianally, perivulvally or on the lower abdomen or groin as an eczematous-looking, thickened patch. The source of the carcinomatous cells in the extramammary form may be apocrine glands but is often undiscovered.

Histological appearance

Histologically clusters of abnormal large clear cells are evident within the epidermis (Figure 9.25). These have to be distinguished from the dysplastic epidermal cells of Bowen's disease, the abnormal melanocytes of a lentigo or superficial melanoma, and the invading abnormal lymphocytes of mycosis fungoides.

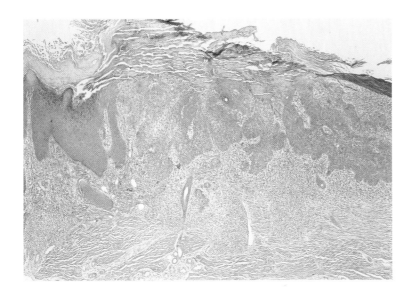

Figure 9.23

Pathology of early squamous cell carinoma. There is massive epidermal hyperproliferation of an irregular kind. Many of the cells are abnormal in appearance (H & E; ×15).

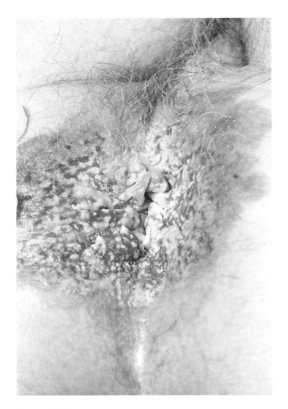

Figure 9.24

Extramammary Paget's disease. Note the eroded appearance in this situation.

Treatment

Every attempt must be made to locate and treat any underlying carcinoma. If none can be found (as in some cases of extramammary Paget's disease) the whole of the involved area should be excised or treated by radiotherapy.

Basal cell carcinoma

Basal cell carcinomas (BCCs, known colloquially as rodent ulcer) are the commonest form of human malignant disease. They are locally invasive and metastasize only rarely. Interestingly, retrospective consideration of lesions that have metastasized failed to identify either clinical or histological features that would pinpoint patients in whom this is a likely occurrence.[30] Although most common in the elderly they are sometimes seen in younger patients. Solar irradiation is the aetiological agent usually responsible, but clearly not the only one, as these carcinomas are not infrequently observed on non-sun exposed sites. They can arise in areas treated by X-rays and from pre-existing naevoid lesions such as naevus sebaceous. They may also be part of an inherited symptom complex known as the basal cell naevus syndrome.[31] Other

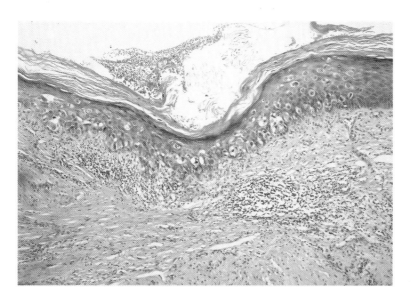

Figure 9.25

Histopathology of Paget's disease. There are many large clear cells invading the epidermis (H & E;×25).

characteristics of the basal cell naevus syndrome include the presence of palmar pits, jaw cysts and bifid ribs. The BCCs in this disorder tend to be pigmented. The syndrome is inherited as an autosomal dominant characteristic.

Clinical types

Nodulocystic

This is the commonest form of basal cell carcinoma. They mostly occur on the face as pearly, greyish, translucent nodules up to 2 cm in diameter (Figure 9.26). They may be crossed by telangiectatic vessels and are sometimes flecked with brownish black pigment. They are often slow growing with a history of gradual increase in size over many years. Sebaceous gland hyperplasia (page 189), non-pigmented compound naevi and benign adnexal tumours are among the lesions that should be distinguished from nodulocystic basal cell carcinoma.

Ulcerative

These may begin as ulcers or develop from large nodulocystic lesions (Figure 9.27). When poor social conditions prevented adequate treatment for the impoverished, these lesions used slowly to erode large areas of the face and were thought to resemble rat bites—hence the name of rodent ulcer. Characteristically the ulcers have a raised and rolled margin.

Pigmented

Some of the nodulocystic variety are uniformly darkly pigmented—to the point of resembling a malignant melanoma (Figure 9.28).

Superficial

This type of lesion occurs mostly on the trunk and limbs. The affected area is usually slightly raised, red and scaling and is often confused with a psoriatic or eczematous patch. The margins are well defined and often very slightly raised and thread-like (Figure 9.29). Superficial basal cell carcinoma can be virtually any size and lesions of 15–20 cm^2 in area are not uncommon.

Morphoeic

The name given to this group of basal cell carcinomas refers to their resemblance to localized

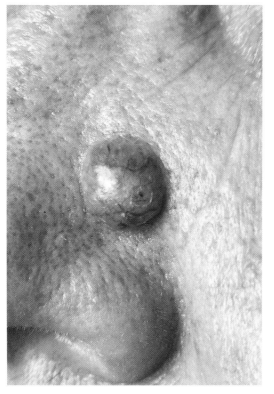

Figure 9.26

Nodulocystic-basal cell carcinoma.

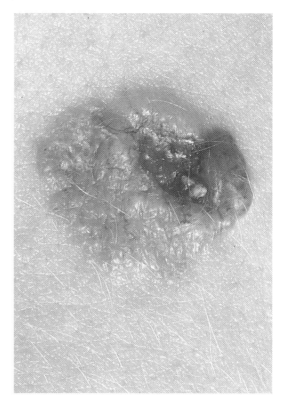

Figure 9.27

Ulcerated basal cell carcinoma.

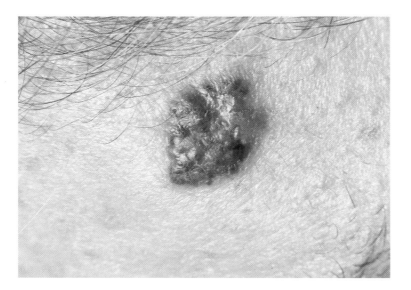

Figure 9.28

Pigmented basal cell carcinoma. This type of lesion is often mistaken for a malignant melanoma.

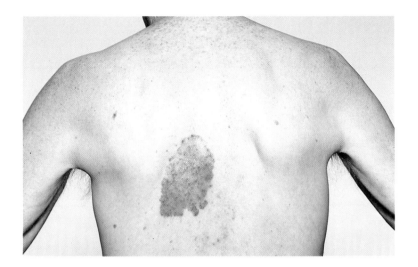

Figure 9.29a

Large superficial basal cell carcinoma.

Figure 9.29b

Detail of 29a, showing raised, pearly edge.

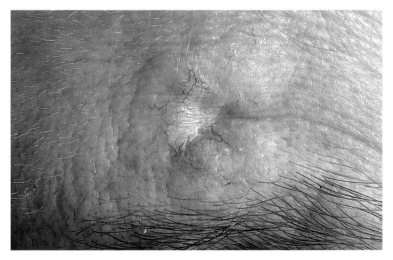

Figure 9.29c

Morphoeic basal cell carcinoma showing irregular scar-like plaque.

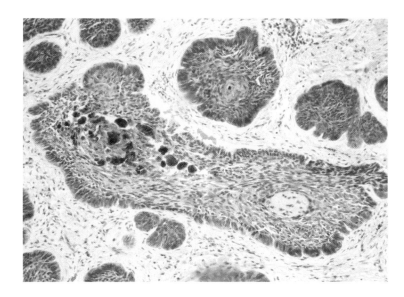

Figure 9.30

Pathology of typical basal cell carcinoma. Note palisaded appearance of lobule containing some basophilic cells. There is also much pigment present in this lesion (H & E; ×150).

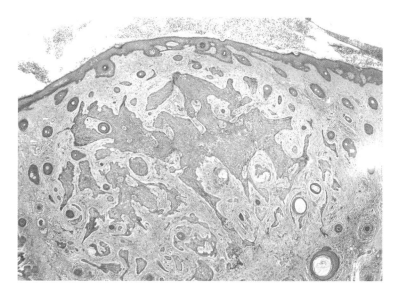

Figure 9.31

Invasive basal cell carcinoma. The tumour tissue is stretched deep into the dermis and is irregular and angular in profile (H & E; ×150).

scleroderma (morphoea). The affected patch is thickened, abnormally firm and pale. This type is the least commonly encountered and the most frequently misdiagnosed.

Pathology of basal cell carcinoma

Rounded lobules of small basaloid epidermal cells characterize the pathology. Typically the outer layer of cells is more columnar and regularly arranged in a palisade fashion (Figure 9.30). There is often mucoid degenerative change within and around the tumour lobules (accounting for the cystic appearance) and a variable degree of melanin pigment production due to the inclusion of melanocytes in the lesion. The lobules of the tumour are often retracted from the surrounding dermis because of dissolving of the mucoid stroma around the tumour lobules as an artefact of the histological technique. Sometimes the tumour masses are not rounded but have other arrangements, such as 'adenoidal', in which glandular structures are simulated or are more aggressive-looking and irregular in outline and appear to infiltrate the dermis (Figure 9.31). In the superficial type the lobules are small and seem to come directly from the interfollicular epidermis. The morphoeic type consists of small columns and cords of the same basal cell carcinoma cells surrounded by a dense fibrous stroma.

There are two main types of lesion to be considered histologically in the differential diagnosis. The first is some type of adnexal tumour, because some hair follicle tumours have similar appearances. The second is squamous cell carcinoma, as in some cases there is an appearance of squamous differentiation within the basaloid tumorous masses.

Treatment

The preferred treatment of this, the commonest form of skin cancer, is surgical removal. In the smallest nodulocystic lesions thorough curettage and repeated cautery at the base is usually sufficient. However, the recurrence rate is higher (5–10%) with this type of treatment. Cryotherapy may be used for some lesions and seems to be especially suitable for the large superficial types. Superficial X-ray therapy is also an adequate way for dealing with the majority of large lesions on the face that cannot satisfactorily be dealt with by surgery. The retinoid drugs have also been used successfully for patients with multiple basal cell carcinoma. Where there are large, infiltrating lesions, the Moh's chemosurgical or microsurgical approach (sometimes called microscopically controlled excision) gives good results.[32] In this technique the tumour is destroyed by a corrosive chemical or by surgical excision and microscopy is used to monitor whether all the tumour has been removed during the operative procedure.

Other types of epidermal malignant lesion

Rarely, malignant lesions arise from eccrine, apocrine and sebaceous gland tissue. They have no particular distinguishing clinical features and are usually diagnosed histologically after removal.

Tumours of melanocytic origin

Benign lesions

The melanocyte is the cell of origin of the various types of naevus cell naevus or mole. Moles tend to disappear gradually during life, but some do remain and can cause difficulties in diagnosis. This applies particularly to the large dermal or compound type of naevus on the face that is either non-pigmented or only slightly pigmented. These are frequently misdiagnosed as basal cell carcinoma. They need no special treatment. Flat junctional naevi normally do not arise in old age and any flat, dark brown or black lesion that appears suddenly after the age of 40 should be regarded as a possible early malignant melanoma or lentigo maligna. The flat, light brown macules that occur on the backs of the hands, the sides of the face and over the upper trunk and are known as senile lentigines must be distinguished from these other, more threatening lesions. Senile or solar lentigines (see page 28) are a difficult group to classify, some appearing to be no more than a form of seborrhoeic wart with a minor degree of wartiness and a more prominent pigment cell component. Others may be true lentigines with focal benign proliferation of pigment cells. It may be especially difficult to distinguish larger flat brown lesions occurring on the side of the face in the elderly. Any lesion that has variation in the degree of pigment and is rapidly enlarging should be regarded with suspicion and biopsied.

Lentigo maligna (Hutchinson's melanotic freckle)

These not uncommon, slowly growing, superficial lesions are seen mainly in patients over the age of 50. They may be regarded as premalignant lesions of melanocytic origin. They occur predominantly but not exclusively on the exposed skin and are most common on the face. It is thought that solar exposure plays the major role in their development.

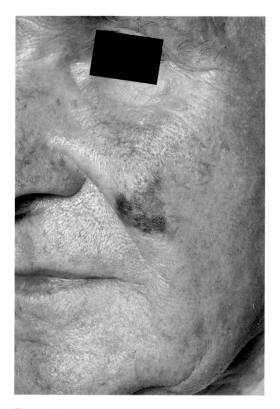

Figure 9.32

Lentigo maligna.

Clinical features

The lesion is typically an irregular flat brown to black freckle and is irregularly dense with a pigment (Figure 9.32). The lesion gradually extends over several years so that eventually quite large areas (eg, 15–20 cm²) may be covered. Lentigo maligna itself does not usually metastasize: however, malignant melanoma not infrequently develops within the lesion and this has all the prognostic implications of this malignancy. The development of malignant melanoma may be recognized by a thickening or appearance of a nodule on the surface, which eventually ulcerates. Lentigo maligna has to be distinguished from the quite common banal flat seborrhoeic warts and senile lentigines. The former have slightly warty surfaces and both usually have a uniform light fawn colour as opposed to the variegate pigmentation of a lentigo maligna.

Histopathology

Large numbers of abnormal clear cells are seen along the basal layers of the epidermis. The degree of cellular atypia is variable but is usually not gross. The cells form small clusters in places and also invade the body of the epidermis. The epidermis itself shows irregular thickening with accentuation of the rete pegs. Melanin pigment is usually shed and engulfed by macrophages in the upper dermis. Lentigo maligna must be distinguished from superficial malignant melanoma on the one hand and banal senile lentigo on the other. When there are many abnormal melanocytes in the epidermis the histological picture may resemble Paget's disease, Bowen's disease or even mycosis fungoides.

Treatment

In many patients with lentigo maligna surgical excision is difficult because of the size and location of the lesion. Despite a reputation for being implacably radioresistant, recent studies show that this is not always the case and that modern radiotherapeutic techniques can ablate many lesions. Cryotherapy has also been used to treat segments of the lesion as there is no objection to letting the treatment span several sessions. The problem with this approach is that the 'tissue iceball' from cryotherapy does not penetrate far into the skin so that abnormal melanocytic cells that have migrated down the sides of follicles may remain visible and allow a recurrence. Topical azelaic acid has also been employed and some success claimed.[32]

Malignant melanoma

Malignant melanoma (MM) excites both fear and fascination: fear because of its unpredictability, its aggressively malignant nature and its increasing incidence in the Western world, and fascination because of the tantalizing closeness researchers have come to unravelling its aetiopathogenesis. The literature on malignant melanoma is enormous and events in this area are moving with a bewildering rapidity. Only the barest outlines of the subject can be included here and for more extensive coverage the reader should consult recent monographs.[33,34] Its incidence ranges from 0.2 per 100 000 in Japan to 40 per 100 000 in Queensland, Australia.[35] In Scotland the incidence between 1979 and 1983 was 4.75 per 100 000 for women and 2.77 for men.[36] It has apparently doubled in each decade in Scandinavia[37] but quadrupled in Arizona[38] and New Mexico[39] in the same period.

MM may appear anywhere on the skin surface but are more common on the upper half of the body. Women develop the lesions more frequently than men by a factor of 2:1 in all countries save those with the highest incidence, such as Australia. They occur at all ages after puberty but are more common after the age of 40.

All the evidence points to the importance of sun exposure as a central aetiological factor but as incidences differ in different countries at the same latitude and the lesion also occurs on the covered parts, there is also the strong suggestion that other factors are important.

Clinical features

About as many malignant melanomata arise from pre-existing melanocytic naevi as *de novo*. Some types of melanocytic naevi are more prone to develop malignant change than others. Giant naevi of the cape or bathing trunk type are notorious in this respect, some 10–20% giving rise to MM. In fact, all congenital naevi (large irregular naevi present at or shortly after birth) seem to possess an increased malignant potential. In addition the dysplastic naevus syndrome has in recent years emerged as an important risk state for MM. Dysplastic naevi differ both clinically and histologically from ordinary moles.[40] They are more irregular in shape and often have irregularities in pigmentation: histologically there is prominent junctional activity and the mole cells may appear abnormal in places. Dysplastic naevi may occur in large numbers and when this

tendency is inherited there is a considerable risk of MM. When the condition is sporadic the risk, although increased, is not as great.

Lesions of MM are basically of two types (or three if lentigo maligna is included)—superficial spreading melanoma (SSM) in which there is a tendency for the malignant growth to take place horizontally and nodular melanoma (NM) where the growth tends to occur vertically. Of the two types the SSM type have a much better prognosis. The clinical types encountered include areas of macular pigmentation, plaques, nodules, exophytic papillomatous lesions, and eroded nodules or plaques (Figures 9.33 and 9.34). The major clinical feature that should lead to the diagnosis being suspected is the development of or increase in brown or brown-black pigmentation in a localized lesion. The pigmentation is often irregular and may even contain non-pigmented areas. The edges of the lesion are usually well defined but are often irregular with areas of pigmentation around the lesion. In late lesions metastatic nodules may arise around the primary MM or may occur at distant sites. The surface may be intact but later becomes roughened, scaling and exudative or even eroded. The rate of growth is extremely variable. A frequent story elicited is that a pre-existing flat (junctional) mole has darkened and enlarged over the previous few months. However, the speed of progress can be frightening, and large exophytic masses can develop very rapidly, often being mistaken for pyogenic granuloma.

Any pigmented lesion can be mistaken for MM and vice versa. The common differential diagnoses are set out in Table 9.2. The lesions that often cause confusion include ordinary moles, seborrhoeic warts, basal cell carcinomata, pyogenic granuloma and histiocytoma.

The prognosis depends on the malignant potential of the lesion and the degree of resistance of the host. Histologically, the prognosis can be estimated most reliably by the depth of penetration into the dermis.[41] The overall prognosis for superficial lesions is about 90% survival for 5 years but is much worse for deep nodular lesions (see Table 9.3). The features that influence prognosis are set out in Table 9.3. Metastasis of MM is both via the lymphatic system and blood borne so that secondary deposits may occur anywhere. Some of the more common sites of spread include the liver, lungs

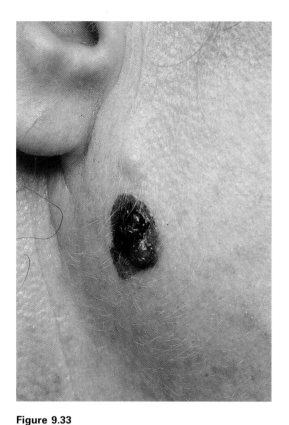

Figure 9.33

Nodular malignant melanoma.

and brain. Metastases are also frequently found in the regional lymph nodes and skin. When there is a heavy tumour load some generalized increase in pigmentation and melaninuria may occur.

Pathology

The essential pathological feature is the marked proliferation of abnormal melanocytic cells in the junctional zone. The abnormal cells, which may closely resemble ordinary mole cells, extend upwards into the epidermis—eventually producing an erosion. They also extend both laterally and downwards (Figure 9.35). Usually the packet-like arrangement of the benign mole becomes distorted or completely lost in sheets and masses of MM cells. The depth of invasion has been found to be the most important prognostic discriminator. A tumour depth of 2.5 mm or more signifies a poor prognosis and is much more significant than any other histological feature, including the number of mitoses seen and the obvious invasion of blood vessels. The degree of cytological abnormality is extremely variable as are the amount of pigment production and the numbers of inflammatory cells around the lesion.

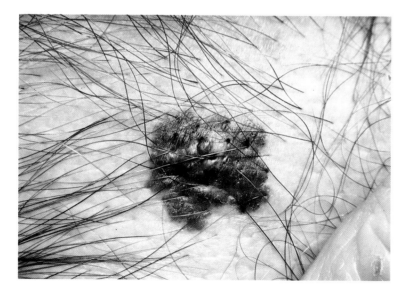

Figure 9.34

Malignant melanoma. This lesion was misdiagnosed as a seborrhoeic wart.

Table 9.3 Main features influencing prognosis of malignant melanoma[a]

Feature	Prognosis
Depth of invasion	The deeper the tumour extends into the skin, the worse the prognosis; thus with a thickness of ≤ 0.85 mm the prognosis for 5-year survival is 99%, for 1.7–3.59 mm it is 81% and for >3.6 mm it is 49%
Lymph node involvement	If nodes are found to be involved microscopically, the prognosis drops dramatically; thus without nodal involvement, the prognosis for 5-year survival is 89%, with one node involvement it is 53% and with 2–3 nodes involved it is 39%
Type of lesion	
Lentigo maligna melanoma	5-year survival is 92%
Superficial spreading melanoma	5-year survival is 91%
Nodular melanoma	5-year survival is 62%
Acral lentiginous melanoma	5-year survival is 79%
Anatomical site, age and sex	In general, lesions on the limbs of women aged <50 have the best prognosis; lesions on the back, male gender and age >50 are adverse prognostic features

[a]Adapted from Rigel DS, Rogers GS, Friedman RJ. The prognosis of malignant melanoma. In: *Melanoma and Pigmented Lesions. Dermatologic Clinics* (1985) 3(2), 309–313.

Treatment

Management depends largely on the stage the lesion has reached. With superficial spreading melanomata and small early nodular MM, wide excision is all that is required. How wide is a matter of some debate.[42] Prophylactic excision of regional lymph nodes is now rarely practised as it seems to have little effect on the ultimate outlook. Immunostimulation of patients with advanced disease with BCG vaccination, transfer factor preparations and thymopoietin analogues has not proved helpful. Chemotherapy with antimitotic or antimetabolite agents rarely prolongs life and often makes patients very unwell in advanced disease.

Merkel cell carcinoma

This is a very uncommon skin tumour deriving from the epidermal Merkel cells which have a neuroendocrine function. It behaves aggressively and in one series survival for 5–6 years was seen in only 2 of 10 patients.[43] The tumour is most common in the elderly (median age cited as 74 by Krasagakis et al[43]) and occurs predominantly in sun-exposed acral areas and on the face. The best treatment appears to be wide excision.

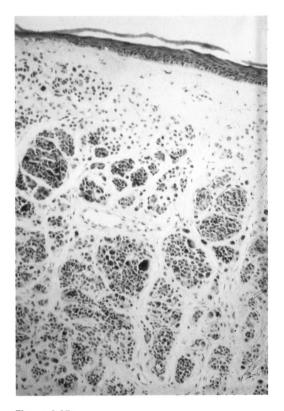

Figure 9.35a

Histopathology of benign melanocytic naevus showing pockets of mole cells regularly faceted together (H & E; ×25).

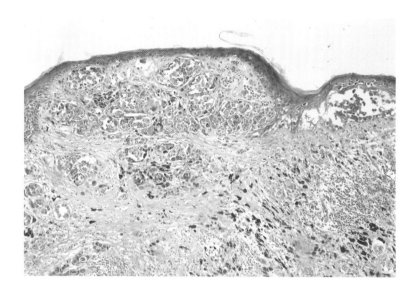

Figure 9.35b

Pathology of malignant melanoma. There are irregular masses of abnormal cells throughout the dermis and marked deposits of pigment (H & E; ×25).

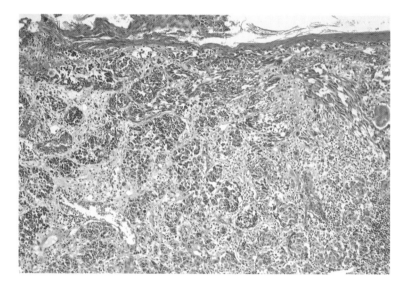

Figure 9.35c

Pathology of malignant melanoma. There is marked 'junction' proliferation of abnormal naevus cells. The upper and mid dermis are filled with irregular pockets of melanoma cells and inflammatory cell infiltrate (H & E; ×25).

Dermal tumours

Histiocytoma (dermatofibroma)

It is not certain whether this extremely common lesion is a true neoplasm or some type of reactive inflammatory abnormality. It is quite common and found most frequently in the middle aged and older age groups.

Clinical features

Solitary lesions may occur but multiple lesions (up to six) are seen frequently. They often arise on the limbs but may occur on the trunk and rarely on the face. Histiocytomata usually present as firm intracutaneous light brown nodules or plaques that are attached to the overlying skin (Figure 9.36). Sometimes they have a warty or roughened surface. They are

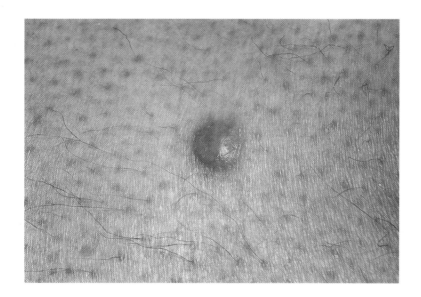

Figure 9.36a

Typical histiocytoma (dermatofibroma).

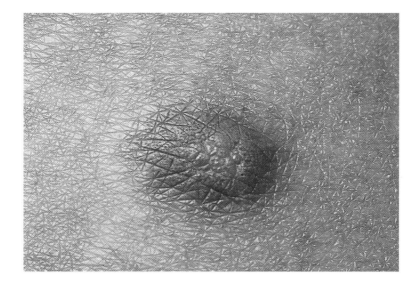

Figure 9.36b

Histiocytoma (dermatofibroma). Note pigmentation.

mostly less than 1.5 cm in diameter. Differential diagnosis includes MM and moles.

Pathology

In the upper and mid-dermis there are whorls and strands of new connective tissue interspersed with blood vessels, fibroblasts and histiocytes. The latter cell type often contains granules of haemosiderin and lipid vacuoles. The nodule does not possess a capsule and merges into the surrounding normal dermis. The overlying epidermis is often markedly thickened (Figure 9.37). In some instances the acanthotic epidermis includes areas of basaloid hyperplasia which may take on the structure of hair follicles and rarely even basal cell carcinoma.[44]

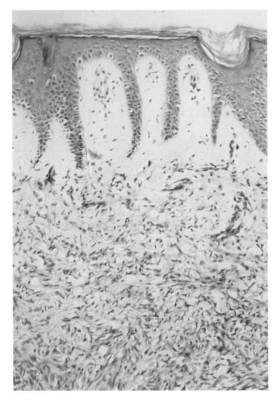

Figure 9.37

Histopathology of histiocytoma showing the edge of the cellular mass with many histiocytic ad fibroblastic cells (H & E; ×90).

Treatment

As these lesions are benign no particular treatment is required. If there is doubt as to the diagnosis or their removal is required for some other reason, simple surgical excision is adequate.

Dermatofibrosarcoma protuberans

This uncommon, slow-growing lesion may resemble a large histiocytoma or is more usually a thickened intracutaneous plaque a few centimetres in diameter. It is regarded as locally invasive only, but is certainly capable of metastasis. It may be difficult to distinguish histologically from a banal histiocytoma, but invasion of the fat and a cartwheeling pattern of the fibroblastic element with abnormal cellular forms usually assist in a correct diagnosis being reached. Wide excision is the treatment of choice, although Moh's micrographic surgery has also been recommended because of the high recurrence rates reported (up to 60%) from surgery.[45]

Fibrosarcoma

True fibrosarcomas of the skin are extremely rare, though occasionally occur as a complication of neurofibromatosis (see below).

Tumours of nerve sheath

Neurofibroma

Solitary neurofibromas are not uncommon but these lesions are probably best known as an important component of the dominantly inherited disorder known as von Recklinghausen's disease or neurofibromatosis. The lesions are skin-coloured or bluish, soft and often papillomatous, but may also be plaque-like or nodular. They are usually small but very large lesions several centimetres across also occur. Histologically they consist of whorls of fibrous structures which sometimes emulate nerves. They do not have a capsule but are quite well defined from the surrounding dermis. They may contain large numbers of mast cells.

Neurilemmoma

This benign nerve sheath tumour is less common than neurofibroma. Clinically it presents as a smooth, soft, solitary, skin-coloured nodule. The histopathological appearance is often distinguished by a peculiar staggered stacking type arrangement of the spindle-shaped cellular elements (Verocay bodies).

Table 9.4 Tumours with a predominant spindle cell component

Tumour	Major histological features	Clinical features
Histocytoma (dermatofibroma)	Whorls of angulated spindle-shaped cells and obvious histiocytic cells containing lipid and pigment	Brownish red, firm, intracutaneous nodules on limbs of middle-aged and elderly
Dermatofibrosarcoma protuberans	Similar to above but much larger and with tendency to infiltrate deeply into fat and with 'cartwheel' pattern	Rare, slowly enlarging nodular plaque
Neurofibroma	Bundles of long spindle-shaped cells occasionally in neural pattern	Multiple soft pedunculated nodules (neurofibromatosis)
Leiomyoma	Bundles of slightly thicker spindle cells with blunt-ended nuclei	Firm intracutaneous pink or brown painful nodules
Keloid scar	Pale highly cellular fibrous tissue with homogenized appearance	Smooth, pink, firm or hard nodules often at site of injury

Leiomyoma

Benign tumours of soft muscle may arise from the muscle coats of small dermal blood vessels (angioleiomyoma) or from the arrector pilores muscle of hair follicles. They mostly occur on the limbs and are often multiple and sometimes present in very large numbers. Clinically they are pink or mauve, smooth and deeply set in the skin (Figure 9.38). Sometimes mechanical stimulation or the cold will make them contract and give rise to pain. Histologically they must be distinguished from other tumours which possess spindle cells as the predominant cellular component, including scars, keloids, neurofibroma, histiocytoma and dermatofibrosarcoma protuberans (Table 9.4). The cells of leiomyoma tend to be broader, have blunter ends and more prominent nuclei than those of neural or fibrous lesions.

Adenoma sebaceum

The term adenoma sebaceum is a complete misnomer, as this cutaneous manifestation of tuberous sclerosis consists of multiple centrofacial

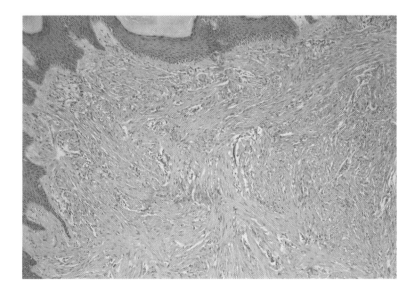

Figure 9.38

Pathology of leiomyoma. There are many plain muscle cells in the subepidermal zone (H & E; ×45).

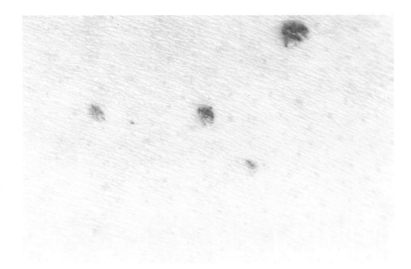

Figure 9.39

Campbell de Morgan spots.

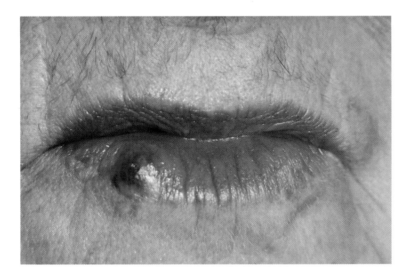

Figure 9.40

Venous lake on lower lip in elderly female patient.

nodules of vascular fibrous tissue. The disorder is dominantly inherited and characterized by neurological abnormalities and other cutaneous anomalies, besides the fibrovascular nodules mentioned above.

Tumours of vascular tissue

Congenital malformations of vascular tissue are not a problem in the elderly, and will not be described.

Campbell de Morgan spots (senile angioma, cherry angioma)

These cherry red, smooth, hemispherical nodules, 1–4 mm in diameter, are very common in the elderly. They are generally multiple and restricted to the trunk (Figure 9.39). Campbell de Morgan spots, as one of their synonyms implies, rarely occur before the age of 50. They cause no symptoms and are usually noted only in the course of examination for an unrelated problem.

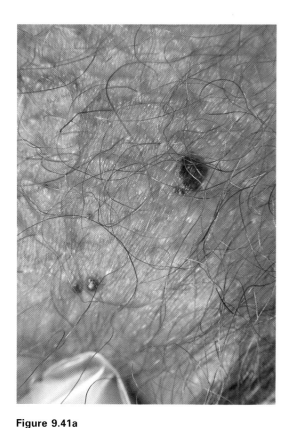

Figure 9.41a

Angiokeratoma affecting the scrotum.

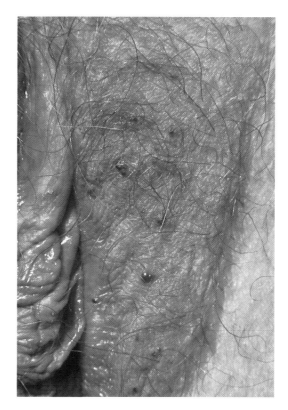

Figure 9.41b

Angiokeratoma affecting the vulva of woman aged 69.

Rarely, very large numbers of tiny lesions appear in a relatively short period. These produce diagnostic confusion owing to their resemblance to the serious congenital metabolic disorder angiokeratoma corporis diffusum (Fabry's disease).[46] Histologically they consist of a mass of endothelial cells containing more or less well-developed vascular channels. They have no medical significance.

Venous lakes

It is not unusual to observe smooth, dark mauve or blue, soft tumours which may reach 1 cm in diameter on the lips in patients over 55 (Figure 9.40). These venous lakes are not true neoplasms, but are sometimes misinterpreted as malignant melanomas. They are due to ectasia of venous channels and are usually asymptomatic.

Angiokeratoma

One type of angiokeratoma has already been briefly mentioned above. Essentially this sort of lesion represents proliferation and dilatation of papillary capillary blood vessels with hyperkeratosis of the overlying epidermis. One variety that sometimes causes alarm to elderly men occurs on the scrotum (angiokeratoma of Fordyce). Lesions are often multiple and present as red, slightly warty nodules. They do not usually cause discomfort. Rarely, similar lesions appear over the vulva in elderly women (Figure 9.41).

Capillary aneurysm

Small red papules consisting of ectatic capillaries occasionally appear quite suddenly and turn black because of thrombosis. They cause alarm because they are often mistaken for malignant melanoma.

Pyogenic granuloma

This odd lesion may appear at any age as a rapidly growing, and sometimes exudative, red nodule over the trunk or limbs. It consists of a mass of immature blood vessels and curious-looking new connective tissue. It is neither pyogenic nor granulomatous.

Spider naevus

This lesion has the peculiar property of appearing only within the drainage of the superior vena cava. It is most common over the face and forearms. The name refers to the appearance of a central vascular 'body' with radiating 'legs'. If large numbers appear in late middle age or in the elderly, they may signify underlying hepatic disease.

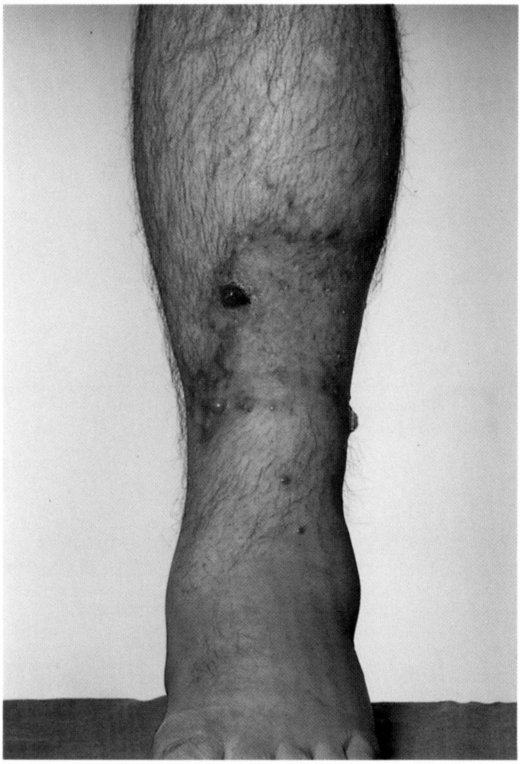

Figure 9.42

Kaposi's sarcoma. There are many purple nodules and brown macules in this patient, who had already had surgery and radiotherapy to the lesions on his leg.

Glomangioma

Glomangioma may be single or multiple. The latter condition is often familial. The lesions arise from the glomus cells of arteriovenous shunts and consist of masses of cuboidal cells and vascular channels. They are small bluish nodules which are occasionally spontaneously painful and exquisitely tender.

Kaposi's idiopathic haemorrhagic sarcoma

Kaposi's sarcoma (KS) has achieved notoriety in recent years as a component of the acquired immunodeficiency syndrome (AIDS). It appears confined to those whose AIDS has been contracted via homosexual contact. Prior to AIDS this multicentric malignant vascular disorder was virtually restricted to elderly subjects who originated from Italy around the Po valley or who were of Jewish origin and came from central Europe, although it also occurred in younger subjects endemically in areas of Uganda and South Africa. It has also been noted as a complication of the immunosuppression in renal transplant patients.

In the classical European type, the typical lesions usually occur on the lower legs at first as mauve or reddish-brown nodules and plaques (Figure 9.42). Flatter, brownish-red macules are also seen. The lesions enlarge and spread and eventually affect internal organs and cause death. Generally in this variety of KS the progress is slow, so that the patient may outlive his disease and die of some unrelated cause. In HIV-associated Kaposi's the individual elements of the disease are the same as in the 'classical' disorder. However, the disease progresses very much more rapidly and may result in death within 12–18 months.[47]

Pathology

The histological picture of KS depends on the stage of the disorder. The diagnostic feature is the presence of abnormal spindle-shaped cells and thin, vascular, slit-like channels. Other stages are marked by granulomatous inflammation or by fibrosis. In most biopsies extravasated red cells and haemosiderin pigment are prominent.

Treatment

Excision or locally destructive measures can be used for isolated lesions in the classical disorder. Larger lesions are profitably treated by radiotherapy. When the disease has spread to the viscera, chemotherapy has proved helpful in some patients. Interferons and IL-2 have also been used to treat severely ill patients with widespread Kaposi's sarcoma.

Angiosarcoma (malignant angioendothelioma)

This is another type of rare malignant vascular disease seen predominantly in the elderly. It often starts on the face or scalp and spreads relentlessly. The lesions are generally large pink or red macules or plaques. Histologically abnormal vascular channels can be found infiltrating the surrounding connective tissue bundles. Eventually metastases develop in the viscera. Generally the disorder is poorly responsive to treatment and is usually fatal in 12–18 months.

Haemangioendothelioma and haemopericytoma

Benign and malignant varieties of these rare vascular tumours are known. They have a variable histological appearance but are characterized by the formation of abnormal vascular channels.

Cutaneous lymphoma

Malignant lymphomas affecting the skin may be seen at all ages, but are more common in the elderly. The subject has become extremely complex and the account given below should be regarded only as a brief overview of the more important aspects. More detailed coverage is available in MacKie.[48]

Mycosis fungoides may arise *de novo* or be presaged by skin disorders which may or may not have the characteristics of malignancy and for which the term premalignant is probably inappropriate. The term parapsoriasis for these disorders has proved so confusing in the past that it is probably best not used at all.

Skin disorders from which mycosis fungoides may arise

Poikiloderma atrophicans vasculare

In this odd skin condition there are areas of atrophy, telangiectasia and reticulate pigmentation in and around the flexures in particular (Figure 9.43). The disorder persists largely unchanged or slowly extending for many years but eventually may transform into mycosis fungoides.

Lymphomatoid papulosis

The relationship of this disease to mycosis fungoides and Hodgkin's disease has been a contentious issue for some time (see also Chapter 10). Histologically bizarre, large

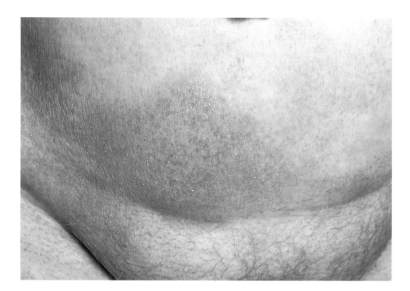

Figure 9.43

Poikiloderma atrophicans vasculare. The affected patch appears atrophic and shows scaling and telangiectasia.

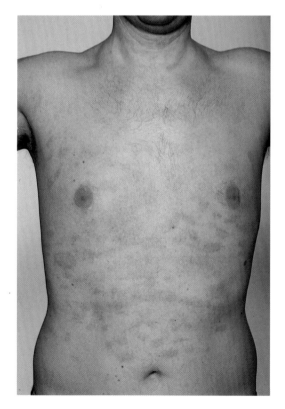

Figure 9.44

Parapsoriasis en plaque. There are many scaling pink areas on the trunk of this patient.

mononuclear cells are evident in the dermal cellular infiltrate but the individual papular and papulonecrotic lesions come and go and the entire disorder may disappear without trace. Furthermore, lymphomatoid papulosis appears to be related to the benign disorder pityriasis lichenoides. None the less, there are patients in whom the disease is a forerunner to mycosis fungoides or Hodgkin's disease.[49]

Pre-mycosis fungoides

Persistent round or irregularly shaped, flat scaling pink patches on the trunk or limbs are not infrequently the first signs of mycosis fungoides. However, they may remain unchanged for very many years and even temporarily disappear. The difficulty is in distinguishing the forerunner lesions of mycosis fungoides from similar appearing quite benign disorders. Parapsoriasis en plaques and xantho-erythroderma perstans are two such benign diseases that are characterized by the presence of well defined, pink or pink-yellow scaling patches on the trunk (Figure 9.44). These diseases persist unchanged for many years with little in the way of symptoms. Histologically they show minor changes of eczema. Unfortunately the histological features of true pre-mycosis fungoides lesions are very little different and several biopsies may be required before anything suspicious is seen. Eventually in some patients with the forerunner disease the individual lesions enlarge and become more numerous and plaque-like, heralding the beginning of frank mycosis fungoides.

Mycosis fungoides

This is the archetypal lymphoma affecting the skin. It is uncommon but by no means rare. The average regional hospital may have 10–20 such patients under its care at any one time. It may occur any time during adult life but is more common in late middle age and the elderly. Mycosis fungoides may start insidiously in the course of one of the predisposing disorders mentioned above or after a predisposing disorder has remitted some time previously, or it may start spontaneously, there having been no previous skin disorder. It is thought to be a neoplastic disorder of lymphocytes of the T-helper cell type.

Clinical features

The disorder is characterized by the appearance of rounded or irregularly shaped, red scaling macules. Pruritus is often a prominent syndrome at this stage. The involved areas enlarge and thicken to produce plaques and eventually tumours, which become eroded (Figure 9.45). Visceral involvement occurs late in the disease. In the later stages, patients become generally unwell and death usually occurs from a secondary infection.

Pathology

There is a band-like subepidermal infiltrate of mixed inflammatory cells, among which are found variable numbers of large, abnormal mononuclear cells that have large convoluted or reniform hyperchromatic nuclei. An important diagnostic feature is the invasion of the epidermis by the abnormal cells (epidermotropism). Often the cells group together to form microabscesses (Pautrier micro-abscesses) (Figure

9.46). The epidermis itself is usually thickened and sometimes psoriasiform and parakeratotic.

Aetiology

The cause is unknown, but it has been suggested that a retro virus infection of lymphocytes is involved. The abnormal cells appear to be abnormal T-helper lymphocytes, although immunocytochemical tests do not always succeed in identifying the abnormal population of cells. It has been suggested that this treatment may delay progression of the disease.[49] Long term remissions can be expected for patients with stage I or II disease.[50] Patients with erythrodermic mycosis

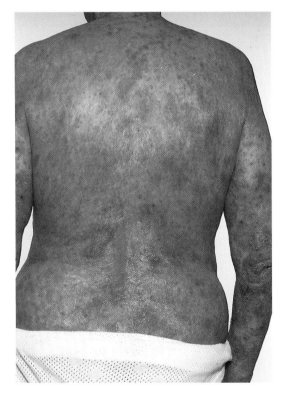

Figure 9.45a

Mycosis fungoides. The lesions are in the early plaque stage and have not yet become nodular, although some are already raised.

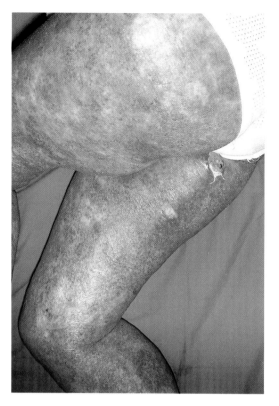

Figure 9.45b

A more advanced stage of mycosis fungoides. Most of the lesions are raised plaques.

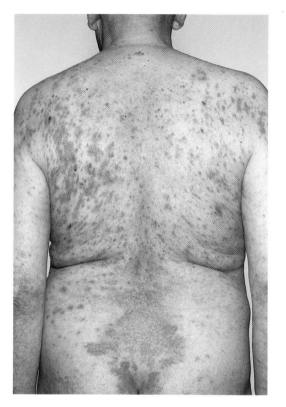

Figure 9.45c

Further patient with mycosis fungoides.

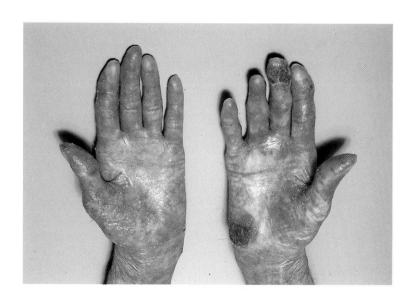

Figure 9.45d

Tumour stage of mycosis fungoides. There are eroded nodules affecting a finger and a hypothenar eminence.

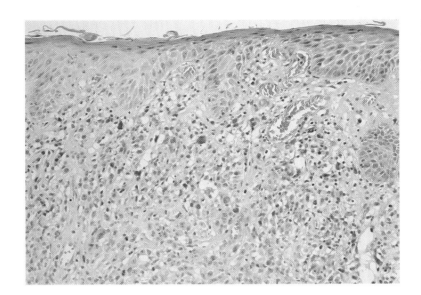

Figure 9.46

Histopathology of mycosis fungoides. Note the large number of cells subepidermally, some of which have abnormal nuclei (H & E; ×90).

fungoides responded well to extracorporeal phototherapy (photopheresis).[51]

Treatment

The most suitable treatment for early stages of the disorder is PUVA (see page 27). This treatment produces remission in most patients and relieves symptoms. Emollients and weak topical corticosteroids are also useful in alleviating discomfort and pruritus. If required, PUVA may be administered on several occasions, but unfortunately the disease usually escapes from control at some stage, necessitating other forms of treatment. Superficial radiotherapy or treatment with electron beams has been found useful for some patients. Combinations of chemotherapeutic agents have also been used in attempts at eradication of the disease and for advanced stages. Thus far the results have been disappointing and are certainly not as good as for those for Hodgkin's disease.

Variants of mycosis fungoides

Sézary syndrome

This rare disorder is an erythrodermic form of mycosis fungoides. Certain areas are especially affected. The face, for example, may be thickened and almost leonine. The palms may also be extremely thickened. Abnormal cells can be found circulating in the blood—so-called Sézary cells (sometimes known as Lutzner cells). These are large mononuclear cells with large, dark, cerebriform nuclei. The progress of this form of the disease tends to be more rapid than the classical type.

Woringer–Kolopp disease

This extremely rare variant is a chronic localized form of the disorder. One solitary, slowly enlarging plaque may be the only sign of mycosis fungoides. Histologically the epidermotropism is very marked, and there is marked epidermal thickening. Some cases have become generalized.

Other types of cutaneous lymphoma

The skin may be involved in almost all types of leukaemia and lymphoma, including Hodgkin's disease on rare occasions, but primary cutaneous lymphoma other than mycosis fungoides is extremely uncommon. Primary cutaneous lymphosarcoma and reticulum cell sarcoma do rarely occur but do not have specific clinical appearances and are diagnosed histologically with difficulty. Some disorders originally believed to represent lymphomas of the skin are now more accurately described as pseudolymphomas. These include Spiegler–Fendt sarcoid, in which there are persistent large papules containing a myriad of lymphocytes. They are now believed to be the result of persistent insect bite reactions and other persistent and highly cellular hypersensitivity reactions. Actinic reticuloid (see page 53) is also quite reasonably regarded as a pseudolymphoma.

Proliferative histiocytic disorders

This group of diseases (known as the histiocytosis X group) is properly regarded as a malignant disease of the reticulo-histiocytic system. The abnormal histiocytic cells often retain in part their phagocytic function. They contain the characteristic Langerhans cell tennis-racket-shaped organelle. The skin is rarely affected in isolation: lesions in bone, liver and bone, in lung and in the central nervous system often accompany cutaneous involvement. Letterer–Siwe disease is essentially a progressive disorder of children and will not be discussed further. Hand–Schuller–Christian disease is more restricted in distribution and less aggressive in speed of progress. It mainly affects young adults and is not seen in the elderly. Eosinophilic granuloma, in which the process is even more slow-moving and localized, may be seen in adult life but rarely in the elderly.

Xanthoma disseminatum

This may not be of the histiocytosis X type, and its true nosological position is unclear. It is an uncommon disorder of adults and the elderly are affected only rarely. Numerous yellowish-brown papules containing a mixture of inflammatory cells and histiocytes and giant cells appear over the trunk, to disappear in the course of some months.

Reticulohistiocytoma

This is another rare disorder that is not related to histiocytosis X. It may occur as a solitary nodule or in a disseminated form. When disseminated it is associated with a destructive small joint arthropathy. The nodules, which are smooth and reddish-brown, contain giant cells and characteristic large cells with ground glass cytoplasm.

Proliferative disorders of mast cells

Mast cell naevus and mastocytosis are disorders of infancy and childhood. However, there is an adult variety that is sometimes seen in the elderly. This unfortunately is known as telangiectasia macularis eruptiva perstans of Parkes Weber![52] Numerous red telangiectatic macules appear over the trunk and limbs. Unlike the juvenile forms, mast cells are not always easy to demonstrate in the lesions. The disorder is persistent and gradually progressive and visceral lesions are not infrequently present.

References

1 Halevy S, Feuerman E J. The sign of Leser-Trelet: a cutaneous marker for internal malignancy. *Int J Dermatol* (1985) **24:**359–61.

2 Kopf A W, Muntzis M, Bart R S. Diagnostic accuracy in malignant melanoma. *Arch Dermatol* (1975) **111:**1291–2.

3 Lever L, Marks R. Pigmented facial macules: a sign of photoaging. In: Marks R, Plewig G, eds, *The Environmental Threat to the Skin*, (Martin Dunitz: London, 1992) 91–6.

4 Ortonne J P. Pigmentary disorders associated with sun exposure. *J Dermatol Treat* (1996) **7**(suppl 2): S7–S8.

5 Desmons F, Breiullard F, Thomas P et al. Multiple clear cell acanthomas [Degos]: histochemical and ultrastructural study of two cases. *Int J Dermatol* (1977) **16:**203–13.

6 Wilson-Jones E, Heyl T. Naevus sebaceous: a report of 140 cases with special regard to the development of secondary malignant tumours. *Br J Dermatol* (1970) **82:**99–117.

7   Lever W F, Schaumberg-Lever G. *Histopathology of the Skin*, 6th Edn. (Lippincott: Philadelphia, 1983).

8   Pinkus H, Mehregan A H. *A Guide to Dermatohistopathology*, 3rd Edn (Appleton-Century-Crofts: New York, 1981).

9   Kumar P, Marks R. Sebaceous gland hyperplasia and senile comedones: a prevalence study in elderly hospitalized patients. *Br J Dermatol* (1987) **117**:231–6.

10 Marks R, Ponsford M W, Selwood T S et al. Non melanotic skin cancer and solar keratoses in Victoria. *Med J Aust* (1983) **2**:619–22.

11 Harvey I, Frankel S, Marks R et al. Non-melanoma skin cancer and solar keratoses. I Methods and descriptive results of the South Wales Skin Cancer Study. *Br J Cancer* (1996) **74**:1302–7.

12 Epstein J H. Photocarcinogenesis, skin cancer and ageing. *J Am Acad Dermatol* (1983) **9**:487–502.

13 Marks R. Premalignant disease of the epidermis—some light on neoplasia. *J R Soc Physicians* (1986)

14 Shahrad P, Marks R. The wages of warmth: changes in erythema ab igne. *Br J Dermatol* (1977) **97**:179–86.

15 Lang P G. Non melanoma skin cancer. In: Thiers B H, Dobson R L, eds, *Pathogenesis of Skin Disease*, (Churchill Livingstone: New York, 1986) 431–2.

16 Marks R, Foley P, Goodman G, Hage B H, Selwood T S. Spontaneous remission of solar keratoses: the case for conservative management. *Br J Dermatol* (1986) **155**:649–55.

17 Tan C Y, Marks R. Lichenoid keratoses. Prevalence and immunological findings. *J Invest Dermatol* (1982) **79**:365–7.

18 Hardie I R, Strong R W, Hartley L C J et al. Skin cancer in Caucasian renal allograft recipients living in a subtropical climate. *Surgery* (1980) **87**:177–83.

19 Schwartz R A. Premalignant keratinocyte neoplasms. *J Am Acad Dermatol* (1996) **35**:223–42.

20 Pearse A D, Marks R. Actinic keratoses and the epidermis on which they arise. *Br J Dermatol* (1977) **96**:45–50.

21 Peck G L. Therapy and prevention of skin cancer. In: Saurat J H, ed, *Retinoids: New Trends In Research & Therapy*, (Karger: Basle, 1985) 345–54.

22 Kingston T, Marks R. Cutaneous neoplasia and the retinoids. In: Cunliffe W J, Miller A J, eds, *Retinoid Therapy: A Review Of Clinical & Laboratory Research*, (MTP Press: Lancaster, 1984) 195–9.

23 Kligman A M, Thorne E G. Topical therapy of actinic keratoses with tretinoin. In: Marks R, ed, *Retinoids in Citaneous Malignancy*, (Blackwell Scientific: Oxford, 1991) 66–73.

24 Jones C M, Mang T, Cooper M et al. Photodynamic therapy in the treatment of Bowen's disease. *J Am Acad Dermatol* (1992) **27**:979–82.

25 Coleman W P, Yarborough J M, Mandy S H. Dermabrasion for prophylaxis and treatment of actinic keratoses. *Dermatol Surg* (1996) **22**: 17–21.

26 Rook A, Whimster I. Keratoacanthoma—a thirty year retrospect. *Br J Dermatol* (1979) **100**:41–7.

27 Editorial: Genital wart virus infections: Nuisance or potentially lethal? *Br Med J* (1984) **288**:735–6.

28 Marks R. Squamous cell carcinoma. *The Lancet* (1996) **347**:737–8.

29 Jones R E, Austin C, Ackerman A B. Extramammary Paget's disease: a critical re-examination. *Am J Dermatopathol* (1979) **1**:101–5.

30 Domarus H V, Stevens P J. Metastatic basal cell carcinoma. *J Am Acad Dermatol* (1984) **10**:1043–60.

31 Mason J K, Helwig E B, Graham J H. Pathology of the nevoid basal cell carcinoma syndrome. *Arch Pathol* (Chicago) (1965) **79**:401–8.

32 Zitelli J A. Mohs surgery concepts and misconceptions. *Int J Dermatol* (1985) **24**:541–8.

33 Hölzle E, Kind P, Plewig G. *Malignant Melanoma Diagnosis and Differential Diagnosis* (Martin Dunitz: London, 1989).

34 MacKie R M. *Skin Cancer* (Martin Dunitz: London, 1989).

35 Armstrong B K. Melanoma of skin. *Br Med Bull* (1984) **40**:346–50.

36 MacKie R M, Soutar D S, Watson A C H et al. Malignant melanoma in Scotland 1979–1983. *Lancet* (1985) **ii**:859–62.

37 Magnus K. Habits of sun exposure and risk of melanoma. *Cancer* (1981) **48**:2329–35.

38 Shreiber M M, Bozzo P D, Moon T E. Malignant melanoma in South Arizona. *Arch Dermatol* (1981) **117**:6–11.

39 Pathak D R, Samet J M, Howard C A et al. Malignant melanoma of the skin in New Mexico 1969–1977. *Cancer* (1982) **50**:1440–6.

40 MacKie R M. Clinical features of cutaneous melanoma and the role of naevi as precursor lesions. In: MacKie R M, ed, *Melanoma*, (W B Saunders: London, 1984) 439–55.

41 Breslow A. Thickness cross sectional area and depth of invasion in the prognosis of cutaneous melanoma. *Ann Surg* (1970) **172**:902–8.

42 Morton D L. Surgical treatment for malignant melanoma. In: MacKie R M, ed, *Melanoma*, (W B Saunders: London, 1984) 517–29.

43 Krasagakis K, Almond-Roesler B, Zouboulis C C et al. Merkel cell carcinoma: report of ten cases with emphasis on clinical course, treatment and in vitro drug sensitivity. *J Am Acad Dermatol* (1997) **36**:727–32.

44 Dalziel K, Marks R. Hair follicle like change over histiocytomas. *Am J Dermatopathol* (1986) **8**:462–4.

45 Gloster H M. Dermatofibrosarcoma protuberances. *J Am Acad Dermatol* (1996) **35:**355–74.

46 Morgan S H, Crawford Md'A. Anderson Febry disease: a commonly missed diagnosis. *Brit Med J* (1988) **297:**872–3.

47 Penneys N S. Cutaneous presentations of malignancy in AIDS. In: *Skin Manifestations of AIDS*, (Martin Dunitz: London, 1990) 95–110.

48 MacKie R M. Lymphomas and leukaemias. In: Champion R H, Burton J L, Ebling F J G, eds, *Textbook of Dermatology*, 5th Edn, (Blackwell Scientific: London, 1992) 2107–314.

49 Roupe G, Sandstrom M H, Kjellström C. PUVA in early mycosis fungoides may give long term remission and delay extracutaneous spread. *Acta Derm Venereol* (Stockh) (1996) **76:**475–8.

50 Hermann J J, Roenigk H H, Huria A et al. Treatment of mycosis fungoides with photochemotherapy (PUVA): long term follow-up. *J Am Acad Dermatol* (1995) **33:**234–42.

51 Duvic M, Hester J P, Lemark N A. Photophoresis therapy for cutaneous T-cell lymphoma. *J Am Acad Dermatol* (1996) **35:**573–9.

52 Czarnetzki B M. Mastocytosis. In: *Urticaria*, (Springer Verlag: Berlin, 1986) 116–21.

10
Skin manifestations of endocrine, neoplastic and nutritional deficiency disease

Physicians are fascinated by this group of disorders. A correct diagnosis is a feather in the professional cap. However, many of the disorders are rare, and it is almost as inconvenient for the elderly patient to be subjected to endless investigation through over awareness of their disorder's existence as to be left alone. Often the internal problems they presage are incurable, and the quality of life remaining is not much improved by treatment.

Skin markers of internal malignant disease

Acanthosis nigricans

This rare disorder is characterized by increased pigmentation and warty hyperplasia of the skin of the flexures. It is often caused by an underlying adenocarcinoma or less frequently some other visceral malignancy but may also be seen as part of an endocrine disorder and the Laurence–Seip lipodystrophy syndrome. It should be distinguished from the more common pseudoacanthosis nigricans seen predominantly in the flexures of the obese (Figure 10.1).

Apart from the flexural changes mentioned above, true acanthosis nigricans is characterized by other signs. There is often some generalized increase in pigmentation and all normally pigmented areas (including seborrhoeic warts) become even darker. There may also be an increase in the number of seborrhoeic warts, and indeed, when there is a sudden outbreak of these warty lesions in the absence of other signs of

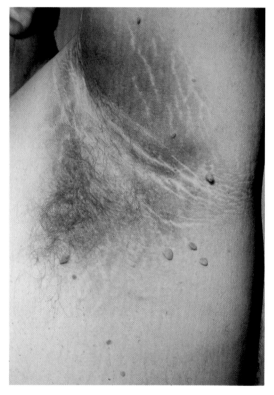

Figure 10.1

Pseudo acanthosis nigricans. There are hyperpigmentation, warty thickening and papillomas in the axillae.

acanthosis nigricans, the condition has been thought to be a forme fruste of acanthosis nigricans and a sign of visceral malignancy (sign of Leser-Trélat[1]). Though this may be the case in some patients, the majority with large numbers of seborrhoeic warts of recent onset are found free from visceral disease after investigation. The palms often show a curious succulent verrucous hypertrophy, and when marked and occurring in isolation the condition has been dubbed 'tripe palms' and found to indicate visceral malignant disease.[2]

The occurrence of acanthosis nigricans in endocrine (and in particular, pituitary) disease has led to the suggestion that the secretion of growth-promoting peptide may be responsible for the pigmentary change and warty hypertrophy found in the disease.[3] However, as yet no particular substance has been incriminated. Many patients with acanthosis nigricans have insulin resistant diabetes but how this fits in with the tissue changes that take place in the skin is unclear.

Treatment must be directed to the underlying disorder. If a malignant tumour is found and successfully removed the skin condition remits, only to relapse when the tumour recurs.

Erythema gyratum repens

This is an extremely rare form of figurate erythema and is almost invariably a sign of malignancy.[4] Classically the appearance is likened to that of wood grain with polycyclic erythematous rings inside which are other concentric rings (Figure 10.2). The lesions are migrating, so that the pattern over the skin slowly alters. The underlying neoplasm in several reported patients has been bronchial carcinoma.

Other types of figurate erythema

The various other types of annular or figurate erythema are not usually indicators of internal malignancy. However, some cases have been reported where simple annular erythema has been a sign of internal cancer. The author remembers vividly one such patient who presented with an odd annular erythema of the shins and on examination was found to have a carcinoma of the rectum (Figure 10.3). Any

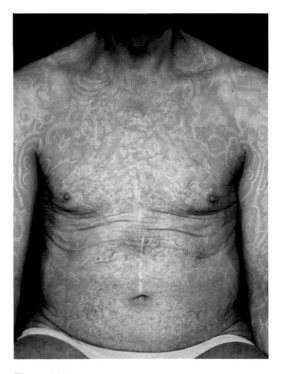

Figure 10.2

Erythema gyratum repens. Note the wood grain type of patterning. This patient of Dr P. Holt was found to have an underlying carcinoma of the bronchus.

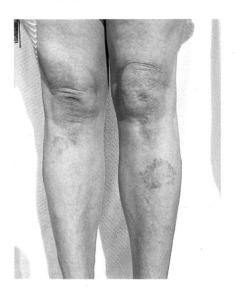

Figure 10.3

Annular erythema on legs of elderly lady who was found on physical examination to have carcinoma of the rectum.

patient past middle age with a persistent or recurrent eruption of this kind should be examined and studied with this possibility in mind.

Dermatomyositis (polymyositis)

Dermatomyositis is a disorder of the autoimmune connective tissue type characterized predominantly by inflammatory changes in skin and muscle. Its exact relationship to visceral malignant disease has been a contentious issue for many years. There can be little doubt that in some older patients dermatomyositis is precipitated by a neoplasm. It is the proportion of cases in which there is such an association that has caused argument.[5] The estimate that 50% of dermatomyositis patients over 50 have underlying cancer is almost certainly too pessimistic. One study shows that the figure in patients over the age of 37 is nearer 37.5%.[6] A wide variety of neoplastic lesions may be associated with dermatomyositis without a preponderance of any one particular type. There have been several cases reported in which the dermatomyositis improved after removal of the tumour—with recrudescence of the disease when metastases appeared.

In patients with dermatomyositis and malignant disease the clinical features of the former do not differ from those of patients without the association. At least they do not differ in type, but clinical experience suggests that dermatomyositis due to malignant disease has a stormier course than when it occurs in isolation.

An immunopathogenesis has been suspected for dermatomyositis as with other autoimmune disorders. Where neoplastic disease appears to have precipitated the disorder it is reasonable to suggest that antigenic stimulation from the tumour is involved and in some way responsible for stimulating the production of autoantibodies.

Necrolytic migrating erythema

There is a strong association between this disorder and certain tumours of the alpha cell system of the pancreas. It is in fact one of the components of the glucagonoma syndrome[7] resulting from a pancreatic alpha cell tumour (or, rarely,

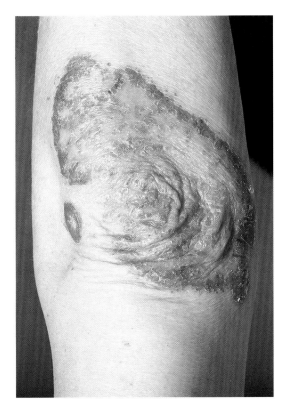

Figure 10.4

Necrolytic migratory erythema. This patient of Dr A. Knight was found to have a glucagonoma. The affected areas were raised at the edges, scaly and erosive.

alpha cell hyperplasia). Other clinical features include a mild diabetes, diarrhoea, weight loss, glossitis and angular stomatitis. Typically the biochemical findings are also characteristic. There is hyperglycaemia from the glucagon stimulated gluconeogenesis, a much raised plasma glucagon (which may have a different molecular weight from normal), and considerably decreased levels of amino acids and zinc in the blood. The rash seen in the course of the disease is variable in its severity but always present. It is particularly marked around the groins and in the facial flexures, but may appear anywhere. The lesions slowly spread, heal and recur. Characteristically the affected areas are red, slightly raised and scaling or erosive or crusted (Figure 10.4). There may be a serpiginous outline

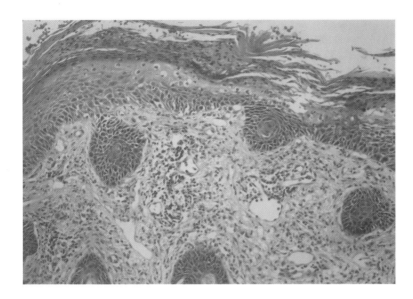

Figure 10.5

Necrolytic migratory erythema. Typical appearance of necrosis on the upper epidermis and parakeratosis (H & E; ×90).

Table 10.1   Causes of acquired ichthyosis

Cause	Notes
Malignant disease	Commonest visceral malignancy responsible is Hodgkin's disease but other types are sometimes responsible[10]
Essential fatty acid (EFA deficiency)	EFA deficiency may be due to faulty parenteral feeding[11] or malabsorption due to intestinal bypass operation Experimental deprivation in small mammals has been used as a model of psoriasis
Blood lipid lowering drugs	The butyrophenones, 7–12 diazocholesterol, Mer 29, have been associated with acquired ichthyosis; the diazocholesterol-treated mouse[13] has been made the basis of a model for ichthyosis
Leprosy	Quite common in the course of lepromatous leprosy undergoing treatment with Dapsone

to the lesions. Biopsy of an affected lesion shows degenerative change in the upper epidermis and parakeratosis (Figure 10.5). The eruption does not seem to be due to the increased levels of glucagon per se but may well be caused by the hypoaminoacidaemia or the low blood levels of zinc.

Several cases have been described in which necrolytic migratory erythema has not been associated with a glucocagoma or alpha cell hyperplasia. Some of these have been associated with a low cirrhosis and low serum zinc with improvement after zinc supplement.[8]

Treatment of the established disorder is difficult; by the time the patient presents there are usually metastases in the liver. Some patients' rashes improve after removal of the pancreatic tumour or courses of chemotherapy, but they generally return as metastases spread.

Acquired ichthyosis

As indicated in Chapter 4, the ichthyotic disorders are usually congenital in origin: when ichthyosis develops in adult life it is often a sign of a serious metabolic disturbance—usually due to a visceral malignancy of some type.[9] The various causes of acquired ichthyosis are set out in Table 10.1. It will be seen that some types of acquired ichthyosis are due to interference with

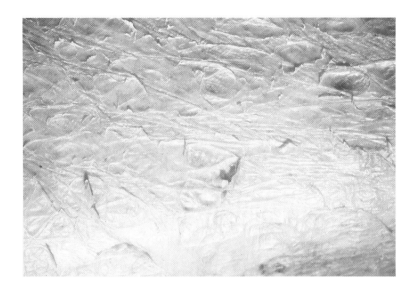

Figure 10.6

Close-up view of skin of patient with acquired ichthyosis. This man's skin problem started at the age of 67. He was found to have reticulum cell carcinoma.

some aspects of lipid metabolism. The metabolic causes for the other provoking agencies for acquired ichthyosis are unknown.

Acquired ichthyosis should be distinguished from the less severe type of roughness and dryness of the skin (xeroderma) seen in the course of many serious wasting diseases, including intestinal malabsorption and renal failure. The reticuloses are the most usual cause of acquired ichthyosis.[9] The associated ichthyosis resembles autosomal dominant ichthyosis but is often quite severe (Figure 10.6). It improves when the reticulosis has been adequately treated by chemotherapy or radiotherapy.

Bullous pemphigoid

This blistering disorder (described more fully in Chapter 6) is sometimes noted in concurrence with a visceral malignancy, and as with dermatomyositis, it is the frequency and specificity of the association that has caused disagreement and debate. Pemphigoid is essentially a disorder of the elderly—the time of life when the discovery of malignant disease coincidentally is not uncommon. For this reason it is difficult to establish in any particular case whether the blistering disorder was causally related to a neoplasm.

Stone and Schroeter found very little difference in the prevalence of neoplastic disease in bullous pemphigoid patients compared with the normal population.[14] Others have suggested that patients with especially severe pemphigoid and who have oral lesions may be likely to have an associated malignancy.[15] It is presumed that when there is a true association, immunopathogenetic mechanisms are involved, such as shared antigens between the tumour and the dermo-epidermal junction. If investigation for a malignant disorder is deemed necessary, it should not delay treatment (see page 000). Rarely, other blistering disorders, including a dermatitis herpetiformis-like picture and a pemphigus vulgaris type of disorder have been found in patients with a neoplasm. The two disorders have been thought to be associated.

Cutaneous metastases[16]

Secondary deposits from internal cancers are not uncommon and it has been suggested that approximately 6% of all metastases are deposited in the skin. Some tumours seem to disseminate to the skin more commonly than others: renal, ovarian, gastric and other gastrointestinal, breast and bronchial cancers are the

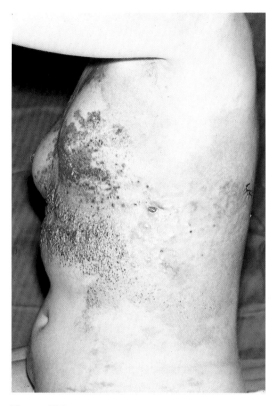

Figure 10.7

Carcinoma en cuirasse due to carcinoma of the breast.

most frequent carcinomata to metastasize to the skin. Melanomatous deposits are also common and are not always pigmented. Deposits of leukaemic cells and lymphosarcoma are also found on the skin,[17] though these diseases more often affect the skin in other ways (see below).

Cutaneous metastases do not have a particularly characteristic appearance and are often removed in the belief that they are simple cysts or histiocytomas or because no clinical diagnosis is possible. They are usually multiple, but solitary lesions are also found. Generally they are asymptomatic, firm intracutaneous nodules and are either pink or skin-coloured. They seem to favour certain sites—the scalp and front of the trunk in particular. Those from the breast and gastrointestinal tract favour the upper trunk. Carcinoma en cuirasse occurs when the dermis and subcutis are extensively infiltrated by metastatic cancer—usually from the breast (Figure 10.7).

Other signs of malignant disease

Erythroderma and exfoliative dermatitis

Universal reddening of the skin with or without scaling is a sign of several unrelated disorders (see Table 10.2) originating in the skin. In some cases, however, there is no primary inflammatory or neoplastic disease of the skin and an erythroderma, with or without accompanying scaliness,

Table 10.2 Causes of erythroderma

Cause	Notes
Psoriasis	Generally supervenes in patients with several plaque type or generalized pustular psoriasis. Scaling may be prominent
Eczema	Erythroderma states may occur in severe atopic dermatitis, severe seborrhoeic eczema and in actinic reticuloid; scaling may be prominent
Pityriasis rubra pilaris	Most adult onset cases are either 'erythrodermic' or nearly so with a few islands of normal skin; scaling is prominent (page 000)
Non-bullous (and bullous) ichthyosiform erythrodema	Generalized erythema in all patients that improves with age; there is also scaling and hyperkeratosis as well as blisters in bullous form (page 00)
Drug eruptions	May start off as maculopapular rash or 'toxic erythema' or be generalized from beginning; toxic epidermal necrolysis is one variety (page 000)
Sézary syndrome	A generalized form of mycosis fungoides in which abnormal circulating mononuclear cells are found (page 00); scaling may be prominent
Erythroderma secondary to reticuloses and leukaemia	No primary cutaneous cause of erythroderma found; scaling not generally prominent

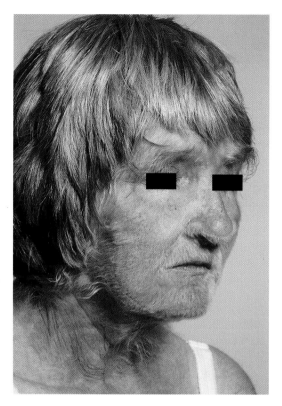

Figure 10.8a

Hypertrichosis lanugosa. Note fine, downy hair over the face, trunk and limbs of this woman who had underlying neoplastic disease.

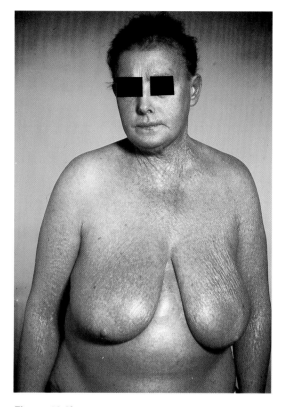

Figure 10.8b

The sudden onset of erythroderma in this woman heralded a lymphoma.

appears to be associated with an underlying neoplastic process elsewhere. The leukaemias and the reticuloses are the usual cause of this odd phenomenon (Figure 10.8). Erythema multiforme may occasionally be associated with underlying malignant disease. Curiously, this is mostly seen after radiotherapy treatment of the neoplasm.

Livedo reticularis

Transient prominence of the subcutaneous venous plexus on the limbs is not abnormal in young women when they are cold. When the prominence is persistent and generalized it indicates either abnormal dilatation and sluggish blood flow in these vessels owing to increased blood viscosity or abnormality of the vessels themselves. The connective tissue autoimmune diseases, such as lupus erythematosus or polyarteritis nodosa, may be responsible. Haematological disorders associated with hyperviscosity states, including polycythaemia rubra vera, myeloma and paraproteinaemias, can also cause this appearance (Figure 10.9).

Hypertrichosis lanugosa

The sudden appearance of a profuse widespread growth of fine hair is a rare sign of underlying neoplastic disease; the cause is unknown.

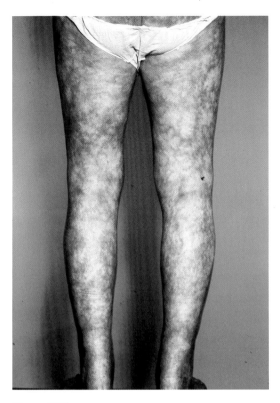

Figure 10.9

Livedo reticularis in an elderly man.

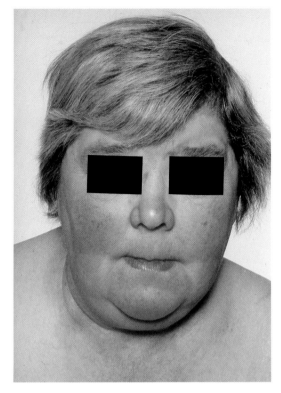

Figure 10.10

Typical 'peaches and cream' complexion in myxoedema.

Pruritus

Persistent severe pruritus without much in the way of the signs of skin disease may occur in polycythaemia rubra vera and in Hodgkin's disease. Less commonly it is a complaint in patients with other types of neoplastic disease.

Tylosis

This is the term used to describe a group of inherited disorders of keratinization characterized by hyperkeratosis of the palms and soles. The details of the clinical appearance and the pattern of inheritance vary in the different varieties. One rare type is inherited in a dominant fashion and is marked clinically by diffuse hyperkeratosis of the palms and soles and the development of carcinoma of the oesophagus.[18] Rarely palmar filiform hyperkeratosis may be indicative of neoplastic disease.[19] Filiform hyperkeratotic spicules appearing over the face and elsewhere has been reported as associated with monoclonal gammopathy.[20]

Carcinoid syndrome

This is the result of hepatic metastases from an argentaffinoma (carcinoid tumour) of the small bowel or from a bronchial carcinoid tumour. Flushing attacks occur and when severe these are accompanied by sweating and anxiety. At one time it was thought that serotonin was responsible but this is now not thought to be the case, and it is believed that kallikrein secreted by the tumour is responsible for the generation of vasoactive peptides (bradykinin in particular) and that these cause the signs and symptoms.[21] Malar erythema and telangiectasia develop after the condition has been present for some time.

Skin manifestations of endocrine disease

These are by no means confined to the elderly but they merit some mention here.

Thyroid disease

The epidermis appears quite responsive to thyroid hormones[22,23] and this accounts for at least some of the changes noted clinically. The roughness and dryness of the skin in myxoedema and the smoothness in hyperthyroidism may be explained in this way. In hypothyroidism there is often a faint yellowish tinge to the skin, said to be due to the deposition of carotenes in the skin. There is also often a reddish blush high on the cheeks, giving the appropriately termed peaches and cream appearance (Figure 10.10). The skin seems dry and may be roughened and the hair tends to be coarse and thinner than normal in myxoedema. In thyrotoxicosis the skin feels warm and moist because of the hyperdynamic circulation and increase in sweating. The hair is fine and difficult to control. In addition, some patients complain of persistent generalized itch—the cause for this is uncertain. Onycholysis occurs in some patients with hyperthyroidism and a diffuse Addisonian type of pigmentation is also seen in a few.

Associated conditions: pretibial myxoedema

In some 1 to 3% of patients with hyperthyroidism an odd condition develops on the front of the shins and occasionally elsewhere, known as pretibial myxoedema. Occasionally it occurs in hypothyroidism and other types of thyroid disorder.[24] In this disorder the local fibroblasts appear to proliferate and become hyperactive, secreting more proteoglycan than fibrous elements. The skin locally thickens into a plaque of variable size and becomes rugose and coarse and the hair becomes thicker over the area—giving a pig-skin or orange peel effect overall (Figure 10.11). A diffuse form affecting the lower legs is also described. The condition is strongly associated with exophthalmos.

Thyroid acropachy

The condition of pretibial myxoedema may spread outside the shins and involve the feet and even the face and hands, where subperiosteal new bone deposition and clubbing of the fingers is characteristic. This condition is known as thyroid acropachy. The cause of this odd localized sort of connective tissue hypertrophy is not entirely clear. Pretibial myxoedema occurs in close association with exophthalmos and it has been suggested that the circulating LATS factor (a polyclonal IgG) could be responsible. However, it has only been seen in 90% of patients with pretibial myxoedema. Certainly serum from thyrotoxic patients has been found to stimulate fibroblasts from the legs alone *in vitro*.[25] The disorder is extremely resistant to treatment although some success has been claimed from the intracutaneous injection of potent corticosteroids or hyaluronidase. Localized PUVA treatment has also been found to be effective in a few patients.

Parathyroid disease

The hypercalcaemia of primary hyperthyroidism rarely gives rise to symptoms in the skin but when due to secondary hyperthyroidism in chronic renal disease can cause intractable pruritus. In hyperparathyroidism the skin tends to be dry and slightly scaly, and there may be sparseness of scalp hair.

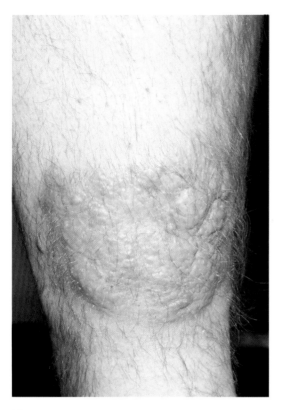

Figure 10.11a

Patch of pretibial myxoedema in an elderly woman who had hyperthyroidism.

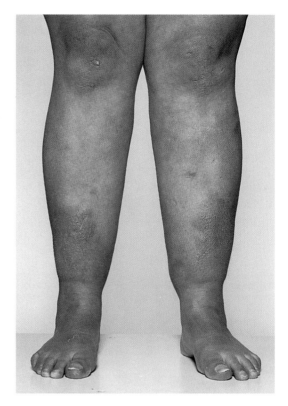

Figure 10.11b

Areas of pretibial myxoedema on both lower legs.

Disease of the adrenal gland

Cushing's syndrome

Whether this disorder is due to an adrenal tumour, hyperplasia or to the therapeutic administration of corticosteroids, the changes that occur in the skin are the same. The glucocorticoids have profound effects on both the epidermis and the dermis. They cause slowing of epidermal cell production, thinning of the epidermis and shrinking of individual epidermal cells.[26] These compounds also have the effect of thinning the dermis owing to their antimitotic and antisynthetic effects on fibroblasts.[27] The net result of glucocorticoid action is skin thinning and this is very obvious in patients with Cushing's syndrome—as it is in patients with

iatrogenic hypercortisonism. The well-known livid facial appearance, especially marked on the cheeks, is due to the skin thinning at a site where the subpapillary venous plexus is nearer the surface than in most other body sites (Figure 10.12). Striae distensae are the results of rupture of the structure of the dermis at sites of maximal stress and appear to represent elastic fibre rupture owing to the stress placed on weakened collagen (Figure 10.13). These lesions are normally evident to some degree in adolescence and pregnancy but are very much more prominent in Cushing's syndrome. In addition, the skin looks thin and the subcutaneous veins are obvious, there is skin fragility to minor trauma and purpuric patches occur after trivial knocks (Figure 10.14).

Apart from the changes due to skin thinning, other signs are found, including acne and hirsuties.

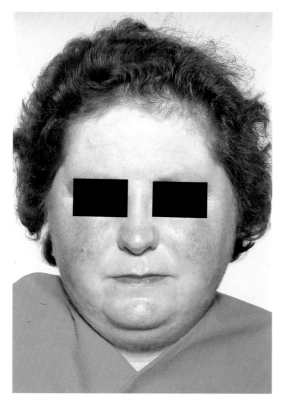

Figure 10.12

This woman's appearance had recently changed and the reddening of the cheeks and slight mooning was found to be due to Cushing's syndrome.

The acne of hypercortisonism is often widespread, affecting the trunk as well as the face, and consists predominantly of small follicular horny papules (Figure 10.15)—the larger and more inflamed lesions rarely occurring. A degree of hirsutism is usually present but variable in degree. The hairiness is not as severe as that seen in a true virilizing syndrome. The excess is mostly of the vellus type, but it is none the less a problem for women, who notice the growth of fine facial hair in particular.

Addison's disease

Hyperpigmentation is the major skin manifestation of destruction of the adrenal cortex, whatever the cause. The pigmentation is generalized but especially noticeable in areas that are normally not or only slightly pigmented, particularly the palmar creases and the buccal mucosa.

Virilizing syndromes

These are uncommon in the elderly. They are due to ovarian tumours, adrenal cortical tumours or adrenal hyperplasia. The skin changes that occur are predominantly hirsuties, acne and thickening of the skin.

Acromegaly

The major external signs of this disorder, which is usually due to an eosinophilic pituitary adenoma, are those of bone overgrowth and skin and subcutaneous tissue hypertrophy. The hands and feet show the changes particularly, becoming enlarged and succulently thickened. Measurement of skin thickness by ultrasound or by an X-ray technique demonstrates thickening of the dermis. The epidermal cells are increased in size and there is an increase in the rate of epidermal cell production.[28] There is an increased rate of sebum secretion and the skin looks greasy. Sweating is also increased in acromegaly and in some patients there is a generalized increase in pigmentation.

Diabetes mellitus

There are several skin disorders that occur more frequently in diabetes than in a control population but are by no means specific to diabetes. Vitiligo is a disorder of pigmentation in which focal degeneration of melanocytes results in sharply defined hypopigmented areas. This disease is much more common in diabetes—particularly in women—some 4.8% of patients with diabetes having vitiligo compared with 0.7% in a control population.[29] Interestingly, it now seems likely that vitiligo has an autoimmune basis and the same is true for diabetes in a substantial proportion of patients. Atherosclerosis and its consequences are certainly more common in diabetes than in a matched

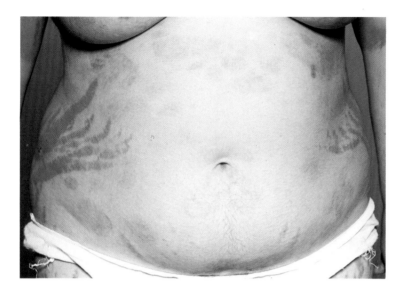

Figure 10.13a

Striae on the trunk due to Cushing's syndrome.

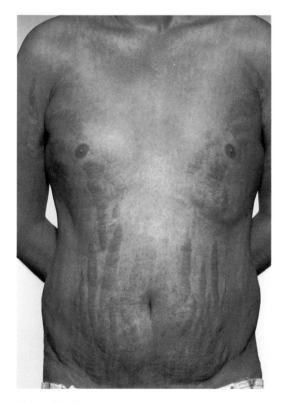

Figure 10.13b

Extensive striae on the trunk of a man treated with systemic steroids.

control population. The resulting ischaemia first produces loss of hair and skin atrophy and later may result in gangrene of a peripheral part such as the heel or one of the toes. The condition is disastrous, being painful and disabling; it usually necessitates amputation (Figure 10.16).

There is a generalized abnormality of the small blood vessels in diabetes due to deposition of glycoprotein in the vessel wall and resulting in narrowing of the lumina and decreased blood flow through them.[30] This tendency to ischaemia seems to predispose to ulceration of the skin from other causes and diminish wound healing capacity. Gravitational ulceration in diabetics is particularly resistant to treatment and prone to secondary infection. Disabling penetrating ulcers may also develop on the soles of the feet after minor injury in those with diabetic neuropathy. It is extremely important that elderly diabetic subjects are aware of the dangers and are carefully instructed in foot care.

The increase in atherosclerotic disease is probably due in part to the hyperlipidaemia that often occurs in diabetes. The appearance of xanthomatous lesions is also a result of the disturbance of lipid metabolism and resultant hyperlipidaemia. Although uncommon eruptive xanthoma is the usual clinical type of disease to develop. Numerous small (2–3 mm in diameter) pinkish-yellow papules appear in the course of a few days or up to

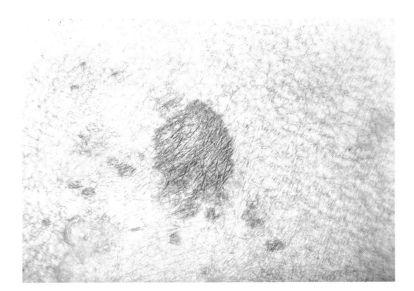

Figure 10.14

Purpura in a patient with Cushing's syndrome.

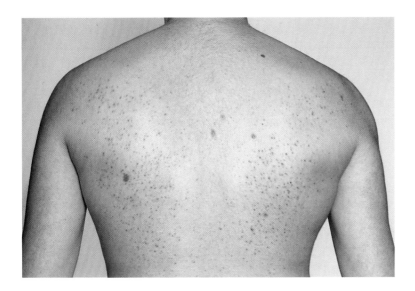

Figure 10.15

Steroid-induced acne in man who had received systemic steroids for lymphoma.

2 weeks. They are particularly numerous on the extensor surfaces of the back and the buttocks. The flexures and buccal mucosa may also be involved. Blood lipid analysis in most patients demonstrates that the triglyceride fraction is increased (type IV). The disorder is usually a complication of the early uncontrolled phase of the disease and the lesions disappear when the diabetes is adequately treated.

Some disorders are so much more frequent in diabetes than in the normal population that they are almost specific to the disease. Necrobiosis lipoidica is one such disorder. In one study some 65% of patients with necrobiosis were found to have diabetes at the time of examination,[31] but others developed the disorder subsequently, so that eventually some 90% or more of patients can be expected either to have or to develop diabetes.

Necrobiosis occurs on the legs in 90% or more of patients who have this disorder, but the skin

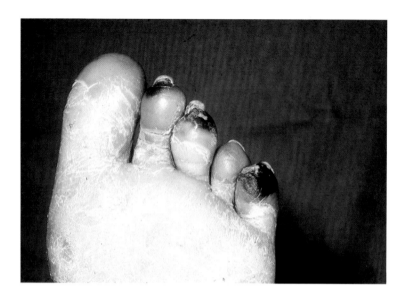

Figure 10.16

Gangrene of the tips of the toes in an elderly man with diabetes. He later had to have his leg amputated.

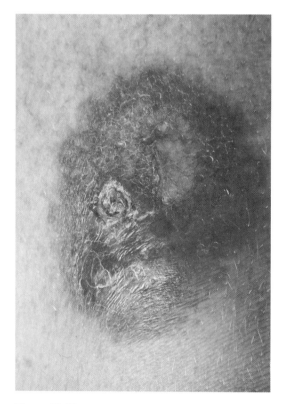

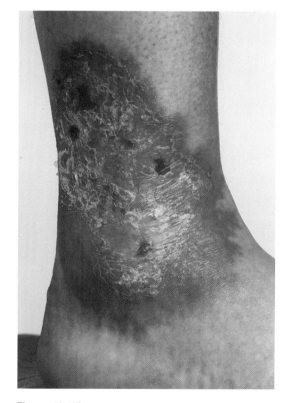

Figure 10.17a

Close-up of patch of necrobiosis lipoidica. Note slight yellowishness of the lesion at one side.

Figure 10.17b

Large patch of necrobiosis lipoidica on the ankle.

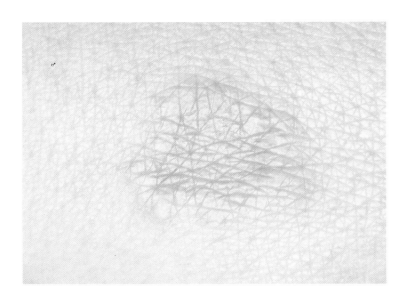

Figure 10.18a

Typical annular lesion of granuloma annulare.

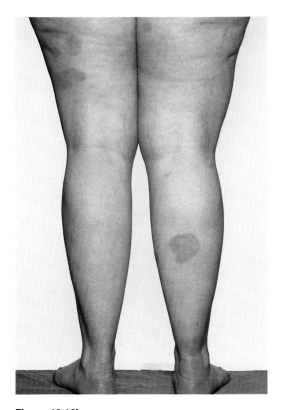

Figure 10.18b

This woman had many flat, red, well-defined macules due to superficial granuloma annulare. She was found to have diabetes.

of virtually any part can be affected. The lesions are yellowish and pink, irregular sclerotic nodules and plaques which occasionally become eroded (Figure 10.17). In many patients the lesions gradually improve so that eventually the affected area becomes atrophic. Unfortunately there is no treatment that can be prescribed with confidence that will alter the natural history of this disorder.

Histologically there are diffuse acellular and disorganized areas in the dermis that are paler but slightly more eosinophilic than usual and which have inflammatory cells surrounding them, including many histiocytes and some giant cells. The cause of the necrobiotic change in the dermis is uncertain but may have an immunopathogenetic basis. Immunoglobulin and complement have been localized in the lesions.[32]

Granuloma annulare is a common disorder characterized by necrobiotic changes in the dermis that are more pronounced than in necrobiosis lipoidica. The disease is common in children and adolescents and is mostly perfectly harmless. The relationship between this disorder and necrobiosis lipoidica is unclear. Some workers have claimed that there is a pronounced disposition to diabetes in patients with granuloma annulare.[33] Others have stated that this is not the case. However, when the disorder is generalized and superficial there does appear to be an association with diabetes (Figure 10.18).[34]

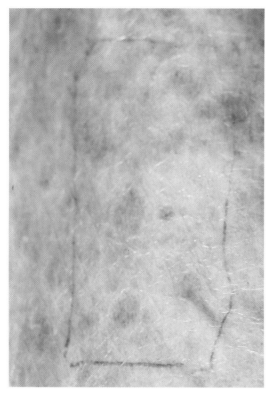

Figure 10.19

Small brown depressed area on shin due to diabetic dermopathy.

Diabetic dermopathy is predominantly seen in younger, male diabetics. It may be an odd reaction to trauma in diabetics but is of unknown cause. Small, pigmented, atrophic depressed areas occur over the front of the lower legs (Figure 10.19).[35] These lesions may also occur to a lesser extent in the normal population, and their significance is uncertain. Occasionally blisters occur in diabetic patients—their cause is unknown (Figure 10.20).

Patients with diabetes appear prone to candidiasis of the perigenital and perianal skin. The resulting localized pruritus may account for the mistaken belief that diabetes is a cause of generalized pruritus. There is no evidence that diabetics suffer more from generalized pruritus than any other group.

Skin stiffness and decreased joint mobility has been noted to occur more frequently in diabetics and has been thought to be due to glycosylation of dermal connective tissue.

The skin in nutritional deficiency disorders

The elderly often exist on a substandard diet deficient in many of the nutrients thought to be essential to maintain health. Protein-containing

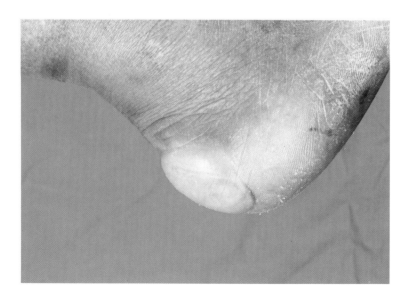

Figure 10.20

Spontaneously appearing blisters on the heel in a diabetic.

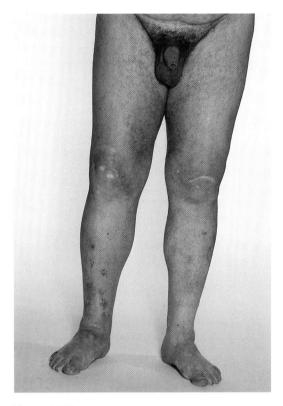

Figure 10.21

The speckled brown staining on this man's thighs was due to punctate haemorrhages, a result of vitamin C deficiency.

foods such as meat, fish, cheese and eggs tend to be too expensive and troublesome to prepare. Confusional states, forgetfulness and dietary fadism are other reasons for an inadequate diet. If insufficient protein is included in the diet over a long period there is a predisposition to osteoporosis and then easily damaged skin which heals slowly after injury.[36] The major causes of osteoporosis, however, are a low calcium and vitamin D intake and deficiency in sex hormone production.

If insufficient fresh fruit and/or vegetables are eaten, vitamin C deficiency occurs and scurvy can develop, as in the patient illustrated in Figure 10.21. In this disorder there is a defect in coagulation and resulting purpura—particularly in a punctate perifollicular pattern on the legs.

In the elderly, iron deficiency is common and may result in anaemia. It has been suggested that iron deficiency can also result in generalized pruritus and some diffuse loss of scalp hair. Despite iron being required for epithelial health, it has never been established that these symptoms can be the result of an iron deficit.

Many of the elderly are also deficient in zinc, and it has been suggested that this may be an important factor in preventing the healing of chronic gravitational ulcers.[37] Zinc supplements, however, do not appear to improve healing[38] and this issue has as yet not been settled. Essential fatty acid deficiency causes an ichthyosis-like picture (see page 230) but this is rarely due to dietary faddism or deprivation. It is mainly the result of parenteral feeding or intestinal bypass operations.

References

1   Halevey S, Fauerman E J. The sign of Leser-Trelet: a cutaneous marker for internal malignancy. *Int J Dermatol* (1985) **24:**359–61.

2   Breathnach S M, Wells G C. Acanthosis palmaris: tripe palms. A distinctive pattern of palmar keratoderma frequently associated with internal malignancy. *Clin Exp Dermatol* (1980) **5:**182–9.

3   Bernstein J E, Rothstein J, Soltani K et al. Neuropeptides in the pathogenesis of obesity associated benign acanthosis nigricans. *J Invest Dermatol* (1983) **80:**7–9.

4   Skolnick M, Mainman E R. Erythema gyratum repens with metastatic adenocarcinoma. *Arch Dermatol* (1975) **111:**227–9.

5   Callen J P. Malignancy in polymyositis/dermatomyositis. In: Sontheimer R J, ed, *Clinics in Dermatology*, (Lippincott: Philadelphia, 1988) 55–63.

6   Braverman I. Connective tissue (rheumatic diseases) In: *Skin Signs of Systemic Disease*, (W B Saunders: Philadelphia, 1981) 255–377.

7   Hashizumet T, Kirya H, Noda K et al. Gluconogoma syndrome. *J Am Acad Dermatol* (1988) **19:**377–83.

8   Sinclair S A, Reynolds N J. Necrolytic migratory erythema and zinc deficiency. *Br J Dermatol* (1997) **136:**783–5.

9   Dykes P J, Marks R. Acquired ichthyosis: multiple causes for an acquired generalised disturbance in desquamation. *Br J Dermatol* (1977) **97:**327–34.

10   Flint G L, Flam M, Soter N A. Acquired ichthyosis. A sign of nonlymphoproliferative malignant disorders. *Arch Dermatol* (1975) **111:**1446–7.

11 Caldwell P D, Johnsson H T, Othersen H B Jr. Essential fatty acid deficiency in an infant receiving parenteral alimentatin. *J Pediatr* (1972) **81:**894–8.

12 Prottey C. Essential fatty acids and the skin. *Br J Dermatol* (1976) **94:**579–85.

13 Elias P M, Williams M L, Maloney M E et al. Drug induced animal models of ichthyosis. In: Maibach H I, Lowe N, eds, *Models in Dermatology*, (Karger: Basle, 1985) 105–26.

14 Stone S P, Schroeter A L. Bullous pemphigoid and associated malignant neoplasms. *Arch Dermatol* (1975) **111:**991–4.

15 Rook A J. A pemphigoid eruption associated with carcinoma of the bronchus. *Trans St John's Hosp Dermatol Soc* (1968) **54:**148–51.

16 Schwartz R A. Cutaneous metastatic disease. *J Am Acad Dermatol* (1995) **33:**161–82.

17 Braverman I. Leukaemia and allied disorders. In: *Skin Signs of Systemic Disease*, 2nd Edn, (W B Saunders: Philadelphia, 1981) 179–96.

18 Harper P S, Harper R M J, Howell Evans A W. Carcinoma of the oesophagus with tylosis. *Q J Med* (1970) **39:**317–33.

19 Kaddy S, Soyer P, Kerl H. Palmar filiform hyperkeratosis: a new paraneoplastic syndrome. *J Am Acad Dermatol* (1995) **33:**337–40.

20 Paul C, Fernand J P, Flageul B et al. Hyperkeratotic spicules and monoclonal gammapathy. *J Am Acad Dermatol* (1995) **33:**346–51.

21 Melmon K L. Kinins: one of many mediators of the carcinoid spectrum. *Gastroenterology* (1968) **55:**545–8.

22 Holt P J A, Marks R. The epidermal response to change in thyroid status. *J Invest Dermatol* (1977) **68:**299–301.

23 Holt P J A, Lazsarus J, Marks R. The epidermis in thyroid disease. *Br J Dermatol* (1976) **95:**513–18.

24 Lynch P J, Maize J C, Sisson J C. Pretibial myxedema and non thyrotoxic thyroid disease. *Arch Dermatol* (1973) **107:**107–11.

25 Cheung H S, Nicoloff J T, Kamiel M B et al. Stimulation of fibroblast biosynthetic activity by serum of patients with pretibial myxedema. *J Invest Dermatol* (1978) **71:**12–17.

26 Marks R, Dykes P J. Steroids, squamous epithelium and psoriasis. In: Wright N A, Camplejohn R S, eds, *Psoriasis: Cell Proliferation*, (Churchill Livingston: Edinburgh, 1983).

27 Dykes P J, Marks R. An appraisal of the methods used in the assessment of atrophy from topical corticosteroids. *Br J Dermatol* (1979) **101:**599–609.

28 Holt P J A, Marks R. Epidermal architecture. Growth and metabolism in acromegaly. *Br Med J* (1976) (6008) 496–7.

29 Dawber R P R. Vitiligo in mature onset diabetes mellitus. *Br J Dermatol* (1968) **80:**275–8.

30 Ajjam Z S, Barton S, Corbett M et al. Quantitative evaluation of the dermal vasculature of diabetics. *Q J Med* (1985) **215:**229–39.

31 Muller S A, Winkelman R K. Necrobiosis lipoidica diabeticorum. A clinical and pathological investigation of 171 cases. *Arch Dermatol* (1966) **93:**272–81.

32 Ullman S, Dahl M V. Necrobiosis lipoidica. An immunofluorescence study. *Arch Dermatol* (1977) **113:**1671–3.

33 Muhlemann M F, Williams D R R. Granuloma annulare and diabetes mellitus—an association. *Br J Dermatol* (1984) **111:**12–13.

34 Haim S, Friedman-Birnbaum R, Shafrir A. Generalised granuloma annulare: relationship to diabetes mellitus as revealed in 8 cases. *Br J Dermatol* (1970) **83:**302–5.

35 Jelnick J E. The skin in diabetes mellitus: cutaneous manifestations, complications and associations. In: Kopf A W, Andrade R, eds, *Yearbook of Dermatology*, (Year Book Medical: Chicago, 1970).

36 McConkey B, Walton K W, Carney S A et al. Significance of occurrence of transparent skin. A study of the histological characteristics and biosynthesis of dermal collagen. *Ann Rheum Dis* (1967) **26:**219–25.

37 Pollack S V. System drugs and nutritional aspects of wound healing. *Clinics in Dermatology, Wound Healing* **2:**68–80.

38 Haley J V. Zinc sulphate and wound healing. *J Surg Res* (1979) **27:**168–74.

11
Vascular disorders and ulceration

Both large and small blood vessels suffer in the ageing process. Structurally, the lumina become narrower and the walls thicker, leading to reduction in blood flow and ischaemia. This process is the result of several disorders, including atherosclerosis and hypertension. Regardless of the cause, the end results involving the skin are similar—the development of ischaemia and tissue necrosis.

Persistent ulceration is the unfortunate result in many instances. The clinical appearance varies to some extent according to the underlying predominant aetiological cause. Despite this, a mixture of pathological processes is usually present.

Regardless of the cause, chronic ulceration of the skin is a miserable condition for the elderly and an enormous drain on personal, community and national resources. The major causes for persistent ulceration are set out in Table 11.1.

The gravitational syndrome

This term is used to describe all the clinical changes consequent on long-standing venous hypertension of the legs. It is preferable to the term stasis syndrome as the overall flow of blood through the venous system may be increased, rather than decreased. It is also preferable to the term varicose, which is descriptive only of the visible superficial dilated veins or varicosities.

Prevalence

There are no reliable estimates of the prevalence of the gravitational syndrome. If we accept the presence of a venous flare and slight transient orthostatic oedema around the ankles with

Table 11.1 The main causes of chronic ulceration of the skin

Type of ulcer	Clinical features	Aetiopathological notes
Gravitational ulcer	Accompanying pigmentation and swelling; mostly on medial aspect of ankle	Long-standing venous hypertension; typically fibrin cuffs develop around small blood vessels
Ischaemic ulcer	Anywhere around ankle and foot; typically painful; atrophic changes in skin surrounding ulcer	Due to either atherosclerosis of larger arteries or less frequently an inflammatory arteritis
Diabetic ulceration	Either perforating ulcer over weight-bearing areas of foot, or ischaemic with infection	Perforating ulcer due to diabetic neuropathy; ischaemic type caused by accelerated atherosclerosis and infection
Decubitus ulcer	Ulcers over pressure areas in paralysed or unconscious patients	Due to pressure necrosis of body parts against unyielding bedclothes
Haematological ulceration	May stimulate ischaemic or gravitational ulcer; often in younger individuals	Due to microthrombi
Neoplastic ulcer	Raised everted margin, gradual enlargement and induration	Either primary or arises secondarily in long-standing ulcer of another cause

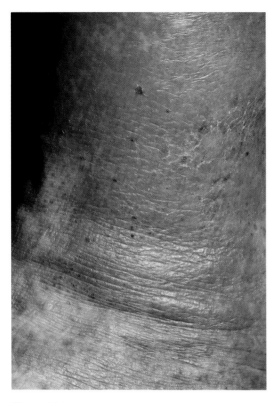

Figure 11.1a

Early gravitational changes affecting the ankle. There is a suffused, slightly eczematous, mauvish area and small visible veins.

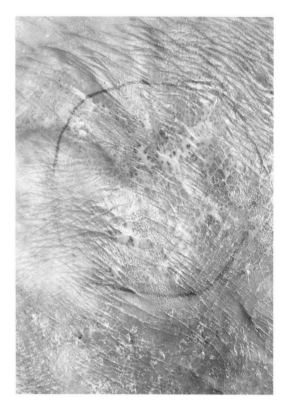

Figure 11.1b

Atrophie blanche in the gravitational syndrome. The small porcelain white, depressed areas are quite typical of this condition.

brownish discoloration as a minimal qualification, the overall prevalence in a European or American population over the age of 50 may amount to 20%, although some 50% may have minor subclinical evidence of venous hypertension. There are some estimates for the frequency of gravitational ulceration which point to a prevalence of approximately 1%.[1] Whatever the exact prevalence, there can be little doubt that the disorder is a monumental medical and social problem for the elderly.[2]

Clinical features

The disorder is essentially one of late middle and old age. It occurs mainly in those who have had a condition further embarrassing an already compromised venous drainage system of the legs. Thus it is more often seen in women who have had multiple pregnancies or venous thrombosis during pregnancy, the obese and those who have had an injury to the lower legs. There may be a heritable component. It has been suggested too that it may be particularly prevalent in tall, hypogonadal men.[3]

The earliest clinical changes include a characteristic form of telangiectasia, in which mauve and blue vessels can be seen tracking around the medial aspect of the ankle and the dorsum of the foot. Brownish discoloration of the skin develops above the medial malleolus: this is due to the deposition of haemosiderin pigment. General thickening and stiffening of the skin follows and may be accompanied by some pitting oedema of the ankle. Sometimes porcelain-white depressed

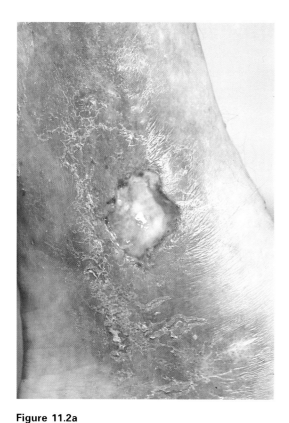

Figure 11.2a

Small gravitational ulcer with a sloughy base.

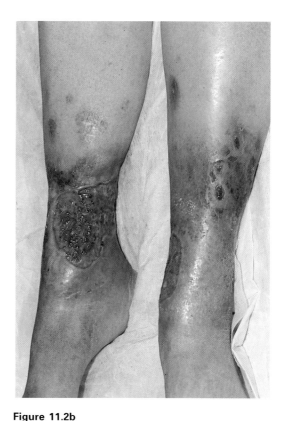

Figure 11.2b

Extensive gravitational ulceration of both legs. Note the hyperpigmentation.

macules are present within the suffused and telangiectatic patches over or just above the malleolus. These areas, known as *atrophie blanche* are thought to be the result of skin infarcts (Figure 11.1). Ulceration of the skin is superimposed on a background of the changes described and usually develops insidiously after a superficial injury to the leg, such as a graze from a supermarket trolley or a scratch from a cat.

Gravitational ulcers mostly develop above the medial malleolus (Figure 11.2) but they eventually extend around the leg to involve the lateral aspect of the ankle as well (Figure 11.3). Occasionally gravitational ulcers begin *de novo* on the lateral side of the leg but these lesions should be regarded with suspicion and considered due to another cause until proven otherwise. The initial erosion typically extends slowly, both laterally and in depth. Gravitational ulcers can reach frightening proportions (Figure 11.4), the worst cases showing almost complete loss of skin in the lower third of the lower leg. Their depth is variable, depending on site, duration and the presence of complicating factors such as infection. The floor of such lesions is also variable, but tends to be pink or red and granular when healing, and flecked with yellow, greenish or greyish slough or pus when static or enlarging. The ulcer edge is usually slightly thickened and irregular. Sometimes two or more small ulcers merge, giving a festooned appearance.

Gravitational ulcers may persist for very long periods—sometimes indefinitely. Even if persuaded to heal by one or several of the therapeutic measures suggested below, they often recur. There are no accurate figures for the likelihood of healing, recurrence or persistence.

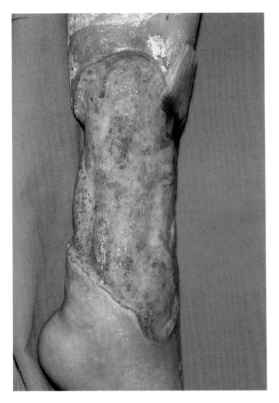

Figure 11.3

Circumferential ulceration in the gravitational syndrome. This woman's ulcer had been present for more than 15 years.

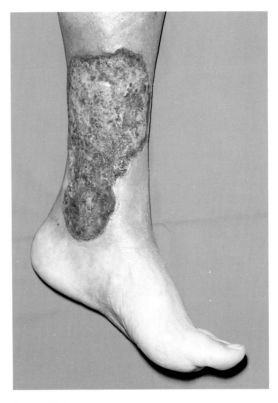

Figure 11.4

There is a very large gravitational ulcer affecting the medial aspect of the ankle. Note the greenish-yellow slough, denoting infection with Gram negative micro-organisms.

Complications

Infection

Gravitational ulcers always carry a heavy, mixed bacterial flora, particularly Gram-negative species—hardly surprising for a large raw area containing tissue debris. In most cases the rich colonization does not seem to have much clinical significance, and it is a vexed question as to whether these resident micro-organisms play any role in the persistence of the lesions.

Some ulcers encounter more virulent micro-organisms and even though there may be little apparent change in the results of bacterial culture, they suffer accordingly. These infected ulcers become exudative and are covered by a mixture of thick grey-green slough and pus. There is often an increase in the size of the lesion and an unpleasant, characteristic pungent stench. The sequence is by no means infrequent and it is fortunate that it can now be treated moderately easily (see later) and does not usually result in the disastrous consequences common in the past. A variety of bacteria may be responsible but *Pseudomonas* species and *Escherichia coli* types are mostly to blame.

Occasionally *Staphylococcus aureus* or streptococci cause a more virulent pattern of infection, with redness and tenderness of the surrounding skin, fever and malaise. Provided that the bacteria responsible are not resistant to most antidotes and that the situation is recognized in good time, this complication is also little more than a minor setback in the overall management.

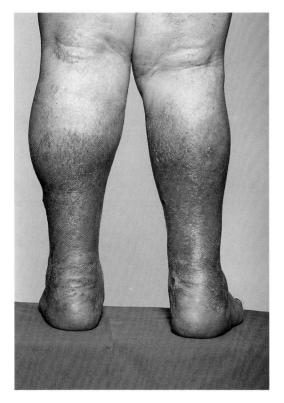

Figure 11.5

Extensive hyperpigmentation of both lower legs with apparent thinning of the ankle areas, giving an almost 'inverted champagne bottle' appearance to the legs.

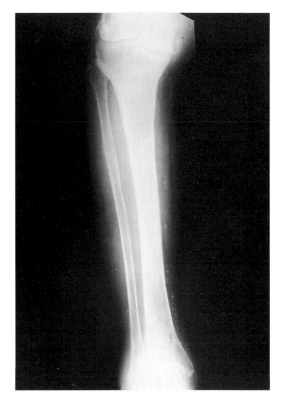

Figure 11.6

X-ray to show flecks of calcium in the subcutaneous tissue. These could be either in the tissue itself or in thrombosed veins.

Of more serious significance is an overwhelming septicaemic infection with one of several virulent Gram-negative microbes (for example, *Pseudomonas* species or *Aerobacter aerogenes*). There may be relatively few local signs in such patients but there is usually a severe systemic disturbance and even cardiovascular collapse. Blood cultures should be performed immediately the condition is suspected to isolate and characterize the appropriate micro-organism.

Infestation

At one time, when social conditions were worse than at present, it was not uncommon to find fly maggots in large gravitational ulcers. This still happens occasionally when the ulcer has been left exposed for long periods and the patient has had inadequate local care, but is more often seen as part of a planned therapeutic manoeuvre to débride the ulcer.

Fibrosis and calcification

Fibroplasia is a regular occurrence in long-standing gravitational syndrome and is due to the tissue damage, hypoxia and fibrin deposition (see later). The condition has come to be known as lipodermatosclerosis or liposclerosis.[4] When pronounced, this leads to constriction of the lower leg, giving it an inverted champagne bottle appearance (Figure 11.5). Calcification of the subcutaneous tissue is a late complication and imparts a woody or even stony, hard feel to the affected limb (Figure 11.6).

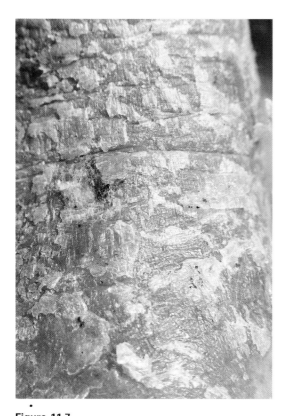

Figure 11.7

Gravitational eczema. There is erythema and scaling.

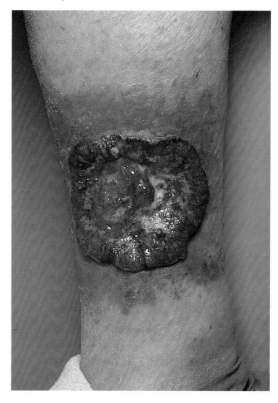

Figure 11.8

Squamous cell carcinoma has developed in this man's gravitational ulcer. Note the exuberant rolled, everted margin.

The mechanical obstruction to healing tissues and blood flow further aggravates the situation and indicates a poor prognosis.

Gravitational dermatitis

In perhaps one-third to a half of patients with the gravitational syndrome, signs of dermatitis appear around the ulcer and elsewhere on the affected lower limb. Generally this amounts to no more than some scaling and pinkness with itching, but in a few unfortunates the rash becomes extensive and severe (Figure 11.7). It then spreads to involve the opposite limb and even the arms and trunk. This was termed autosensitization eczema, but many cases are now recognized as being the result of allergic contact dermatitis to one of the topical medicaments being used[5] (see page 39).

Neoplastic change

In contrast to the above complications, neoplastic change in a gravitational ulcer is extremely uncommon. In most cases squamous cell carcinoma is the type of neoplasm involved, but basal cell carcinoma has also developed in some ulcers. It should be suspected if the ulcer has a raised and rolled edge (Figure 11.8).

Anaemia

Many patients with long-standing gravitational ulceration have a significant degree of anaemia. This is usually normochromic normocytic in type, but may be hypochromic. It has been assumed that the chronic ill health and tissue destruction in the ulcerated area is responsible

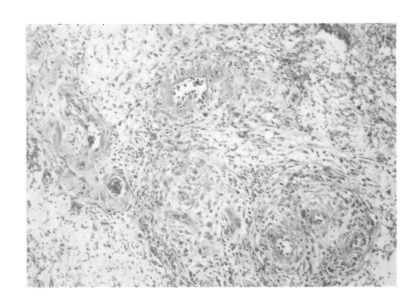

Figure 11.9

Pathology of area near gavitational ulcer. Note the numerous thickened blood vessels and marked mixed inflammatory cell infiltrate (H & E; ×90).

and that this in some way interferes with haematopoiesis.

Aetiology, pathology and pathophysiology

The ultimate cause of the gravitational syndrome is venous hypertension in the venous system of the lower limbs. The visible varicosities and telangiectatic venules in the subcutaneous tissue are also signs of venous hypertension but are themselves not responsible for the changes of liposclerosis on the ulceration, making the older term varicose ulceration inappropriate. Indeed, ulceration may be seen in the absence of varicosities. Despite the varicosities, there is no evidence for venous stasis, and some older studies found a higher blood oxygen content in venous blood and an increased rate of venous return suggesting that arteriovenous shunting had occurred. More recent techniques have failed to confirm the presence of shunts.

The venous hypertension is the result of venous valvular incompetence and an ineffective calf muscle pump[6] stemming from previous phlebothrombosis and inadequate calf muscle development. Other factors including multiparity, congenital venous disorders, obesity and male hypogonadism may also play a role.

Whatever its cause, the venous hypertension results in exudation across the walls of the venous ends of the capillaries and the deposition of a pericapillary fibrin cuff.[4] This in turn prevents adequate perfusion of the tissues and causes hypoxia and tissue inanition, despite the relatively high volume blood-flow rate.[6] There also appears to be a defect in the removal of the fibrin from around the small vessels as there is decreased fibrinolytic activity in the walls of the veins involved.[7] It has also been suggested that the extravascular fibrin traps growth factors and other substances making them unavailable for the maintenance of tissue integrity and predisposing to ulceration.[7]

A striking feature of biopsies from areas affected by the gravitational syndrome is the profusion of thick-walled capillaries throughout the dermis. Extravasated red cells and deposits of haemosiderin in macrophages are also prominent (Figure 11.9). The large number of small blood vessels, free red cells, haemosiderin, fibrosis and inflammation may simulate the pathology of idiopathic haemorrhagic sarcoma (Kaposi's sarcoma) and for this reason the picture has come to be known by some as pseudo-Kaposi's disease. Presumably these numerous small vessels result from the persistent venous hypertension, although the mechanism is uncertain. As mentioned previously, a fibrin cuff surrounds many of the small vessels (Figure 11.10). A large number of inflammatory cells and fibrosis are also obvious in most tissue samples and these probably arise from the

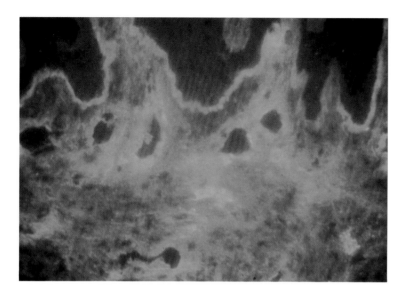

Figure 11.10

Immunofluorescence photomicrograph. The tissue has been stained with a fluorescein labelled antifibrin antibody and the fluorescence can be seen around many of the small vessels, demonstrating the presence of perivascular fibrin deposits (original magnification ×90).

tissue damage caused by the hypoxia and infection. In long-standing ulcers, deposits of calcium are found amidst the fibrosis.

At the edge of the ulcerated area the epidermis is thickened and irregular. At times the thickening may be extreme and give rise to the picture of pseudoepitheliomatous hyperplasia. Occasionally small protrusions of epidermis can be observed arising from the edge of the ulcer and tracking to the surface of the ulcer. These are attempts at re-epithelialization and are more prominent when the ulcer is in a healing phase.

Treatment

The treatment of the gravitational syndrome requires knowledge of the natural history and the pathogenesis of the disorder as well as experience. It has to be remembered that in our present state of knowledge very little can be done to remove the basic haemodynamic fault, that is, the venous hypertension, but there are measures available that can improve it and may diminish its effects.[8]

The pre-ulcerative stage

At this stage of the disorder every effort should be made to reduce the hypertension.

Surgical treatments are much less in vogue at the time of writing than they once were. Removal by stripping of the obvious varicosities may improve the appearance of the legs but does nothing for the haemodynamic situation. Tying off perforating veins that communicate between the deep and superficial venous systems has some theoretical value but rarely produces much clinical improvement. Major venous reconstructions may be suitable for some patients but require a surgeon with a special interest in the problem.

Attempts to improve drainage by periods of rest with the legs elevated are universally praised as a useful measure, and despite a lack of objective clinical evidence, do seem to have a beneficial effect. However, recumbency has been noted to improve tissue oxygenation in the legs.[9] The same is true for instructions to the patient to improve the calf muscle pump by judicious exercise. A further measure for which there is more evidential support is pressure bandaging to prevent a backflow of venous blood into the tissue of the skin. Various ways of doing this include binding the lower leg to just above the knee with firm elastic bandages or elasticated crepe bandage and elasticated stockings. A large number of bandages and stockings are available for this purpose and the dressing chosen depends on the experience and preference of the clinician involved. Some stipulate just how much pressure is applied by the bandage.

A device that supplies a ripple or wave of skin support by a mechanically driven pneumatic device has been tried. The idea is ingenious but as yet there is little evidence to suggest that results are better than with other forms of external support.

Efforts have been made to reduce the amount of pericapillary fibrin as this appears to be a fundamental fault causing tissue hypoxia. The anabolic steroids have the effect of increasing tissue fibrinolysis, and favourable results have been obtained with stanozolol by mouth in combination with support bandaging.[10] The optimal length of this treatment and whether it gives long-term benefit have not as yet been determined.

Another aspect of the treatment of the pre-ulcerative stage of the disorder concerns weight reduction. Many patients with the gravitational syndrome are considerably overweight, and there can be little doubt that successful dieting is of assistance. This is never easy in the elderly, but the effort is worthwhile and this should be emphasized to patients. Ankle oedema due to the disorder itself or to other causes should be treated with diuretics. Any measure that can help reduce the increased intracutaneous pressure will be of assistance.

Attention to other aspects of general health is also of major importance. Any underlying cardiorespiratory or haematological disorder must be treated concomitantly, as their presence will worsen the tissue hypoxia.

Patients with the gravitational syndrome should be told to avoid trauma to their ankles and to wear comfortable thick socks if possible, as minor cuts and abrasions will often lead to the next and more difficult stage of ulceration.

Treatment of gravitational ulcers

At the outset a warning must be issued—the numbers and range of treatments for ulcers is amazing. The profusion of these is the result of none being particularly effective and there being inadequate methods for their assessment. In few other areas of medicine is it as difficult to design a clinical trial that can withstand proper critical appraisal. The heterogeneity of ulcers with regard to size, site, duration, infection and other complications as well as the real difficulty of assessing improvement confound most clinical trials of treatments for leg ulcers. A further important observation is that although some local treatments may assist, there do not appear to be any that help all patients or that actually speed the processes of wound healing in the ulcer.

Local ulcer treatments may be divided into dressings and local applications, but often these two types are used together. The dressings are mostly designed to be non-adherent so that when they are removed they do not take with them new, delicate epithelium. Several dressings are described as 'biological'. These are based either on pig skin or on a plant product such as seaweed.

In most cases dressings are designed to be occlusive, as occlusion is one of the few positive benefits that dressings can offer. Ideally dressings should also inhibit microbial growth and prevent bacterial invasion of the raw area. Many dressings are impregnated with chemotherapeutic agents for this purpose. Provided that the antimicrobial compound does not sensitize (neomycin, Soframycin® and Vioform® are unsuitable because of this), does not damage healing tissues (many of the 'vital' dyes have this disadvantage) and has a broad spectrum of antimicrobial activity, the inclusion of such a material is an advantage. Povidone-iodine and silver sulphadiazine are two such suitable compounds. Topical mupirocin is specially useful for patients with infection by *Pseudomonas* micro-organisms.

Absorbency of dressings is another aspect to be considered. Absorption of exudate is desirable as this will assist in removing tissue debris, bacterial products and mediators that cause pain. The ulcer–dressing interface should not be allowed to remain soaked in fluid in these circumstances.

The comfort, cost and overall convenience of dressings must also be taken into account. Dressings that easily conform to the contour of the leg are justifiably popular, as are individually packed dressings.

The frequency with which a dressing should be changed is an important consideration. There is no universal formula—changes should be made according to the amount of exudate from the lesion, the patient's symptoms and the experience of the medical attendant. Changes less frequent than twice weekly are more often than not a sign of the ostrich attitude, that what cannot be seen is of little importance, rather than an informed attempt at healing. Daily changes probably indicate an overoptimistic attitude, suggesting that frequent inspection is itself therapeutic.

Removal of exudate, pus and slough is usually attempted by bathing of the affected area in saline, povidone-iodine preparations, dilute potassium permanganate solution (1 in 8000) or dilute hydrogen peroxide (10 volumes per cent). Eusol and hypochlorite solutions are antibacterial but are irritant and may harm new tissues; they should no longer be used. When soaking and bathing are not effective, various other methods have been used. These include an enzyme preparation of streptokinase and streptodornase, which is believed to liquefy tissue debris and bacteria but not living tissue, and seems to be useful in some patients. Dextran monomer beads have also been advocated for the same purpose, but they are very difficult to use and are expensive. Sugar and honey are traditional applications to open wounds that are again in vogue. There is some evidence that these materials are antibacterial and may decrease slough. Benzoyl peroxide lotion may also be helpful in removing slough and debris. There are numerous other topical agents with an antimicrobial action that have been promoted for the treatment of ulcerated areas. Those that contain corticosteroids should not be used as they can impede ulcer healing. As stated above, sensitizing compounds and agents that can harm delicate tissues should also be avoided. If there is obvious infection of the ulcer, surrounding erythema and an increase in pain, the appropriate systemic antibiotics should be administered.

Grafting

If an ulcer appears clean, shows signs of granulation, but is slow to heal, pinch grafting can speed the process of re-epithelialization. Split skin samples are taken aseptically from the lateral aspect of the thigh and fragments (0.5 × 0.5 cm approximately) are placed on the cleaned ulcer bed. Although healing may be speeded in this way, recurrence of ulceration is heartbreakingly frequent. Rarely, other types of grafting and surgical excision of the ulcer are attempted, but such an approach is not often justified. Application of skin grown *in vitro* and subsequently freeze dried has been tried by several groups; opinion seems divided as to its usefulness.

Prognosis

Regardless of treatment, once the ulcer is healed, further ulcers occur only too frequently either at the original site or in adjoining areas. The precise chances of this happening do not appear to have been computed but a reasonable estimate would be that less than one-third of patients with a gravitational ulcer stay healed and do not develop further lesions.

Ischaemic ulceration

This condition is most commonly the result of atherosclerosis, but can also be caused by diseases affecting the smaller blood vessels, including polyarteritis nodosa, thromboangiitis obliterans and lupus erythematosus.

Clinical features

A major distinguishing factor between this form of ulceration and gravitational ulceration is its very painful nature. Another major discriminant is the site of ischaemic ulceration. Areas such as the heel, the dorsum of the foot and toes and the lateral aspect of the lower leg are not infrequently involved (Figure 11.11).

The ulcer itself, when the result of atherosclerosis, typically has a dark red, mauve or blackish base without the moist granulations often seen in gravitational ulceration. The surrounding skin is cool or cold to the touch. In most cases it is preceded by a diminished blood supply to the skin and this results in trophic changes. The skin appears smooth and shiny and may have lost its usual complement of terminal hairs. Oedema of the skin or ankle oedema are uncommon accompaniments and help differentiate the ulcer from

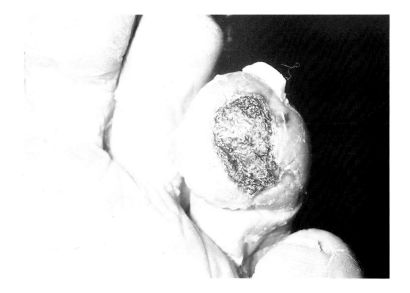

Figure 11.11a

Ischaemic ulceration affecting a toe due to atherosclerosis.

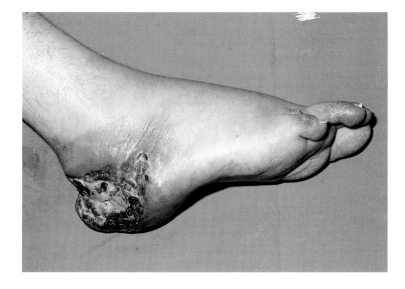

Figure 11.11b

Ischaemic ulceration affecting the heel in an elderly man who had a collagen vascular disease.

gravitational ulcers. Brownish staining and dilated venules are not seen and are also useful discriminants. Confirmation that there is ischaemia of the skin of the affected area can be obtained by measurement of skin blood flow using the laser Doppler flow technique or one of the other methods available.[11] Thermometry can also be helpful but as there is no direct relationship between blood flow and the skin temperature this cannot be used to gauge the severity of

the disorder. Infra-red thermography will assist in delineating the area affected by the reduction in blood flow and can indicate the site of the vascular obstruction.

When the ischaemia is due to an embolus that has lodged in a distal arterial conduit, tissue necrosis starts abruptly and at the periphery of the affected limb. If collateral vessels manage to open in time, much of the necrosis may be avoided, although it is common for ulceration to develop at the point at which the blood supply was most precarious before the event.

Focal ischaemic necrosis also occurs in the collagen vascular disorders. It may occur on the hands in Raynaud's syndrome and this will be described later. In polyarteritis nodosa, thromboangiitis obliterans and lupus erythematosus, areas of skin necrosis may develop suddenly in the course of the disease, preceded by painful mauvish-blue swellings. The accompanying systemic disorders and the characteristic evolution, plus the laboratory findings (see Chapter 7), usually serve to distinguish these conditions.

Treatment

In contrast to the gravitational syndrome, the most appropriate treatments for ischaemic ulceration due to atherosclerosis are surgical. The surgical approach adopted depends on a host of variables, including the general condition of the patient, the likelihood of surgical success and the experience of the surgeon. Endarterectomy, arterectomy with insertion of prostheses, and bypass operations may be used according to the circumstances. If there is no hope of success, amputation may be required. Grafting may be appropriate if the vascular supply is adequate. Sympathectomy (either surgical extirpation of the ganglia or chemical destruction) may help a few patients but its effects are unpredictable and anyway are relatively short-lived.

Pharmacological treatments designed to improve the blood supply to the skin are rarely of much avail. Drugs such as inositol nicotinate, the hydroxyethyl rutosides, pentoxyphylline, eicosanoids including prostaglandin E1 and prostacyclin analogues and ketanserin are rarely of assistance for chronic ischaemic disease of the skin due to atherosclerosis.

The local care of ischaemic ulcers is similar to that described above for gravitational ulcers, save that support bandaging to decrease venous hypertension in the skin and subcutaneous tissues should not be employed.

Ulceration in diabetes

The skin of the feet and lower legs is peculiarly prone to ulceration in diabetes. Atherosclerosis is more common, so that ischaemic ulceration often occurs. In addition, in many diabetics the small blood vessels of the skin tend to be thickened but to have a decreased luminal area and diminished blood flow, making ulceration more likely.[12] Ulcers in diabetics are at risk from serious infections because of the predisposition of diabetics to this type of complication. When this happens extensive tissue necrosis can spread rapidly and precipitate diabetic coma. Ulceration may also occur owing to the development of diabetic neuropathy and hypoaesthesia. Perforating ulcers develop as a result, affecting the tissues over the bony prominences of the feet (Figure 11.12). They are painless but penetrate deeply and can be very destructive.

Treatment

Once ulceration in a diabetic has occurred the treatment does not differ from treatment of this condition in the non-diabetic, save that infection must be rapidly and vigorously treated. Perforating ulcers should be treated by prevention of weight bearing on the affected part as well as prevention of any mechanical trauma to the area. Those who care for diabetics are aware of the dangers of these complications and attempt to educate patients in foot care. Unfortunately adequate control of the diabetes and even appreciation of the problems and dangers by the patients do not completely eliminate the possibility of ulcers developing.

Decubitus ulcers

Decubitus ulcers are areas of ischaemic necrosis of the skin that develop over bony prominences of the dependant parts in paralysed, extremely weak or unconscious patients. They are quite common in the elderly—for example, it has been found that they occur in some 20% of those aged over 60 taken into an orthopaedic ward.[13]

Clinical features

The most usual sites affected are the contact area of the sacral region and over the ischial tuberosities (Figure 11.13). Several others are

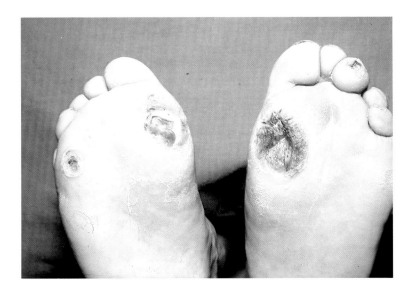

Figure 11.12

Bilateral perforating ulcers of the soles of the feet in a patient with longstanding diabetes and diabetic neuropathy.

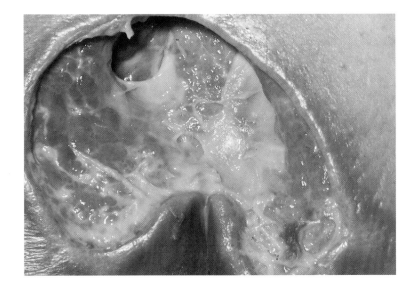

Figure 11.13

Severe decubitus ulcer in a paralysed patient.

susceptible to decubitus ulceration, including the backs of the heels, the back of the head, the scapular region and the elbows. Typically such lesions develop in quadriplegics and those who are comatose for long periods, but they may also occur in the very sick patient who is literally too weak to move, and in paraplegics. The first signs of the development of an ulcer are bluish or mauve areas on the sites at risk. Ulceration follows shortly after and may enlarge to expose deep tissue and even bone, and cover large areas with frightening rapidity.

Pathogenesis, prophylaxis and treatment

The cause of decubitus ulceration is the ischaemia caused by unrelieved pressure on the small blood vessels supplying the skin and subcutaneous tissues. Normally voluntary or reflex movements ensure that pressure on any one skin site is not maintained unrelieved for long periods. Paralysis, unconsciousness or inanition may prevent this and allow ischaemic changes to occur.

Maceration of the skin predisposes to decubitus ulceration by softening the stratum corneum barrier. Certain types of bed linen and beds seem to predispose to this unpleasant complication. Any surface that is rough and may abrade the skin contributes to the likelihood of the development of an ulcer. Similarly, surfaces that encourage a shearing stress between the skin and the bedding surface increase the tendency to ulceration.

All medical and nursing staff who are responsible for the care of patients who may develop decubitus ulceration should be aware of the factors that encourage the development of these lesions and be constantly on the lookout for the earliest signs. Regular turning and meticulous nursing care of the pressure points on the body are required, but even with devoted care it may not be possible to prevent ulcers with this practice alone. A variety of beds and bedding have been promoted to aid in the prophylaxis. Sheepskin or lamb's-wool underblankets, pneumatic devices (ripple beds) to alternate the sites at which skin contact is made and water beds have all been in vogue with various units at different times.

Our ability to keep patients with devastating injury and disease alive for long periods has increased, but our capacity to prevent decubitus ulceration has not kept pace. Consequently this type of ulcer is of major importance and has commanded a not inconsiderable amount of attention from researchers.[14]

Once developed, decubitus ulcers are extremely difficult to heal, if, as is usually the case, the immobility of the patient is unchanged. Dressings of the types described in the section on gravitational ulceration may be used, as may topical antiseptics or desloughing agents, but these can do no more than keep the area clean. The only effective remedy is to keep the area free from further pressure to allow whatever healing capacity is present to function.

Haematological ulceration

Patients of any age with sickle cell disease, thalassaemia and with essential thrombocytopaenic purpura sometimes develop ulceration of the lower legs. Presumably the basis of these lesions is ischaemia of the skin due to microthrombi in vessels supplying the skin or reduction in the rate of flow below critical values due to increased blood viscosity in the cutaneous vasculature. These lesions may occur on either the medial or lateral aspects and have no particular identifying clinical features. The possibility of ulceration of this type should always be considered in someone who may have a haemoglobinopathy or a disorder of platelets.

Pyoderma gangrenosum

This is a rare and serious form of ulceration that occurs in approximately two-thirds of patients in association with ulcerative colitis, Crohn's disease, multiple myeloma or rheumatoid arthritis, although sometimes no underlying disease can be detected.[15] It may occur anywhere on the skin surface but seems to be more frequent on the lower limbs and trunk. Lesions usually begin as swollen mauve or purple areas, which break down into ulcers and spread with horrifying rapidity (Figure 11.14). One or several lesions may appear simultaneously. The edges of the ulcers of pyoderma gangrenosum often have a characteristic bluish or mauve appearance and overhang the ulcerated areas. These ulcers may heal spontaneously and unexpectedly almost as rapidly as they develop, but some persist for long periods. Histologically no characteristic features have been identified, despite intensive searching. Treatment should be directed at the underlying disease, if any is present, and should be consistent with the nature of the ulcers themselves, using the same principles as outlined for gravitational ulceration. If the lesions become life threatening, other measures should be tried, although reports do not suggest that any one modality is consistently successful. Steroids and immunosuppressive agents, dapsone, thalidomide, Minocycline, cyclosporin, pentoxifylline, potassium iodide and plasmapheresis all have their advocates.

Rheumatoid ulceration

Apart from pyoderma gangrenosum, lesions due to vascular inflammation may occur in patients

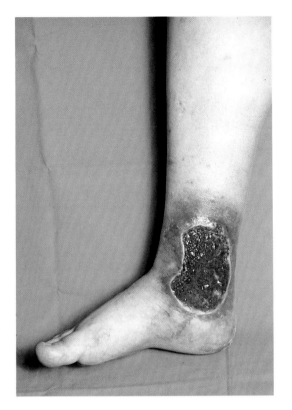

Figure 11.14

Pyoderma gangrenosum in a patient who had Crohn's disease. Note the suffused margin and inflammatory change around the ulcer.

with severe and long-standing rheumatoid arthritis. Small lesions of this type are not uncommon around the fingers and over the lower legs. Occasionally the small areas of infarction spread to produce large ulcers which may be quite intractable to local treatments and which can be confused with other forms of ulceration.

Corticosteroid treatment of rheumatoid arthritis over long periods causes considerable thinning, easy bruising and extreme skin fragility. The most minor injuries can produce frightful wounds and be extremely difficult to heal.

Neoplastic ulceration

Squamous cell carcinoma and basal cell carcinoma may occur either as a complication of long-standing ulceration of another cause or as a *de novo* event. When the lesions occur on the lower legs it is unfortunately often the case that they are not recognized as early as they might be. This is especially true when a neoplasm arises in a long-standing ulcer, as the initial signs of the complication may not differ greatly from the usual appearance. Typically the edges of a malignant ulcer have a raised and everted border. Later, the base of the lesion also becomes raised above the skin surface and the whole area becomes indurated. Later still, secondary nodules occur around the lesion and secondary deposits are found in the inguinal nodes. Although most lesions of squamous cell carcinoma are easily eradicated, this is not so with large ulcerative lesions of the lower leg, and the author knows of several cases where unfortunately the lesion disseminated widely and caused death.

Because of the situation and size of this type of lesion the treatment options are limited. They usually rest between radiotherapy and amputation or palliative chemotherapy.

Functional vascular disorders

Cold extremities

Elderly patients frequently complain that their hands and feet are always cold. In part this is due to the diminished capacity for the peripheral vasculature to vasodilate. The diminished cardiac output and rate of blood flow to the limbs contribute to the diminished blood flow to the skin of the hands and feet. It should also be remembered that the elderly may find difficulty in maintaining the normal body temperature in cold weather because of the drop in metabolic rate. The social circumstances of patients with this complaint should be checked as the cause may often be ascribed partly to inadequate clothing and heating at home. There are often few, if any, physical signs accompanying the complaint. In other cases, the hands and fingers may be bluish, pale and cool to the touch. The skin of the hands frequently has an atrophic, dry appearance.

The complaint of cold hands has to be distinguished from Raynaud's syndrome (see below) in which the symptom is episodic and accompanied by a characteristic series of colour changes. The complaint needs a sympathetic hearing, for unless some obvious social deficit or vascular complaint can be identified there is little that can be offered.

Raynaud's syndrome[16]

This complaint may be observed at any age from adolescence onwards and appears most frequently in young or middle-aged women. The disorder is due to episodic digital arterial vasospasm, causing attacks of intense pallor of the fingers, followed after some minutes by a red and then a mauve or purple discoloration. Usually not all fingers are affected, and often only a segment of an affected finger is involved. Typically attacks are precipitated by any sudden drop in ambient temperature, but emotion or mechanical stress may also be responsible, and they may even occur spontaneously in some patients.

Raynaud's syndrome often appears to develop as an isolated complaint without any obvious precipitating cause, but in an appreciable proportion of sufferers it develops as a consequence of underlying connective tissue disorder, particularly systemic sclerosis (see Chapter 7), an orthopaedic problem such as cervical rib, chronic mechanical trauma (as with workers with drills), a hyperviscosity syndrome or a dysproteinaemia.[17]

When the condition is severe and long-standing, dystrophic changes occur in the affected fingers. The skin becomes shiny and smooth and the nails look lustreless and ridged. In the most severe cases, which are mostly associated with systemic sclerosis, the fingers become tapered and areas of necrosis appear at the finger tips which may develop into frank gangrene of portions of the digits (Figure 11.15).

Treatment consists of careful advice on avoidance of drops in temperature and carrying heavy articles, and the use of warm gloves for the mildly affected individual. For other patients various drugs have been used with some degree of success claimed for them all.[17] They include smooth muscle relaxing agents such as Hexopal®, topical glyceryl trinitrite and nifedipine, mediator blocking agents and analogues such as reserpine, prostaglandin E1, prostacyclin and ketanserin and miscellaneous drugs such as pentoxyphylline, hydroxyethyl rutosides, stanozolol and naftidrofuryl. Electrically heated gloves seem to help some patients and sympathectomy gives relief to others.

Minor structural vascular disorders

Campbell de Morgan spots (cherry angiomata)

Bright red hemispherical nodules 1–3 mm in diameter appear over the trunk in perhaps a quarter of subjects over the age of 55 or 60 (Figure 11.16). In most cases they are multiple. They seem to have no particular significance and cause no symptoms. Histologically they consist of a mass of endothelial cells arranged in clumps or organized into vascular lumina. Their cause is unknown. Rarely they appear to occur in small epidemics.[18]

Angiokeratomata

There are several types of angiokeratomata which, as the name suggests, are vascular malformations with a hyperkeratotic covering. The only variety seen at all frequently in the elderly is that seen over the scrotum. The appearance may cause alarm, but they have no sinister implication and cause no symptoms. Rarely they are also seen on the vulva in elderly women (see Chapter 9).

Spider naevi

These lesions, which appear in areas of the body drained by the superior vena cava, have a central feeding arteriole and radiating vascular 'legs'. They are more common in young women, especially during pregnancy. When many occur in the elderly they may be a sign of hepatic cirrhosis (Figure 11.17).

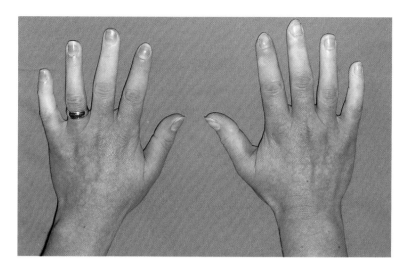

Figure 11.15

Raynaud's phenomenon. This patient had several attacks a day. The white appearance of the fingers is well seen.

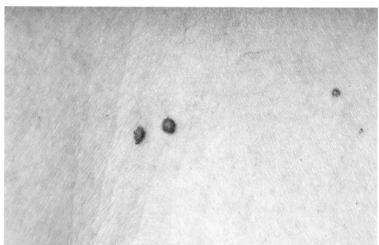

Figure 11.16

Campbell de Morgan spots (senile or cherry angiomata).

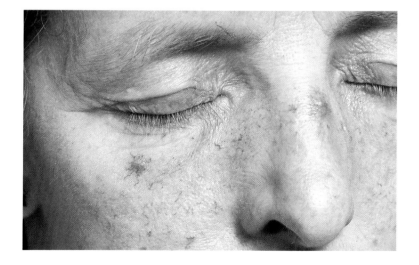

Figure 11.17

Spider naevi on the face in an elderly woman.

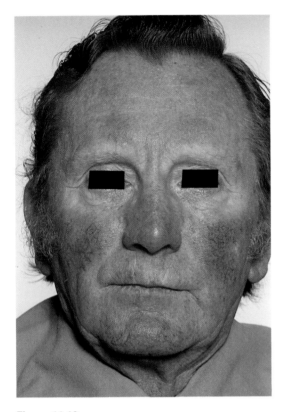

Figure 11.18

Telangiectasia on the face.

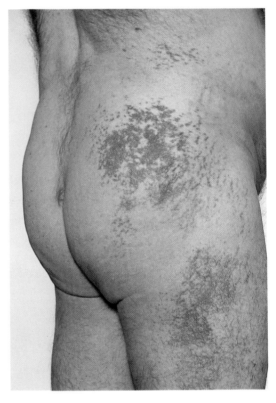

Figure 11.19

Arborizing telangiectasia affecting the buttocks in an elderly man.

Telangiectasia

The term telangiectasia means the presence in the skin of visible small blood vessels which normally cannot be seen. There are different types, and the significance of the appearance depends upon the particular variety.

Telangiectasia due to dermal damage

When the perivascular connective tissue is damaged the venous plexuses in the dermis become dilated and visible. This mechanism

accounts for the facial telangiectasia seen in the elderly—the dermal damage being caused by solar elastotic degeneration (Figure 11.18) (see page 000). Telangiectasia of a similar sort may also be seen due to dermal atrophy after long-term use of potent topical corticosteroids and as a physical sign in poikiloderma (see page 000).

Telangiectasia due to venous obstruction

Portal hypertension from cirrhosis, portal vein thrombosis or lymph node enlargement in the porta hepatis causes varices and telangiectasia at the junction between the portal circulation and the systemic venous damage. These are obvious as oesophageal varices, as haemorrhoids and as visibly enlarged vessels around the umbilicus.

When there is obstruction to either the superior or inferior vena cava, telangiectasia may become evident at sites where the venous drainage between the two systems overlaps, and particularly around the bottom of the rib cage.

Venous hypertension as part of the gravitational syndrome also results in an abnormal number of small veins around the ankles being visible.

Telangiectasia of unknown cause

Essential familial telangiectasia is an uncommon form that appears to be inherited. In this condition there is striking telangiectasia of the facial skin. Arborizing telangiectasia is an odd condition in which areas of telangiectasia appear anywhere on the trunk or limbs (Figure 11.19). The visible vessels appear to run parallel to each other but in no particular orientation with regard to the body.

Livedo reticularis

This term refers to the appearance of a network of mauve or blue broad lines on the skin, and seems to be due to dilatation and pooling of blood of a subcutaneous venous plexus. The condition is often most marked over the thighs but may also appear elsewhere on the limbs and even over the trunk. In its mildest form it is a normal finding, particularly in young women. When persistent, widespread and marked it may indicate either a connective tissue disorder, such as lupus erythematosus or polyarteritis nodosa, or a hyperviscosity syndrome.

References

1 Callam M J. Prevalence of chronic leg ulceration and severe chronic venous disease in western countries. *Phlebology* (1992) **7**(suppl 1): 6–12.

2 Negus D. Venous insufficiency. *J R Soc Med* (1985) **78**:870–2.

3 Monk B E, Pembroke A C. Hypogonadism with leg ulceration. *Clin Exp Dermatol* (1983) **8**:437–8.

4 Burnand K G, Whimster I, Naidoo A et al. Pericapillary fibrin in the ulcer bearing skin of the leg: the cause of lipodermatosclerosis and venous ulceration. *Br Med J* (1982) **285**:1071–2.

5 Cameron J. The importance of contact dermatitis in the management of leg ulcers. *J Tissue Viability* (1995) **5**:52–5.

6 Browse N L. Venous ulceration. *Br Med J* (1983) **286**:1920–22.

7 Falanga V, Eaglestein W H. The 'trap' hypothesis of venous ulceration. *Lancet* (1993) **341**:1006–8.

8 Falanga V, Eaglestein W H. *Leg and Foot Ulcers: A Clinician's Guide* (Martin Dunitz: London, 1995).

9 Dodd H J, Gaylarde P M, Sarkany I. Skin oxygen tension in venous insufficiency of the lower leg. *Proc R Soc Med* (1985) **78**:373–6.

10 Burnand K, Lemenson G, Morland M et al. Venous lipodermatosclerosis: treatment by fibrinolytic enhancement and elastic compression. *Br Med J* (1980) **280**:7–11.

11 Burcher A J. Laser Doppler measurement of skin blood flux. In: Serup J, Jemec G B E, eds, *Handbook of Noninvasive Methods and the Skin*, (CRC Press: Boca Raton, 1995) 399–404.

12 Ajam Z S, Barton S, Corbett M et al. Quantitative evaluation of the dermal vasculature of diabetes. *Q J Med* (1985) **54**:229–39.

13 Roberts B V, Goldstone L A. A survey of pressure sores in the over 60s on two orthopaedic wards. *Int J Stud* (1979) **16**:355–64.

14 Morison M, Moffatt C, Bridel-Nixon J, Bale S. Pressure sores. In: *Nursing Mangement of Chronic Wounds*, (Mosby: London, 1997) 153–75.

15 Powell F C, Su D, Perry H O. Pyoderma gangrenosum: classification and management. *J Am Acad Dermatol* (1996) **34**:395–409.

16 Blunt R, Porter J. Raynaud's sydrome. *Semin Arthritis Rheum* (1981) **10**:282–308.

17 Dowd P M. The treatment of Raynaud's. *Br J Dermatol* (1986) **114**:527–83.

18 Seville R H, Rao P S, Hutchinson D N et al. Outbreak of Campbell de Morgan spots. *Br Med J* (1970) **1**:408–9.

12
Treatment of skin disorder in the elderly

Differences between treatment for skin disorder in the mature adult and in the elderly stem from several separate issues. The first concerns compliance.

Compliance

At all ages compliance with treatments for any disease is likely to fall short of the prescribing physician's requirements. When these instructions are complex, distasteful, unaesthetic or simply uncomfortable, compliance is correspondingly worse. If the patient has difficulty hearing the instructions given because of otosclerosis, or difficulty in understanding due to cerebral atherosclerosis, he or she cannot hope to follow the advice proffered. Frequently the elderly patient, wanting to please, will nod appreciatively at the earnest young doctor without actually hearing or understanding a significant proportion of what is said. It should also be appreciated that some elderly patients have fixed their understanding of the world at an earlier age. Modern metaphors and fashionable phrases may be totally meaningless. Simply worded, straightforward explanations and instructions should be given. It takes sympathy and skill to prevent this difficulty in communication.

Regrettably, many of the elderly are seriously financially embarrassed. While it is inappropriate to discuss the socio-economic causes of this problem here, it is appropriate to remind the reader that what appears to be a trivial expense, such as a bus fare to attend the clinic or a special soap, may in reality be crippling for a pensioner. In the very poorest of elderly patients there may be inadequate home heating and bathing facilities.

Many patients unlucky enough to be in this position retain a fierce pride and are very reluctant to admit that they have such problems. Sensitivity is needed in the detection of this type of problem. It is not enough to know the dose and routes of administration of appropriate drugs: it is also important to know of the most suitable social agencies and the ways in which they can be of some assistance to distressed patients.

Compliance can also be affected by physical factors. There is decreased limb flexibility and a reduction in general mobility in old age so that an otherwise fit elderly patient may have difficulty treating areas of skin on the feet or the back with a cream or ointment. If, in addition, the patient has arthritis, or some other painful neuromuscular disorder, they may find it impossible to shampoo or apply a scalp treatment. Often spouses or friends can give some help in the application of topical agents to the skin of the back, but many elderly people live alone and have no one who can assist. Thus, there are many reasons for elderly patients not following a recommended treatment regimen, varying from the psychological to the physical. Failure to comply must always be considered when a skin disorder in an elderly patient does not respond to treatment.

Cosmetic considerations

It should not be thought that vanity decreases proportionately with advancing years[1]: there is tremendous variability. Some elderly women—and men too—retain a touching pride in their appearance and are intolerant of even minor blemishes. Others seem less concerned and will uncomplainingly harbour unpleasant tumours and ulcers on visible sites for long periods. However, this apparent lack of concern may in reality be fear of the nature of the lesion and its treatment.

Requests for the removal of seborrhoeic warts, skin tags, ancient hairy moles and other minor benign tumours should be handled sympathetically, remembering that a relatively small alteration in appearance may have enormous significance for the supplicant. Minor benign tumours and cysts and localized, non-progressive dermatoses in elderly patients often stimulate little interest in the dermatologist. Regrettably the attitude often seems to be that it is acceptable for the older segment of the population to carry around unaesthetic skin disorders. The reverse should be the case. Anything that can be done to improve the self regard of the elderly should be pursued. When appropriate they should be encouraged to care about their appearance and to have disfiguring disorders treated.

Xerosis and pruritus in the elderly

The skin of the elderly patient tends to be slightly flaky, rough and itchy. This xerosis is worse in the winter and in low humidity. It is particularly a problem in individuals who spend a large proportion of their time in centrally heated, air-conditioned buildings. The winter in the north eastern United States supplies the classic environment for this problem. The tendency to xerosis aggravates all dermatoses in which there is scaling and should be remembered in prescribing for this group of skin disorders. Greasy ointments rather than lotions and creams are often better tolerated because of their emollient properties. In addition, it is useful to add an emollient separately to the materials prescribed. Emollient cleansing agents also help, as will advice concerning bathing.

Because of the accompanying itch there is a tendency for physicians to prescribe antihistamines; there is no evidence that antihistamines are helpful for pruritus unless this is caused by histamine release, as for example in urticaria.

The older antihistamines such as diphenhydramine have the additional unwelcome effect of producing sedation and sometimes confusional states in the elderly.

Responsiveness to treatment

As a broad generality the skin of older subjects is far less responsive to any stimulus. There is considerable support for this statement with regard to chemical and mechanical traumata.[2–4] The responsiveness to beneficial and therapeutic stimuli is intrinsically harder to compare with that of younger subjects, but clinical observation suggests that it too is decreased in the elderly. Certainly, elderly patients with psoriasis and eczema seem to take longer to improve with treatment than do younger subjects.

Surgical treatments

With the depressed rate of wound healing in the elderly patient,[5,6] complete restoration of function may never occur with some sorts of wounds in the very old. Areas that are fat and droop in folds owing to loss of mechanical integrity of the dermis and the subcutis locally, such as the lateral aspect of the upper arms and the lower abdomen, are notoriously poor at healing. The lower legs and back are other areas that may give rise to problems in healing after surgery. Where the skin incised is involved by solar elastotic degeneration, broad and irregular scars may form. At the time of surgery haemostasis may be difficult to obtain in sun-damaged skin, because of the telangiectatic vessels that course through the abnormal tissue. For the same reason the site of the incision may develop unpleasant bruising. Great care should be taken in the suturing of wounds in older patients. The gaps between interrupted sutures should be smaller than is usual in young patients, and subcuticular sutures may be required in circumstances where they are not usually required in other age groups. Similarly, attention should be paid to the dressings used. Some degree of pressure on the wound to prevent bruising is often helpful—although occlusion of an already compromised blood supply must be avoided.

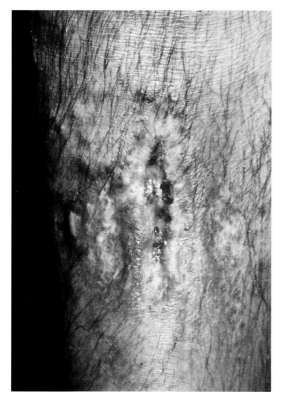

Figure 12.1

The skin of this patient's leg split after removing a plaster. It had been treated for a long period with a potent topical corticosteroid.

Particular care should be taken with patients on long-term systemic steroids for conditions such as rheumatoid arthritis. Elderly patients on steroids can sustain extremely severe injuries to the skin following relatively minor wounds (Figure 12.1) and these can be very difficult to heal.

When planning treatments for melanoma or less aggressive types of skin cancer in an elderly patient there is an understandable tendency to suggest less extensive and maybe less curative types of operation than for younger patients. This may be justified if the lesion has progressed to an advanced stage, or if the individual is very frail and has several other disorders concomitantly. It is hardly every justified just on the basis of age alone. It is often not appreciated that from the actuarial point of view an individual of 80 has a life expectancy of 12 years and at the age of 70 an expectation of 17 years. This should not be taken to indicate that humanity and compassion are of no account when planning surgical treatments, but that it is reasonable to plan curative procedures in elderly patients, as they may have many years of reasonable quality life ahead.

Treatment of concomitant disease

It is uncommon to see a patient with a gravitational ulcer in the eighth decade who does not also have some other medical problem. The presence of arthritis, chronic myocardial and/or respiratory disease and cerebrovascular disorders may all complicate the management of patients with the gravitational syndrome (see pages 245). The same is true for patients with other skin disorders. Firstly the presenting condition may be aggravated and resolution may be delayed by the presence of underlying disease. For example, anything that causes tissue hypoxaemia will delay the healing of ulcers. The presence of underlying disease may also dictate whether one or another treatment is prescribed for the presenting complaint. Methotrexate for psoriasis in the presence of hepatic cirrhosis, or systemic corticosteroids for generalized eczema in the presence of chronic congestive cardiac failure, exemplify the therapeutic dilemmas that may arise. Care must also be taken to ensure that any drugs prescribed do not interact with other drugs being taken for pre-existing conditions.

Hospital inpatient treatment for the elderly

Close supervision of skin disease in the elderly patient is rarely possible except when the patient is admitted to hospital. Physical infirmity, difficulty in using public transport or in finding relatives or friends to accompany patients make repeated clinic attendance very difficult. For this reason if the facilities are available and the social situation appropriate, consideration should be given to admission for treatment of stubborn skin disorders that could be more easily managed at home in younger individuals. However, before admission arrangements are made, sympathetic account should be taken of the patient's concern over a remaining spouse, friend or even a pet left alone at home. Elderly patients are often very fearful of going into hospital. They associate hospitals with severe illness and dying, often because they have recently lost close relatives in hospital. Careful detailed explanations may allay their fears and even a visit to the ward on which they will stay can give more confidence.

Before elderly people are admitted, consideration should be given to the home to which they will return and how they will cope after their inpatient sojourn. It should also be remembered that removal from the familiar environment of the home and at the same time being plunged into the terrifying authoritarian, high technology world of the hospital can cause depression and disorientation in the elderly. Nevertheless, inpatient treatment by sympathetic staff can end a distressing dermatosis and greatly shorten the total period of treatment necessary.

Day hospital rehabilitation for geriatric patients has become popular for patients who do not need treatment supervision over the whole day. If this facility exists and dermatological treatment can be given in the unit, this is an ideal solution for some patients. Patients with stubborn psoriasis or gravitational ulcers may do as well in a day hospital as in a traditional inpatient unit. Unfortunately a recent study suggests that this type of treatment is no less costly than formal hospitalization.[7]

Responsiveness to medication

Corticosteroid treatments

The corticosteroids are an important group of anti-inflammatory agents that provide relief from symptoms and can, on occasion, prove life-saving. Interestingly a recent survey in the USA showed that dermatologists were 3.9 times more likely to prescribe very high potency steroids than were other physicians.[8] It is important that their potential for unpleasant side-effects, as well as their therapeutic usefulness, is understood by

Table 12.1 Potencies of topical corticosteroids and examples

Category	Examples
Weak	Hydrocortisone (1%)
Moderately potent	Clobetasone-17-butyrate (0.05%)
	Desoxymethasone (0.05%)
Potent	Betamethasone-17-valerate (0.1%)
	Fluocinolone acetonide (0.025%)
	Triamcinolone acetonide (0.1%)
	Desoxymethasone (0.25%)
Very potent	Clobetasol-17-propionate (0.05%)
	Halcinonide (0.1%)

those who employ them. The details of their mode of action are not well characterized. It is known that they have a membrane stabilizing effect[8] and an antimitotic effect for fibroblasts, lymphocytes and epidermal cells.[9] They also stimulate the production of a peptide inhibitor of phospholipase A2 (Lipocortin)[10] and inhibit the production of pro-inflammatory prostaglandins. In addition they have many antisynthetic actions and a vasoconstrictor effect.[11] For a detailed review see Marks and Dykes.[12] The topical corticosteroids are by convention divided into weak, moderately potent, potent and very potent groups (Table 12.1). In general, the weakest preparation that produces adequate relief of symptoms and signs should be prescribed if a corticosteroid preparation is indicated.

Many of the actions of corticosteroids on the skin seem broadly similar to those of ageing. They produce thinning of both the epidermis and dermis, cause a reduction in size of epidermal cells and diminish the rate of epidermal cell division. Luckily these atrophogenic effects of corticosteroids do not seem to exaggerate the ageing process in most cases. Skin thinning studies monitored by an ultrasound method of skin thickness measurement[13] demonstrated that the skin of elderly subjects was less affected by potent topical corticosteroids than that of younger individuals (Black and Marks, unpublished observations). None the less, unpleasant petechiae and increased skin fragility can be induced by prolonged use of topical corticosteroids in old age. When used mistakenly in the treatment of rosacea, they have the effect of increasing the redness and telangiectasia,

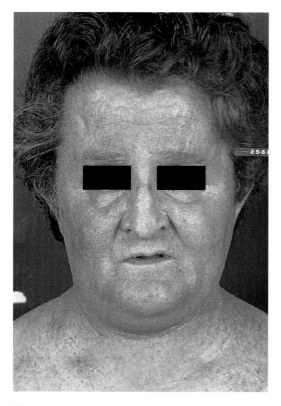

Figure 12.2a

Cushingoid facies. This woman had been using large quantities of potent topical corticosteroids.

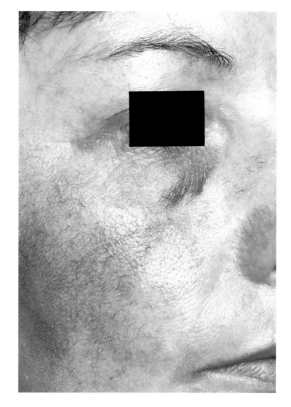

Figure 12.2b

There are telangiectasia and erythema on this woman's cheek—in addition there is an area of purpura below her eye. Overall she had been using a potent topical corticosteroid on her face for the previous two years.

producing a quite characteristic picture (Figure 12.2).

The eczematous diseases are the prime indication for the use of corticosteroids and they can give welcome relief of symptoms in these conditions (see Chapter 3). As with all potent drugs, they should be prescribed only when there is no simpler remedy and for the shortest time possible.

Treatments with systemic retinoids

The retinoid group of drugs have profound effects on epidermal differentiation, although the biochemical mechanisms underlying these effects are not completely characterized.[14] They are prescribed where there is either a primary defect in keratinization or where, as in psoriasis, the underlying disorder causes a defect in keratinization.[15] They are also used in the treatment of malignant and premalignant disease of the skin (see page 196).[16] Acitretin is the most frequently employed retinoid in the elderly in Europe. Isotretinoin is of more use for acne. The commonest disorder for which etretinate is prescribed is psoriasis, and in particular, pustular psoriasis. The drug has proved of great value in patients with severe and widespread disease. It may be of particular use in combination with PUVA or topical dithranol. Patients in need of systemic treatment and who cannot tolerate methotrexate are a group for whom etretinate

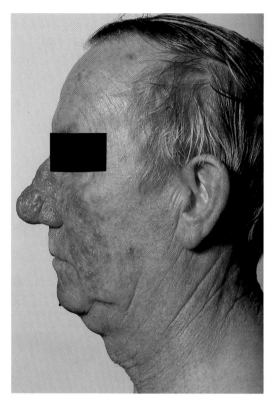

Figure 12.3a

Severe papular rosacea

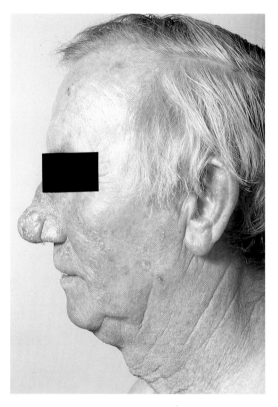

Figure 12.3b

The same patient after two months' treatment with isotretinoin, 1 mg/kg/day. Note the improvement in appearance.

has proved especially helpful. Whatever the indication for the use of acitretin in the elderly, the tolerance is somewhat less than in younger age groups. The dryness and cracking of the lips does not trouble such patients as much as the mild generalized dryness of the skin and the itchiness that occur in a substantial proportion of patients (Figure 12.3). Although many will soldier on uncomplainingly in the knowledge that the treatment will benefit them, some just cannot tolerate the discomfort.

Treatment with methotrexate and immunosuppressive drugs

These drugs are used in the treatment of severe psoriasis, connective tissue diseases and the lymphoproliferative disorders, including mycosis fungoides. It must be remembered that the immune defences are already depressed in the elderly and consequently especial care has to be taken to ensure that geriatric patients treated with these drugs do not succumb to overwhelming infection. In this context the altered pharmaco-dynamics of the elderly patient must be taken into account when the dose is calculated. Depressed renal function may dictate that only very small doses of methotrexate are prescribed.

Phototherapy

Treatment by UVR has become increasingly popular since the early 1970s. Oral PUVA, bath PUVA, UVB treatment and narrow band UVB all have their advocates and detractors. There is no doubt that where the patient can attend for the radiation treatment these phototherapies are often the best option—especially in chronic recalcitrant psoriasis and T-cell lymphoma. Unfortunately the spectre of neoplastic disease from over enthusiastic use of PUVA haunts us increasingly.[17] It must also be remembered that elderly patients often cannot tolerate being stuck in a 'PUVA box'.

Conclusions

Treatment of skin disease in the elderly follows the same general principles as for any other age group. There are none the less special points worth bearing in mind, many of which I have tried to include above. Some of these relate to difficulty in following the treatment regimen suggested and some (such as the altered pharmacodynamics in the elderly) are concerned with changes in the skin in old age. Whatever else is true, experience, patience and sympathy are mandatory components of management of skin disorder in this elderly age group.

References

1   Graham J A, Kligman A M. Physical attractiveness, cosmetic use and self perception in the elderly. *Int J Cosmetic Sci* (1985) **7:**85–97.

2   Grove G L, Duncan S, Kligman A M. Effect of ageing on the blistering of human skin with ammonium hydroxide. *Br J Dermatol* (1982) **107:**393–400.

3   Tuft L, Heck V M, Gregory D C. Studies in sensitisation as applied to skin test reactions. *J Allergy* (1955) **26:**359–66.

4   Bettley F R, Donnaghue E. The irritant effect of soap on the normal skin. *Br J Dermatol* (1960) **72:**67–76.

5   Schneider E L. In vivo vs in vitro cellular ageing. In: Bergson D, Harrison D E, Paul N W, eds, *Genetic Effects in Ageing*, (Alan R Liss: New York, 1976) 159–69.

6   Kligman A M. Perspectives and problems in cutaneous gerontology. *J Invest Dermatol* (1979) **73:**39–46.

7   Tucker M A, Davison J G, Ogle S A J. Day hospital rehabilitation—effectiveness and cost in the elderly: a randomised controlled trial. *Br Med J* (1984) **289:**1209–12.

8   Weissman G, Goldstein I M. Effects of steroids on lysosomes. In: Wilson L C, Marks R, eds, *Mechanisms of Topical Corticoid Activity*, (Churchill Livingstone: Edinburgh, 1976) 128–35.

9   Marks R, Williams K. The action of corticosteroids on the epidermal cell cycle. In: Wilson L C, Marks R, eds, *Mechanisms of Topical Corticoid Activity*, (Churchill Livingstone: Edinburgh, 1976) 39–46.

10 Blake Pepinsky R, Sinclair L F. Epidermal growth factor dependent phosphorylation of lipcortin. *Nature* (1986) **321:**81–4.

11 McKenzie S W, Stoughton R B. Methods of comparing percutaneous absorption of steroids. *Arch Dermatol* (1962) **86:**608–10.

12 Marks R, Dykes P J. Steroids, squamous epithelium and psoriasis. In: Wright N A, Camplejohn R S, eds, *Psoriasis, Cell Proliferation*, (Churchill Livingstone: Edinburgh, 1983) 327–35.

13 Tan C Y, Statham B, Marks R et al. Skin thickness measurement by pulsed ultrasound: its reproducibility, validation and variability. *Br J Dermatol* (1982) **106:**657–67.

14 Marks R, Pearse A D, Hashimoto T et al. Overview of mode of action of retinoids. In: Cunliffe W J, Miller A J, eds, *Retinoid Therapy*, (MTP Press: Lancaster, 1984) 91–9.

15 Lowe N J, Marks R, eds, *Retinoids: A Clinician's Guide*, 2nd Edn (Martin Dunitz: London, 1998).

16 Marks R, ed. *Retinoids In Cutaneous Malignancy*, (Blackwell Scientific: Oxford, 1991).

17 Lever L, Farr P M. Skin cancers or premalignant lesions occur in half of high dose PUVA patients. *Br J Dermatol* (1994) **131:**215–19.

ACKNOWLEDGEMENTS

I gratefully acknowledge the help of my colleagues in gathering material for this book and coping with my bad temper during the writing. I am also grateful to my family, who have hardly seen me; and finally to my publishers for their forebearance.

The author and publishers acknowledge with thanks:
Professor Richard Morton and the Department of Media Resources, Professor Ralph Marshall and the Staff of the Department of Medical Illustration, University Hospital of Wales, Cardiff, for their generous assistance with the illustrations and Dr A. Frazer of the University Hospital of Wales for loan of and permission to reproduce Figure 5.15.

The following are sources of the line illustrations:
Tan, C.Y., Marks, R. and Payne, P., 'Comparison of xeroradiographic and ultrasound detection of corticosteroid induced dermal thinning', *J Invest Dermatol (1981) 76 No 2: 126–128* (Figure 1.1).
Marks, R., 'Measurement of biological ageing in human epidermis', *B J Dermatol (1981) 104: 627–633* (Figure 1.5).

Index